Management of Localized Pancreatic Cancer

Susan Tsai • Paul S. Ritch
Beth A. Erickson • Douglas B. Evans
Editors

Management of Localized Pancreatic Cancer

Current Treatment and Challenges

Springer

Editors
Susan Tsai
Division of Surgical Oncology
Department of Surgery
The Medical College of Wisconsin
Milwaukee, WI, USA

Paul S. Ritch
Division of Medical Oncology
Department of Medicine
The Medical College of Wisconsin
Milwaukee, WI, USA

Beth A. Erickson
Department of Radiation Oncology
The Medical College of Wisconsin
Milwaukee, WI, USA

Douglas B. Evans
Department of Surgery
The Medical College of Wisconsin
Milwaukee, WI, USA

ISBN 978-3-319-98943-3 ISBN 978-3-319-98944-0 (eBook)
https://doi.org/10.1007/978-3-319-98944-0

This Springer imprint is published by the registered company Springer Nature Switzerland AG
The registered company address is: Gewerbestrasse 11, 6330 Cham, Switzerland

Preface

For over three decades, the survival for patients with pancreatic cancer has been stagnant, and the lack of progress offered little hope for patients afflicted with this disease. However, recent improvements in our understanding of tumor biology have impacted our clinical management of the disease. Moving away from a Halstedian approach to cancer management has allowed for more innovative approaches to treatment sequencing, which has in turn resulted in dramatic improvements in overall survival for patients with localized disease. Similarly, there has been an evolution in our understanding of the management of advanced pancreatic cancer as well. Along with a movement away from single-drug regimens towards multi-drug therapies, there is a growing appreciation of the impact of specific somatic and germline mutations on chemotherapeutic sensitivity. As with other solid tumors, the fundamental understanding of the genetic predeterminants of the disease continues to evolve to allow us to better understand disease subtypes and develop a tailored approach for each. These changes have ushered in a new age of hope for patients and their families.

We have created this handbook as a resource for the practicing clinician. The authors represent a diverse group of experts who have endeavored to provide a practical evaluation of the available data and provide insights into the complexities of multimodality management of pancreatic cancer. We are indebted to the exceptional contributions of the authors and reflect their ongoing commitment to the advancement of care for this disease.

We are at an exciting time where clinical medicine and translational science are converging to allow for unprecedented advancements in the care of cancer patients. We look forward to future developments in the area of pancreatic cancer to build upon our current successes and catapult us into a new era of discovery.

Milwaukee, WI, USA

Susan Tsai
Paul S. Ritch
Beth A. Erickson
Douglas B. Evans

Contents

Contributors

Chad A. Barnes, MD Department of Surgery, The Medical College of Wisconsin, Milwaukee, WI, USA

Mariana I. Chavez, MD Department of General Surgery, The Surgical Clinic, Nashville, TN, USA

Kathleen K. Christians, MD Division of Surgical Oncology, Department of Surgery, The Medical College of Wisconsin, Milwaukee, WI, USA

Callisia N. Clarke, MD Division of Surgical Oncology, Department of Surgery, The Medical College of Wisconsin, Milwaukee, WI, USA

Kulwinder S. Dua, MD, DMSc Department of Medicine, Division of Gastroenterology and Hepatology, The Medical College of Wisconsin, Milwaukee, WI, USA

Beth A. Erickson, MD, FACR, FASTRO Department of Radiation Oncology, The Medical College of Wisconsin, Milwaukee, WI, USA

Douglas B. Evans, MD Department of Surgery, The Medical College of Wisconsin, Milwaukee, WI, USA

Ben George, MD Division of Medical Oncology, Department of Medicine, The Medical College of Wisconsin, Milwaukee, WI, USA

Jennifer L. Geurts, MS Department of Surgery, The Medical College of Wisconsin, Milwaukee, WI, USA

William A. Hall, MD Department of Radiation Oncology, The Medical College of Wisconsin, Milwaukee, WI, USA

Michael Holt, MD Department of Radiology, The Medical College of Wisconsin, Milwaukee, WI, USA

Ashley N. Krepline, MD Department of Surgery, The Medical College of Wisconsin, Milwaukee, WI, USA

Naveen M. Kulkarni, MD Department of Radiology, The Medical College of Wisconsin, Milwaukee, WI, USA

Gwen Lomberk, PhD Division of Research, Departments of Surgery and Pharmacology and Toxicology, The Medical College of Wisconsin, Milwaukee, WI, USA

Paul S. Ritch, MD Division of Medical Oncology, Department of Medicine, The Medical College of Wisconsin, Milwaukee, WI, USA

Flavio G. Rocha, MD Department of Surgery, Virginia Mason Medical Center, Seattle, WA, USA

Kara Sonntag, RD, CSO, CD Froedtert Health, Food and Nutrition Services, Milwaukee, WI, USA

Susan Tsai, MD, MHS Division of Surgical Oncology, Department of Surgery, The Medical College of Wisconsin, Milwaukee, WI, USA

Raul Urrutia, MD Departments of Surgery and Biochemistry, The Medical College of Wisconsin, Milwaukee, WI, USA

The Future of Multidisciplinary Care in Pancreatic Cancer

1

Susan Tsai and Douglas B. Evans

Introduction

Over the past two decades, cancer care has evolved from a physician-specific approach, in which cancer care providers existed in relative isolation and interacted with other specialists when their expertise in the management of the cancer patient had been exhausted, to a disease-specific approach, whereby multidisciplinary teams of physicians converge to develop and coordinate a care plan for each individual patient at the time of diagnosis. Such care teams have developed to facilitate patient-centered care. Intended consequences of multidisciplinary care have included improved patient and physician communication, coordination of care (whether the treatments are intended to be in series or parallel), and reduced fragmentation of services as patients move from one treatment modality to the next. There is now clear evidence that multidisciplinary care is associated with better clinical and process outcomes for cancer patients, decreased time from diagnosis to start of treatment, and improved patient survival [1, 2]. Current multidisciplinary pancreatic cancer teams frequently including medical oncologists, radiation oncologists, and surgeons, as well as abdominal imaging specialists, pathologists, gastroenterologists with expertise in advanced endoscopy, and genetic counselors, who collectively are able to select the best treatment options for each patient. As our understanding of the interaction between host (patient) factors and tumor biology/natural history has evolved, the management of pancreatic cancer has shifted away from a physician specialty-centric approach to one that focuses on all aspects of patient care, often including the sequential delivery of oncologic therapies. In the very near future (and right now at some larger centers to include our own), the limitation of available treatments may be dictated by patient factors, and multidisciplinary teams will need to expand to include the expertise of dietitians, psychologists, endocrine specialists, and geriatric specialists to fully realize a patient-centered care model (Fig. 1.1).

S. Tsai (✉)
Division of Surgical Oncology, Department of Surgery, The Medical College of Wisconsin, Milwaukee, WI, USA
e-mail: stsai@mcw.edu

D. B. Evans
Department of Surgery, The Medical College of Wisconsin, Milwaukee, WI, USA

Moving Beyond a Physician (Specialty)-Centric Approach

Patients with pancreatic cancer have historically been treated with up-front surgical resection, likely influenced by the Halstedian paradigm of

S. Tsai et al. (eds.), *Management of Localized Pancreatic Cancer*,
https://doi.org/10.1007/978-3-319-98944-0_1

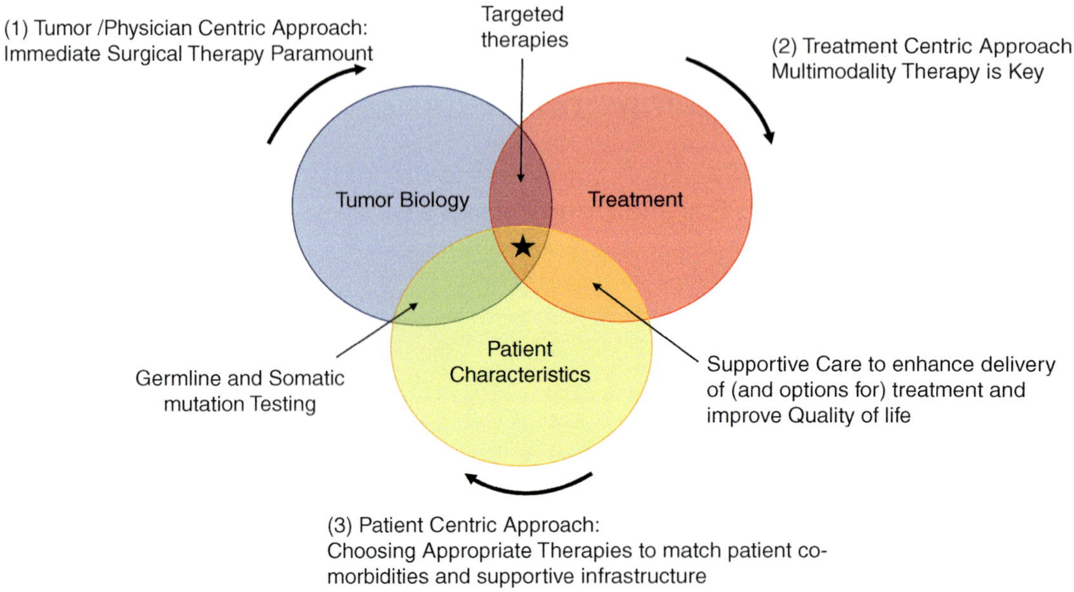

Fig. 1.1 Interrelationship of tumor-, treatment-, and patient-specific factors in the management of pancreatic cancer

cancer progression, whereby cancer spreads from the primary tumor to regional lymph nodes and only afterward to distant sites. Following such reasoning, surgical extirpation of a localized tumor would prevent cancer dissemination and metastatic tumor progression. However, decades of surgical experience have demonstrated that surgical resection alone, even with the addition of adjuvant therapy, provides a limited median survival benefit of only 20–24 months for patients with localized pancreatic cancer [3]. Indeed, the vast majority of patients with presumed localized pancreatic cancer succumb to metastatic disease after a curative-intent surgery [4]. Despite the optimization of surgical technique and perioperative management over the past three decades, little progress has been made to improve the limited survival of patients with localized pancreatic cancer who receive surgery [5, 6]. The development of metachronous distant tumor metastases in the majority of patients for whom local-regional tumor control was achieved, supports an alternative paradigm of cancer progression, whereby systemic metastases may be present even in the absence of radiographic or pathologic (node negative) evidence of disease. This hypothesis, first proposed by Bernard Fisher as an alternative to the Halstedian theory of cancer, was developed from observations in the laboratory involving tumor metastasis in animal models of breast cancer. In pancreatic cancer, preclinical models of genetically engineered mice also support the hypothesis that pancreatic cancer has a proclivity for early metastases, which can occur before a visible tumor may be present in the pancreas [7]. As such, there is an evolving recognition that pancreatic cancer is a systemic disease at the time of diagnosis, even among patients with apparent localized disease, and "a chance to cut" is not necessarily a chance to cure [8, 9].

For patients with localized pancreatic cancer who undergo a margin negative (R0) resection, most will experience disease recurrence, and the overall median survival is approximately 20 months [5]. Most notably, within 6 months of successful surgery, up to 60% of patients who underwent curative-intent surgery have already experienced disease relapse, as reported in the CONKO-001 trial [10]. Therefore, radiographically occult micrometastatic disease may be present in the majority of patients with pancreatic cancer at the time of diagnosis. The benefit of adjuvant systemic therapy was first demonstrated in the CONKO-001 trial, which compared adjuvant gemcitabine to observation in patients with resected pancreatic cancer. This study reported a median overall survival of 22.8 months with gemcitabine as compared to 20.2 months in the observation (surgery alone) group [3]. More recently, the ESPAC4 trial, which compared adjuvant gemcitabine to adjuvant gemcitabine and capecitabine, demonstrated a median overall survival of 25.5 months and 28.0 months, for the two arms, respectively [11]. It is important to note that the modest benefit of adjuvant therapy appears to be stage independent, further supporting the hypothesis that metastatic disease progression occurs early (regardless of nodal status) in this disease.

Although universally recommended, the feasibility of delivering adjuvant therapy to patients with pancreatic cancer in the postoperative setting remains problematic. Approximately 50% of patients will fail to receive any adjuvant therapy following pancreatectomy due to surgery-associated complications, delayed recovery, or failure to return to an adequate baseline performance status acceptable for systemic therapy [12, 13]. Indeed, one of the problems with the interpretation of adjuvant therapy trials is the selection bias introduced by the trial design itself. In order to be enrolled in a trial of adjuvant therapy for operable pancreatic cancer, patients must survive the operation, recover within 2–3 months, have no evidence of early disease recurrence, and have a performance status acceptable for the delivery of systemic therapy. As the toxicity profile of planned adjuvant therapy increases, the selection bias is further exaggerated. This was recently demonstrated in the PRODIGE trial reported at the ASCO 2018 where patients in the control arm (adjuvant gemcitabine) had a median survival of 35 months compared to 26 months (with the same treatment) in ESPAC4 [14]. The selection bias was likely due to the fact that the experimental arm (in PRODIGE) involved adjuvant mFOLFIRINOX – medical oncologists knew that patients would need to be particularly robust to handle this treatment after a pancreatectomy. While those who received mFOLFIRINOX experienced a very favorable survival duration, this lucky subset may represent only a tiny percentage of all patients who undergo a pancreatectomy for pancreatic cancer. Acknowledging that surgery alone is an insufficient therapy to achieve long-term disease control and understanding that surgical resection may unintentionally impede the delivery of future systemic therapies, treatment sequencing which specifically relies on the delivery of adjuvant therapy has been called into question. Commitment to a surgery-first approach may be attractive to surgeons and rewards technical proficiency with respect to local disease management, but does not provide a treatment strategy which reliably delivers systemic therapy for a disease which many clinicians and scientists now agree is distinguished by early metastatic disease.

Era of Neoadjuvant Therapy: Adopting a Patient-Centric Approach

In light of the limitations of a surgery-first approach for patients with localized pancreatic cancer, a logical alternative is to deliver preoperative (neoadjuvant) therapy before surgery. Advantages of a neoadjuvant strategy include (1) early treatment of presumed micrometastatic disease, (2) the ability to minimize stage misclassification by providing a time interval during which indeterminate lesions (that may be metastases) can be better characterized through serial radiographic imaging, and (3) theoretical efficacy of radiation in a non-hypoxic environment. Initial neoadjuvant trials required additional expertise in the management of patients with pancreatic cancer to include the talent of abdominal radiologists, advanced endoscopists, and cytopathologists. First, since treatment would precede an operation, it was necessary to develop a clinical (as opposed to pathological) staging system in order to provide an objective, CT-based anatomic staging system which could assess the efficacy of a therapeutic intervention. When such assessments are performed over serial time points, they provide important insights into tumor biology, response to therapy, and more accurately predict the utility of surgical resection. Second, a tissue diagnosis was required prior to treatment, which historically necessitated percutaneous biopsy with the incumbent risk of peritoneal seeding. This risk could be abrogated with an endoscopic approach. This would require the expertise of an advanced endoscopist to obtain the sample and a cytopathologist to interpret the specimen. Currently, tissue diagnoses can be obtained in almost all patients using endoscopic ultrasound-guided fine needle aspiration, and associated procedural complications are very rare. Finally, patients with tumors in the head of the pancreas frequently require decompression of biliary obstruction with endobiliary stenting. Stent-related morbidities, including cholangitis due to stent occlusion during neoadjuvant therapy, occur in up to 15% of patients and require prompt recognition [15]. However, the use of metal endobiliary stents rather than polyethylene (plastic) stents has reduced stent-related complications [16]. With these issues addressed, neoadjuvant therapy could be implemented in patients with localized pancreatic cancer.

In the early experience with neoadjuvant therapy, approximately 30% of patients with localized PDAC developed metastatic disease progression after a short course of neoadjuvant therapy [17, 18]. Importantly, the patients who were able to complete all intended neoadjuvant therapy and surgery experienced median overall survivals up to 44 months [17, 19, 20]. Such survival durations far exceeded that of a surgery-first approach and suggested that multimodality neoadjuvant therapy may be more effective at eradicating micrometastatic disease than adjuvant therapy; indeed, the sequencing of therapies may matter and effect the host-tumor relationship and tumor response. These early successes spurred an intense debate regarding the optimal treatment sequencing for patients with pancreatic cancer, due to the lack of level III evidence to support a survival benefit. More recently, the PREOPANC trial randomized patients with resectable and borderline resectable pancreatic cancer to either upfront surgical resection followed by adjuvant gemcitabine or preoperative gemcitabine-based chemoradiation, surgery, and adjuvant gemcitabine [21]. An intention to treat analysis demonstrated an improved overall survival among patients treated with perioperative therapy as compared to a surgery-first approach ($p = 0.07$). In addition, a planned subset analysis of just patients who underwent resection demonstrated that the patients who received a perioperative/neoadjuvant approach had a significantly greater overall survival than patients who received upfront surgical resection (42.2 vs. 16.8, $p < 0.001$).

As acceptance of neoadjuvant treatment grows, additional efforts have been directed at improving outcomes for the proportion of patients who develop metastatic disease progression during neoadjuvant therapy. Such disease progression, which occurs despite the receipt of systemic therapy, is due to chemotherapeutic resistance and may be potentially prevented by administering a more effective first-line chemotherapeutic agents. We recently reported the first neoadjuvant trail utilizing molecular profiling to guide chemotherapeutic selection in patients with localized pancreatic cancer [22]. Among 130 patients, 82% of patients were able to complete all intended neoadjuvant therapy and surgery, including 92% of patients with resectable disease and 74% of patients with borderline resectable disease. Because of the increased proportion of patients who were able to complete all intended therapy, the median overall survival of *all* 130 patients was 38 months, and the median overall survival for the 107 patients who completed all intended neoadjuvant therapy and surgery was 45 months [17, 18]. These encouraging findings suggest that real-time prospective molecular profiling may allow for optimal selection of neoadjuvant therapy for patients with localized pancreatic cancer. In the future, an approach which leverages both tumor-specific and treatment-specific approaches and capitalizes on the growing availability of molecular techniques will be needed to guide targeted therapies.

Future of Multidisciplinary Care: Incorporating a Patient-Centric Approach

Tremendous efforts are underway to better understand pancreatic cancer biology and to guide the treatment selection for all patients. Gone are the days of a one-size-fits-all approach to this disease, and the last frontier may be the ability to best predict and meet the needs of each individual patient. This will require improved understanding of individual patent characteristics (immunity and physiologic reserve), refinement of treatment monitoring, innovative approaches to treatment delivery, and improved supportive care. The most compelling example of this is the recent recommendation to include germline genetic testing for all patients with pancreatic cancer [23]. This change occurred as a result of recent studies which demonstrated that approximately 5–10% of patients with pancreatic cancer have disease-associated germline mutations which may not be reliably identified through personal and family history [24]. The identification of BRCA2, BRCA1, PALB2, and MMR gene mutations has important therapeutic implications. This is the first step towards a standardized approach to incorporate individual patient characteristics into multidisciplinary care.

Current neoadjuvant therapy is generally delivered as a prescriptive therapy, where patients are required to undergo multiple therapies in sequence. There is a lack of consensus around what the most effective treatment regimen may be, with controversy regarding the type of systemic therapy delivered, the utilization of radiation therapy, and the plan, if any, for additional adjuvant therapy [25]. It is important to note that neoadjuvant therapy was first conceived in an effort to accurately identify those patients who would evidence disease progression during/after neoadjuvant therapy and thereby avoid the morbidity of surgery, when an operation would provide no clinical benefit. Therefore, the historic threshold for proceeding with surgery after neoadjuvant therapy has been the absence of disease progression rather than the presence of a treatment response. In fact, the primary tumor may not significantly change following neoadjuvant therapy, and occult micrometastases, even if unresponsive to induction therapy, may still not be radiographically apparent at the time of preoperative restaging. The inability to accurately assess response to neoadjuvant therapy, as distinct from disease stabilization, is likely responsible for the early postoperative recurrence seen in some patients who have received neoadjuvant therapy. There is growing evidence that normalization of CA19-9 levels in response to neoadjuvant therapy is an important prognostic marker [26]. Novel clinical trials which prioritize changes in CA19-9 to guide adaptive modification of neoadjuvant treatment over prescriptive, static regimens are ongoing (NCT03322995).

As with other solid tumors, an evolution in treatment sequencing to include total neoadjuvant therapy may also occur in pancreatic cancer. With more extended neoadjuvant therapies, cumulative toxicities are inevitable. As therapies are increasingly tailored to each patient's tumor, it will be equally important that treatment sequencing be tailored to each patient, including patients of all ages, with a variety of medical comorbidities, and with family/social infrastructure varying from robust to unfortunate. It is unrealistic to assume that all patients can tolerate all therapies. In anticipation of the need for increased supportive care, multidisciplinary teams will need to expand to include the expertise of dietitians, psychologists, endocrine specialists, and geriatric specialists to fully realize a patient-centered care model.

Conclusions

The next decade will witness an intense focus on the many new therapeutic options available for patients with pancreatic cancer. For such patients, they will realize this opportunity only if they have been properly cared for at the time of diagnosis – to include accurate staging, tumor biopsy, endobiliary stenting, diabetes management, and genetic counseling. This will require the expertise that exists at a high-volume cancer center (to accurately stage and prepare the patient for treatment, to include review of clinical trial options). Pressure applied to physicians to keep patients in "their system" for the entire continuum of diagnosis and treatment, rather than offer them referral to a center who can do it better, should be discouraged. As we are entering a new era of physician employment, we will face new challenges in inter-system collaboration, and patients may get caught in the middle. For every million population, there are only 150 patients with pancreatic cancer. It is unrealistic to think that all hospital systems will have the physician expertise and breadth of services needed to develop complex treatment recommendations for patients with pancreatic cancer. Physicians in competing health systems must work together to find that sweat spot for optimal patient care wherein patients receive the expertise of the regional high-volume center and the convenience and compassion of their local physicians. Working together for the good of the patient may be as challenging as finding the optimal therapy.

References

1. Horvath LE, Yordan E, Malhotra D, et al. Multidisciplinary care in the oncology setting: historical perspective and data from lung and gynecology multidisciplinary clinics. J Oncol Pract. 2010;6(6):e21–6.
2. Newman EA, Guest AB, Helvie MA, et al. Changes in surgical management resulting from case review at a breast cancer multidisciplinary tumor board. Cancer. 2006;107(10):2346–51.
3. Oettle H, Neuhaus P, Hochhaus A, et al. Adjuvant chemotherapy with gemcitabine and long-term outcomes among patients with resected pancreatic cancer: the CONKO-001 randomized trial. JAMA. 2013;310(14):1473–81.
4. Gnerlich JL, Luka SR, Deshpande AD, et al. Microscopic margins and patterns of treatment failure in resected pancreatic adenocarcinoma. Arch Surg. 2012;147(8):753–60.
5. Winter JM, Cameron JL, Campbell KA, et al. 1423 pancreaticoduodenectomies for pancreatic cancer: a single-institution experience. J Gastrointest Surg. 2006;10(9):1199–210; discussion 1210–1191.
6. Winter JM, Brennan MF, Tang LH, et al. Survival after resection of pancreatic adenocarcinoma: results from a single institution over three decades. Ann Surg Oncol. 2012;19(1):169–75.
7. Rhim AD, Mirek ET, Aiello NM, et al. EMT and dissemination precede pancreatic tumor formation. Cell. 2012;148(1–2):349–61.
8. Sohal DP, Walsh RM, Ramanathan RK, Khorana AA. Pancreatic adenocarcinoma: treating a systemic disease with systemic therapy. J Natl Cancer Inst. 2014;106(3):dju011.
9. Tuveson DA, Neoptolemos JP. Understanding metastasis in pancreatic cancer: a call for new clinical approaches. Cell. 2012;148(1–2):21–3.
10. Oettle H, Post S, Neuhaus P, et al. Adjuvant chemotherapy with gemcitabine vs observation in patients undergoing curative-intent resection of pancreatic cancer: a randomized controlled trial. JAMA. 2007;297(3):267–77.
11. Neoptolemos JP, Palmer DH, Ghaneh P, et al. Comparison of adjuvant gemcitabine and capecitabine with gemcitabine monotherapy in patients with resected pancreatic cancer (ESPAC-4): a multicentre, openlabel, randomised, phase 3 trial. Lancet. 2017;389(10073):1011–24.
12. Mayo SC, Gilson MM, Herman JM, et al. Management of patients with pancreatic adenocarcinoma: national trends in patient selection, operative management, and use of adjuvant therapy. J Am Coll Surg. 2012;214(1):33–45.
13. Wu W, He J, Cameron JL, et al. The impact of postoperative complications on the administration of adjuvant therapy following pancreaticoduodenectomy for adenocarcinoma. Ann Surg Oncol. 2014;21(9):2873–81.
14. Conroy T, Hammel P, Hebbar M, et al. FOLFIRINOX or Gemcitabine as adjuvant therapy for pancreatic cancer. New Eng J Med. 2018;379(25):2395–406.
15. Pisters PW, Hudec WA, Lee JE, et al. Preoperative chemoradiation for patients with pancreatic cancer: toxicity of endobiliary stents. J Clin Oncol. 2000;18(4):860–7.
16. Aadam AA, Evans DB, Khan A, Oh Y, Dua K. Efficacy and safety of self-expandable metal stents for biliary decompression in patients receiving neoadjuvant therapy for pancreatic cancer: a prospective study. Gastrointest Endosc. 2012;76(1):67–75.
17. Evans DB, Varadhachary GR, Crane CH, et al. Preoperative gemcitabine-based chemoradiation for patients with resectable adenocarcinoma of the pancreatic head. J Clin Oncol. 2008;26(21):3496–502.
18. Varadhachary GR, Wolff RA, Crane CH, et al. Preoperative gemcitabine and cisplatin followed by gemcitabine-based chemoradiation for resectable adenocarcinoma of the pancreatic head. J Clin Oncol. 2008;26(21):3487–95.
19. Christians KK, Heimler JW, George B, et al. Survival of patients with resectable pancreatic cancer who received neoadjuvant therapy. Surgery. 2016;159(3):893–900.
20. Cloyd JM, Katz MH, Prakash L, et al. Preoperative therapy and pancreatoduodenectomy for pancreatic ductal adenocarcinoma: a 25-year single-institution experience. J Gastrointest Surg. 2017;21(1):164–74.
21. Van Tienhoven G, Versteijne E, Suker M, Groothuis KB, Busch OR, Bonsing BA. Preoperative chemoradiotherapy versus immediate surgery for resectable and borderline resectable pancreatic cancer (PREOPANC-1): a randomized, controlled, multicenter phase III trial. J Clin Oncol. 2018;36(18_suppl; Abstr LBA4002).
22. Tsai S, Christians KK, George B, et al. A phase II clinical trial of molecular profiled neoadjuvant therapy

for localized pancreatic ductal adenocarcinoma. Ann Surg. 2018;268(4):610–9.
23. Pancreatic Adenocarcinoma. NCCN Clinical Practice Guidlines in Oncology (NCCN Guidelines) 2018. http://www.nccn.org/professionals/physician_gls/pdf/pancreatic.pdf.
24. Hu C, Hart SN, Polley EC, et al. Association between inherited germline mutations in cancer predisposition genes and risk of pancreatic cancer. JAMA. 2018;319(23):2401–9.
25. Tsai S, Evans DB. Therapeutic advances in localized pancreatic cancer. JAMA Surg. 2016;151:862.
26. Tsai S, George B, Wittmann D, Ritch PS, Krepline AN, Aldakkak M, Barnes CA, Christians KK, Dua K, Griffin M, Hall WA, Erickson BA, Evans DB. Importance of normalization of CA19-9 levels following neoadjuvant therapy in patients with localized pancreatic cancer. Ann Surg. 2018; https://doi.org/10.1097/SLA.0000000000003049. [Epub ahead of print] PMID: 30312198.

2 Clinical Staging of Pancreatic Cancer with MDCT and MRI

Naveen M. Kulkarni

Introduction

Pancreatic cancer is the fourth leading cause of cancer death in the United States, with an overall 5-year survival rate of only 7%, when accounting for all stages [1–4]. The poor prognosis of pancreatic cancer relates to its propensity to infiltrate critical vascular and neural structures near the pancreas and is associated with an aggressive disease biology with early metastatic spread, particularly to the liver and peritoneum (Fig. 2.1). As a result, approximately, 40–50% of patients who are considered to have localized, operable pancreatic cancer will have a microscopically positive (R1) resection after surgery [5]. Patients with incomplete/margin positive resection [residual microscopic (R1) or residual macroscopic (R2)] have survival rates similar to patients with metastatic disease, and hence, would not benefit from surgery [6–9]. Cross-sectional imaging plays an essential role in the clinical staging of pancreatic cancer and assists in allocating patients into the appropriate management group.

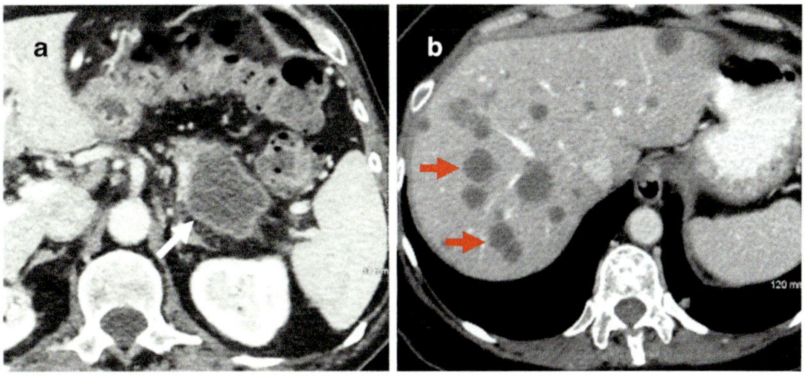

Fig. 2.1 Metastatic pancreatic cancer at presentation. (**a**, **b**) Portal venous phase axial MDCT images through the pancreatic tail and liver shows large pancreatic tail mass (white arrow) and multiple liver metastases (red arrows)

N. M. Kulkarni (✉)
Department of Radiology, The Medical College of Wisconsin, Milwaukee, WI, USA
e-mail: nkulkarni@mcw.edu

S. Tsai et al. (eds.), *Management of Localized Pancreatic Cancer*,
https://doi.org/10.1007/978-3-319-98944-0_2

Staging and Resectability

To understand the clinical significance of cross-sectional imaging in the management of pancreatic cancer, it is important to be familiar with the staging system/resectability criteria for pancreatic cancer. Multiple staging systems from a variety of different societies and institutions have been described [10–14]. The American Joint Committee on Cancer (AJCC) TNM staging has been used to characterize the pathologic stage of pancreatic cancer. This system assesses the status of the primary tumor (T), lymph nodes (N), and metastases (M) with an aim to define tumor stages and provide prognosis based on gross *pathologic* characteristics [15]. With the advent of neoadjuvant therapies for pancreatic cancer, alternative staging systems were developed based on *preoperative* clinical parameters to more accurately categorize the probability of surgical resection based on anatomic factors an the ability to achieve a complete surgical resection, to include the extent of peripancreatic and perivascular invasion. This classification of tumor-mesenteric vessel relationship is a critical component in surgical planning and is not addressed in the AJCC staging system. In order to define the resectability status of pancreatic cancer, additional classification systems have been described. Depending on the tumor location, relationship with peripancreatic vessels, and presence/absence of metastatic disease, published guidelines generally agree on four clinical stages: (1) resectable, (2) borderline resectable, (3) locally advanced [unresectable], and (4) metastatic [unresectable]. Although there is a close agreement on what constitutes resectable and unresectable (locally advanced and metastatic) disease, the definition of borderline resectable disease is more variable (Table 2.1) [16]. Differences in surgical experience, as well as imaging practices and interpretation, contribute to these varying definitions of borderline resectable category. Patients with borderline resectable disease were previously considered as poor candidates for resection; but with improved neoadjuvant therapy, there is growing consensus to offer surgery as a part of multimodality therapy [10, 14]. Irrespective of the classification system used, cross-sectional imaging provides the most objective means to preoperatively stage the pancreatic cancer.

Table 2.1 Definitions of resectability between different classification systems [10–14]

Stage	Anatomy	MCW	NCCN (2017)	MDACC	AHPBA/SSO/SSAT
Resectable	Artery (CA, SMA, or HA)	No involvement	No involvement	No involvement	No involvement
	Vein (SMV, PV, or SMV-PV confluence)	• No involvement • If involved, ≤50% circumference narrowing of vein	• No involvement • ≤180° contact without vein contour irregularity	• No involvement • Abutment (provided vein is patent)	No involvement

Table 2.1 (continued)

Stage	Anatomy		MCW		NCCN (2017)	MDACC	AHPBA/SSO/SSAT
Borderline resectable	Artery	CA	Abutment		• Abutment • Encasement [no involvement of aorta and GDA]	Abutment	Uninvolved
		SMA	Abutment		Abutment	Abutment	Abutment
		HA	Short segment abutment/encasement without involving CA or HA bifurcation		Contact without extension to CA or HA bifurcation	Abutment or short segment encasement	Abutment or short segment encasement
	Vein (SMV, PV, or SMV-PV confluence)		>50% narrowing[a]		• Contact >180°[a] • Contact ≤180° with contour irregularity or thrombosis of vein[a] • Contact with IVC	• Abutment with impingement and narrowing[a] • Segmental venous occlusion[a]	Abutment, encasement, or short segment occlusion[a]
Locally advanced	Artery		Type A	Type B	Encasement of CA, SMA and HA without options for reconstruction		
		CA	Encasement but no extension to aorta[b]	Encasement and extension to aorta			
		SMA	Encasement (>180° but ≤270°)	>270° encasement			
		HA	Encasement and extension to CA[b]	Encasement with extension beyond bifurcation of proper HA			
	Vein (SMV, PV, or SMV-PV confluence)		Occlusion without options for reconstruction				
Metastatic	Evidence of peritoneal and distant metastases						

Abutment is defined as ≤180° contact with vessel and encasement indicates >180° involvement

MCW Medical College of Wisconsin, *NCCN* National Comprehensive Cancer Network, *MDACC* MD Anderson Cancer Center, *AHPBA* American Hepato-Pancreato-Biliary Association, *SSAT* Society for Surgery of the Alimentary Tract, *SSO* Society for Surgical Oncology

CA celiac axis, *SMA* superior mesenteric artery, *HA* hepatic artery, *GDA* gastroduodenal artery, *SMV* superior mesenteric vein, *PV* portal vein

[a]Amenable for safe and complete resection and venous reconstruction

[b]Amenable for celiac resection (with or without reconstruction)

Cross-Sectional Imaging Techniques

During the initial evaluation of patients with pancreatic cancer, obtaining a high-quality cross-sectional imaging is one of the most important components of the workup. A pancreatic mass can be seen on abdominal ultrasound and routine contrast-enhanced computed tomography (CT) may be performed for the evaluation of abdominal pain or sometimes is detected as an incidental finding. However, these studies are not adequate for the staging of pancreatic cancer. A dedicated pancreatic protocol performed as a biphasic technique and scan parameters optimized for detection and staging is essential [17, 18].

Multidetector Computed Tomograph (MDCT)

When pancreatic pathology is suspected, a biphase pancreatic CT protocol should be performed on multidetector scanner (64-detector row or greater is preferred). Neutral oral contrast such as water is used to distend stomach and duodenum to provide optimal visibility of periampullary and pancreatic head pathology (Fig. 2.2). Positive oral contrast should be avoided as it obscures the periampullary region and could impair the visibility of subtle pancreatic head abnormalities secondary to beam-hardening artifacts from contrast pooling within the stomach and duodenum. This also interferes with three-dimensional (3-D) CT post-processing. Multi-phase pancreatic CT is done with rapid injection of intravenous nonionic iodinated contrast (3–5 mL/s). Rapidly injected contrast bolus causes intense pancreatic enhancement enabling distinction of a hypovascular cancer (as is characteristic of pancreatic cancer) from the enhancing normal pancreas. The first part of biphasic pancreatic protocol is acquired during the pancreatic (late arterial) phase, approximately 40–50 seconds after the start of contrast injection. The latter hepatic (portal venous) phase optimizes enhancement of the liver and portomesenteric vasculature and is typically acquired 65–75 seconds after contrast injection. For the pancreatic phase, upper abdomen, including the pancreas is scanned, and the hepatic phase should include entire abdomen and pelvis (Table 2.2) [19–23].

The MDCT images are acquired using thin collimation (0.5–0.6 mm thickness) in a relatively short and comfortable breath hold time to obtain motion-free images. With new MDCT scanners, isotropic volume acquisition (identical resolution in all three planes) allows generation of high-quality multiplanar and curved-planar reformatted images, and 3-D reconstruction of mesenteric vessels [maximum intensity projection (MIP) and volume rendering (VR)] which provides an excellent view of vascular anatomy (Fig. 2.3) and tumor-vessel relationship. Three-D reconstructions offer certain unique advantages over the axial image: (1) better display of tumor encasement/abutment of vessels which may not be seen in the standard axial plane, (2) 2-D and

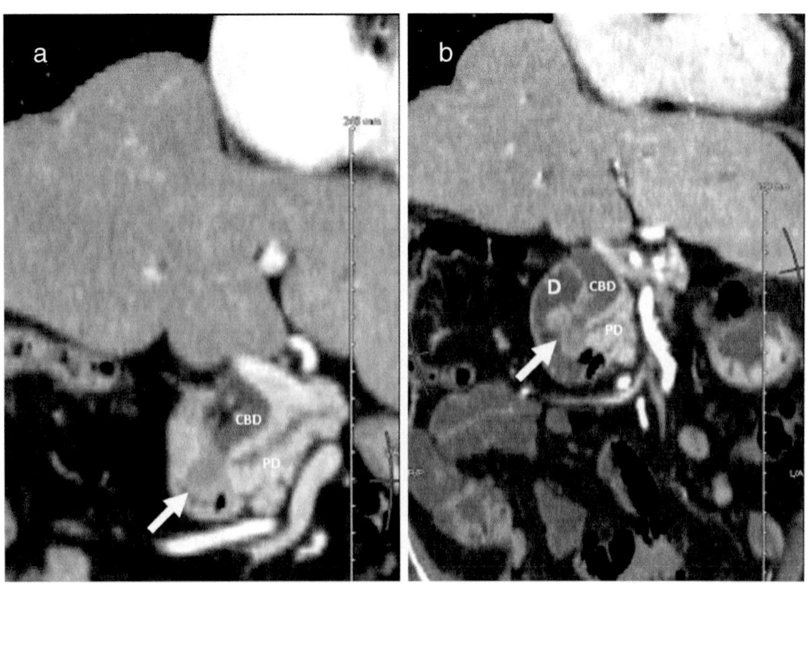

Fig. 2.2 Ampullary tumor on two different studies from the same patient (acquired 4 weeks apart). (**a**) Oblique coronal image from routine contrast-enhanced MDCT shows dilated common bile duct and pancreatic duct and suspected periampullary tumor (white arrow). (**b**) Repeat dual-phase pancreatic MDCT with neutral oral contrast (water) resulted in sufficient duodenum (D) distension confirming bilobed ampullary tumor (white arrow)

Table 2.2 MDCT protocol for evaluation of pancreatic adenocarcinoma [11, 20]

Parameters	Technical aspects	Comments
Scan type and acquisition	Multidetector row CT with thinnest possible section thickness	Scanner with 64-slice or greater is preferred
Oral contrast	Neutral agent (water) should be used	Positive oral contrast can limit assessment of periampullary region and pancreatic head
Contrast-enhanced phases and acquisition timing	Pancreatic phase: 40–50 s Portal venous phase: 65–70 s (Iodinate contrast agent with high iodine content, >300 mg I/ml at injection rate of 3–5 ml/s is preferred)	Pancreatic phase is ideal for assessment of primary tumor and portal venous phase for evaluating metastases
Standard reconstructions	Axial: 2–5 mm thickness MPR (Coronal and sagittal): 2–3 mm	May vary between institutions
Additional reconstructions	MIP, VR, oblique MPR, and CPR (These are always reviewed in conjunction with standard reconstructions)	MIP & VR: for vascular maps Oblique MPR and CPR: to view structures like blood vessel or pancreatic duct which lie or course in a nonstandard plane

MPR multiplanar reformats, *MIP* maximum intensity projection, *VR* volume rendered, *CPR* curved planar reformats

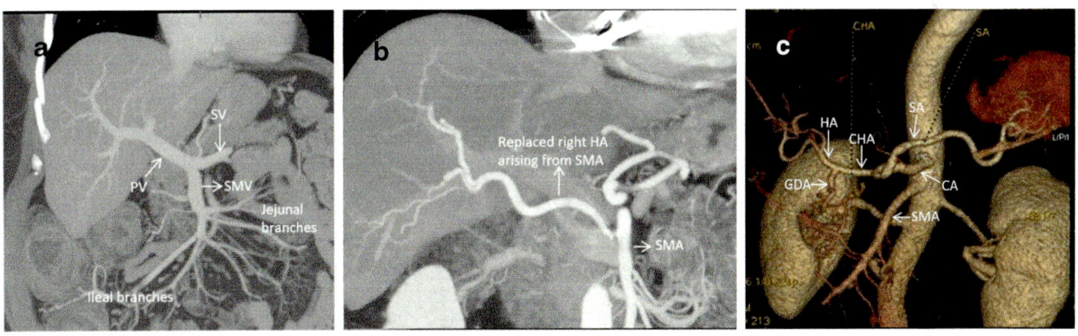

Fig. 2.3 Different post-processing tools to display 3-D anatomy of central mesenteric vasculature relevant to pancreatic imaging. (**a**) Normal coronal maximum intensity projection (MIP) of mesenteric venous systems. (**b**) Coronal MIP shows replaced right HA arising from the SMA. (**c**) Normal volume rendered (VR) image displays important peripancreatic arteries. (PV portal vein, SV splenic vein, SA splenic artery, SMV superior mesenteric vein, SMA superior mesenteric artery, CA celiac axis, CHA common hepatic artery, HA hepatic artery, GDA gastroduodenal artery)

3-D views of variations to mesenteric arterial anatomy and length of vascular involvement, and (3) perineural spread of the tumor [24–28].

The pancreatic phase maximizes the detection of a pancreatic cancer and allows for characterization of the tumor to nearby arterial structures, whereas the hepatic phase is ideal for detecting liver, peritoneal, and lymph node metastases, as well as tumor involvement of venous structures (Figs. 2.1 and 2.4). The visibility of pancreatic cancer is enhanced due to its hypoattenuating appearance on the background of enhancing normal pancreas; this is seen in approximately 90–95% of patients on the pancreatic phase (Fig. 2.4). Often, secondary findings like contour deformity and/or dilatation of either the pancreatic or common bile duct or both (the "double-duct sign") can be seen (Fig. 2.5). 3-D curved-planar reformatted images along the length of the pancreas can better outline subtle degree of dilated pancreatic duct to localize site of obstruction when pancreatic mass is radiographically occult. Such secondary signs are useful in localizing isoattenuating pancreatic cancer

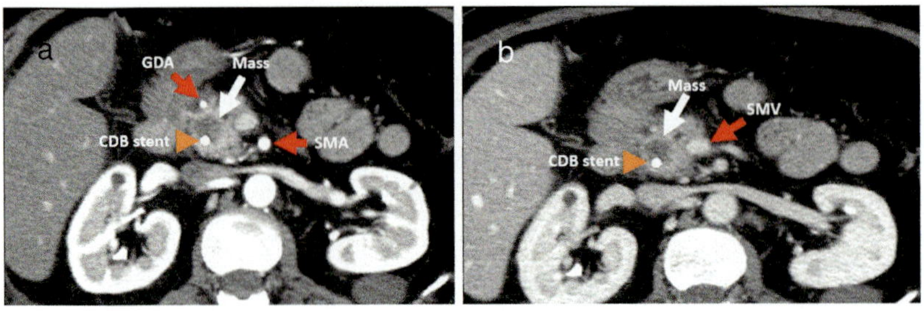

Fig. 2.4 Example of resectable pancreatic cancer. Axial pancreatic phase (**a**) and portal venous phase (**b**) images show hypovascular mass (white arrow) confined to the pancreatic head and without involving peripancreatic vessels (red arrows). (SMV superior mesenteric vein, SMA superior mesenteric artery, GDA gastroduodenal artery, CBD common bile duct)

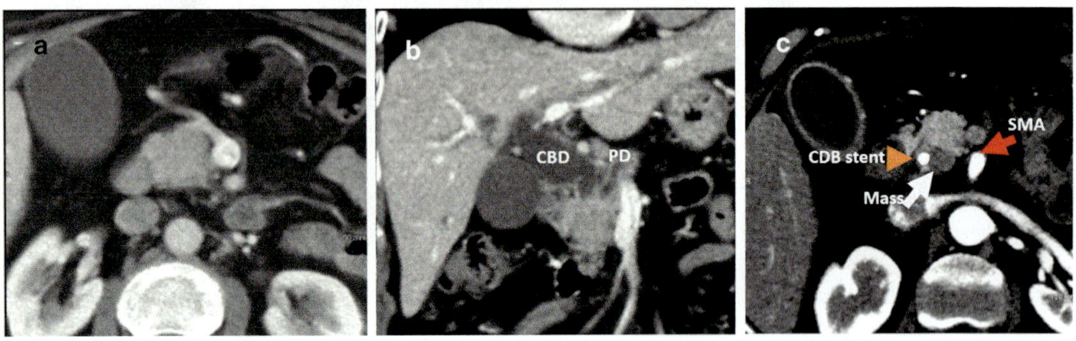

Fig. 2.5 Importance of secondary signs in identifying small pancreatic cancer. (**a**, **b**) Portal venous phase axial and coronal MDCT images from a routine study done for the workup of jaundice shows "double-duct" sign and no visible pancreatic mass. (**c**) Dedicated study with MDCT pancreatic protocol clearly shows small pancreatic head mass (white arrow) on the arterial phase. Small pancreatic cancer can be isodense to normal parenchyma on the portal venous phase and may only be seen on the pancreatic phase, highlighting the importance of dual-phase acquisition. (CBD common bile duct, PD pancreatic duct)

(in roughly 5–10% of cases), especially when they are small (measuring ≤2 cm) and non-contour deforming (Fig. 2.6). In the absence of a visible pancreatic mass, secondary signs should prompt further evaluation with either MRI or endoscopic ultrasound [22, 29–33].

Emerging CT technologies are also being explored for their use in pancreatic imaging. Dual-energy CT is a novel imaging method that simultaneously acquires images with two X-ray beams. Dual-energy CT data can be processed to reconstruct images at multiple different energies, and the lower energy images can identify small pancreatic cancers due to inherent high image contrast. Dual-energy CT also allows reconstruction of iodine images which have high contrast-to-noise ratio and are less prone to artifacts, thus improving the visibility of even small lesions. Studies have shown that using dual-energy CT rather than standard CT could improve lesion detection and lesion characterization. In recent years, this technology has received more attention and support for its use in the detection and staging of pancreatic cancer (Figs. 2.7 and 2.8). A detailed discussion of dual-energy CT technology is beyond the scope of this chapter, and the technology is still evolving requiring standardization and inclusion into the standard imaging guidelines [34–36].

Magnetic Resonance Imaging (MRI)

Unlike MDCT pancreatic protocol, which is relatively standardized, MRI protocol for pan-

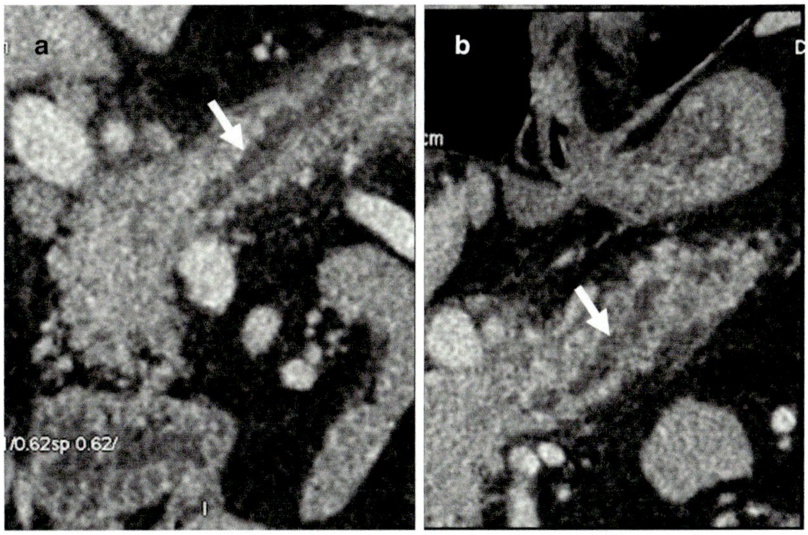

Fig. 2.6 Example of an occult pancreatic mass causing obstruction and dilatation of upstream pancreatic duct. (**a**, **b**) Curved planar reformatted (CPR) images in two different views show dilated pancreatic duct (white arrow) with abrupt cutoff, although a discrete mass is not identified. This was eventually confirmed to result from a small pancreatic cancer by EUS and sampling

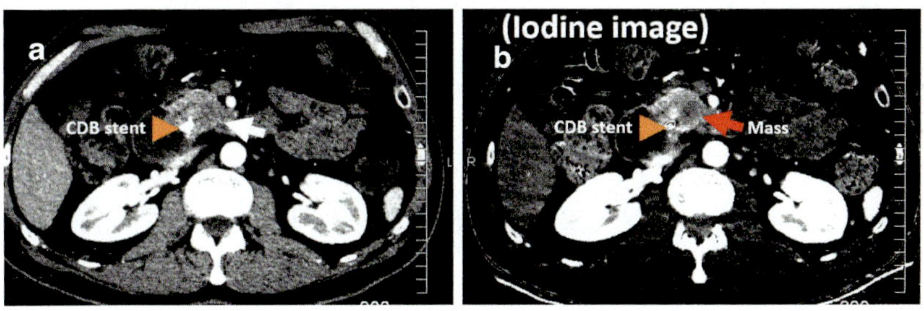

Fig. 2.7 Improved detection of pancreatic cancer with dual-energy CT. (**a**, **b**) Standard contrast-enhanced image (**a**) shows vague hypodensity within the pancreatic head (white arrow). Iodine image (**b**) clearly shows a small pancreatic head mass (white arrow) signifying its role in improved lesion detection. Also note the benefit of iodine image in decreasing artifact from common bile duct stent (arrowhead)

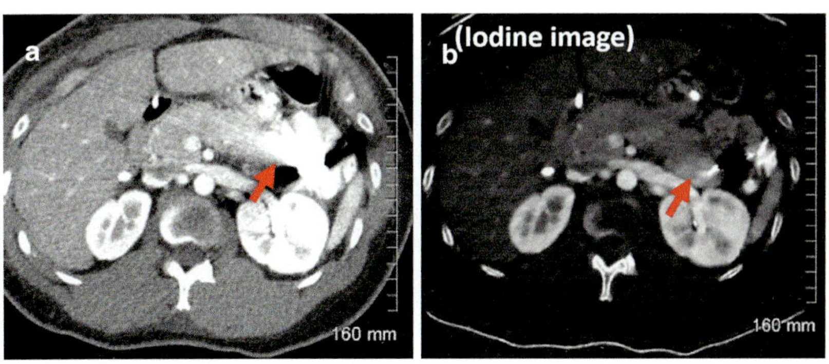

Fig. 2.8 Artifact reduction with DECT. (**a**, **b**) Axial contrast-enhanced DECT images obtained during the portal venous phase of contrast enhancement. Dense artifacts emerging from surgical clips in left upper quadrant is substantially reduced on iodine image (red arrow) thus improving visibility of the pancreatic body and tail

creatic imaging may have some degree of variability across different institutions. In general, the optimal MRI technique uses a combination of sequences obtained in axial and coronal planes, which are designed to provide the highest level of contrast resolution for the pancreas and ductal anatomy. Standard sequences include T2-weighted imaging with and without fat suppression, T1-weighted in-phase and opposed-phase images, T2-weighted MR cholangiopancreatography (MRCP), fat-suppressed T1-weighted gradient echo images without and with gadolinium contrast (acquired in late arterial, portal venous, and delayed phases), and diffusion-weighted imaging (DWI) to image the pancreas, peripancreatic tissue, and liver (Fig. 2.9). The contrast kinetics of the pancreatic (late arterial) and portal venous phases are similar to MDCT with the late arterial phase most suitable for the detection of pancreatic masses and portal venous phase most suitable to evaluate liver lesions/metastases. To achieve optimal evaluation and best possible images without artifacts that result from movement or breathing, scanners with high-strength magnetic field (≥1.5 Tesla) should be used. Table 2.3 summarizes pancreatic MRI protocol used at our institution [37–40].

T1-weighted imaging is the most important sequence in the detection of pancreatic cancers. Due to fibrotic nature, pancreatic cancers appear hypointense (dark) relative to enhancing parenchyma which appears hyperintense (bright) on the pancreatic phase (Fig. 2.9). Even without intravenous gadolinium contrast, the pancreatic

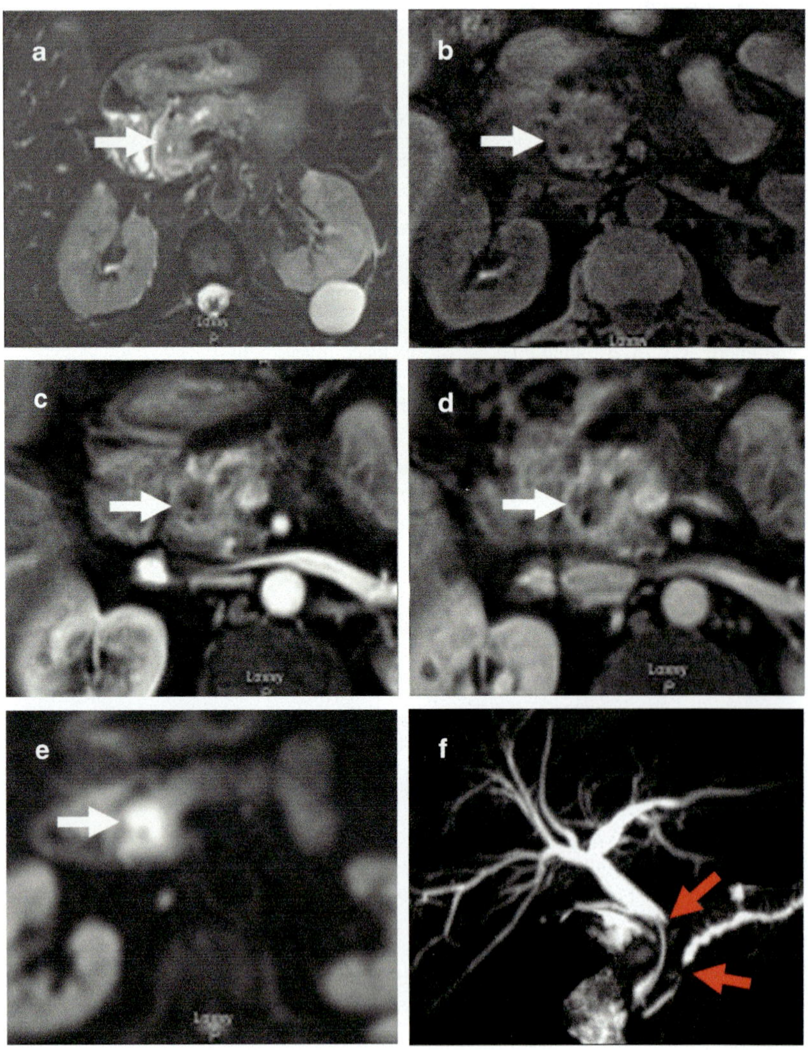

Fig. 2.9 Typical appearance of pancreatic cancer on MR. (**a**, **b**) The pancreatic head mass (white arrow) is isointense to parenchyma on T2-weighted image (**a**) making it difficult to perceive and hypointense on pre-contrast T1W image (**b**) making it visible even without gadolinium contrast agent. (**c**–**e**) Post-contrast and diffusion-weighted imaging (DWI) confirms the presence of mass which is hypointense on the pancreatic (**c**) and portal venous (**d**) phases and hyperintense on DWI (**e**). MRCP image (**f**) displays abrupt cutoff of the pancreatic duct and common bile duct (red arrows) (CBD contains a stent)

Table 2.3 MRI protocol for evaluation of pancreatic adenocarcinoma [11, 20]

Sequence	Plane	Role
T2W single shot (SSFSE or HASTE)	Coronal with or without axial (<6 mm)	To evaluate pancreaticobiliary ductal system and overall anatomy
T2W with fat suppression	Axial (6 mm)	Evaluation of metastasis and cystic pancreatic lesion. Less useful in pancreatic adenocarcinoma
T1W in-phase and opposed-phase gradient echo	Axial (4 mm)	Characterize intracellular fat (such as focal fatty infiltration that can mimic as pancreatic mass on MDCT)
MRCP	Coronal (<3 mm)	Pancreatic and biliary ductal system
Diffusion-weighted imaging	Axial (<6 mm)	Asses pancreatic mass and metastases
Pre- and post-dynamic contrast (gadolinium)-enhanced T1W 3-D fat-suppressed gradient echo (pancreatic, portal venous and equilibrium phases)	Axial (3 mm)	Pancreatic adenocarcinoma is detected using unenhanced and early enhanced T1W sequence Portal venous and delayed phases are best for detecting lymphadenopathy, liver, and peritoneal metastases

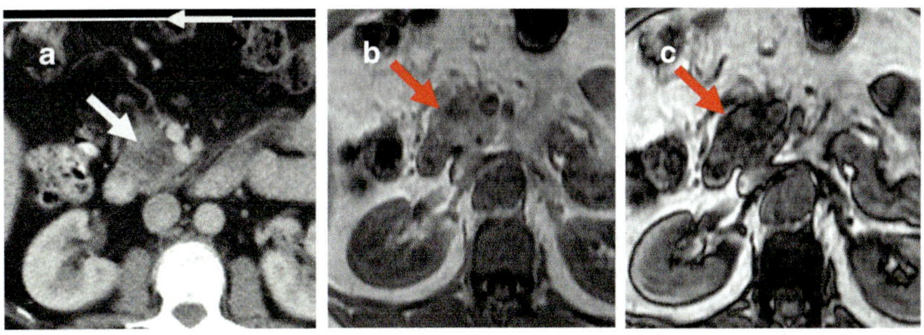

Fig. 2.10 Characterization of pancreatic focal fatty infiltration mimicking as lesion on MDCT. (**a**) Portal venous phase axial MDCT image at the level of pancreatic head shows indeterminate low attenuation lesion (white arrow). (**b**, **c**) Axial T1- weighted in-phase (**b**) and out-of-phase (**c**) images confirm that abnormality in question is focal fatty infiltration (red arrow) as suggested by signal drop on the out-of-phase image. This example highlights the benefit of MRI as a problem-solving tool

cancer can be localized on T1-weighted sequence due to the differences in tissue contrast between hypointense pancreatic mass and intrinsic T1 hyperintensity of the pancreas (secondary to rich acinar protein). The conspicuity of pancreatic cancer is further increased with the use of a fat suppression technique that nulls surrounding extracellular/macroscopic fat. A variant of T1-weighted sequence (in-phase and opposed-phase/chemical shift imaging) is particularly used to detect intracellular fat. These fat suppression techniques are important in characterizing focal pancreatic fat which can mimic pancreatic mass on MDCT (Fig. 2.10) [41–44].

T2-weighted sequence [also referred to as "fluid sensitive" sequence] has variable appearance of pancreatic cancer and is influenced by the degree of pancreatic atrophy. However, T2-weighted images are useful in detecting liver metastases, characterizing pancreatic cystic lesions, and MRCP imaging to map the pancreatic and biliary ductal anatomy. Diffusion-weighted imaging (DWI) is a variant of T2-weighted imaging and a functional MRI technique that assesses motion of water molecule in biologic tissues. Pancreatic cancer and metastases have restricted water motion and appear hyperintense on DWI (Figs. 2.9 and 2.11). Because of false-positive and false-negative findings (related to tumor necrosis and less fibrous tumors), DWI alone is not used to characterize lesions. It is always reviewed in conjunction with T2-weighted and portal venous phase images to

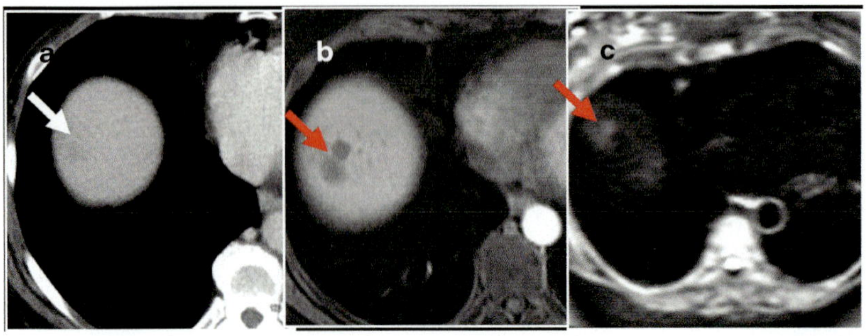

Fig. 2.11 Advantage of MRI over MDCT in assessing liver metastases. (**a**) Portal venous phase axial image at the level of hepatic dome shows indeterminate liver lesion in segment VII (white arrow). (**b**, **c**) Axial contrast-enhanced T1-weighted (**b**) and DWI (**c**) images at the same level shows two distinct liver lesions consistent with metastases (red arrows). Not show here, contrast-enhanced CT underestimated additional liver metastases

improve the sensitivity of MRI in detecting pancreatic tumor and metastases [37, 45–47].

Although MDCT is the preferred technique in the initial staging of pancreatic cancer, MRI can be a useful alternate modality. MRI is equivalent to MDCT for detection and assessment of local disease although it is also easier to identify and grade subtle degrees of vascular involvement on MDCT due to better resolution. MRI best serves as an adjunct tool when confronted with indeterminate findings on MDCT (such as characterizing small pancreatic masses or indeterminate liver lesions) or when contrast-enhanced CT is not possible due to severe allergy to iodinated contrast agent. NCCN guidelines recommend imaging with CT (preferred) or MRI using dedicated pancreatic protocol, while the International Study Group of Pancreatic Surgery (ISGPS) recommends evaluation with pancreatic CT. At our institution, all suspected cases of pancreatic cancer are initially imaged with MDCT for clinical staging; MRI is used as an adjunct problem-solving tool [11, 38, 48–50].

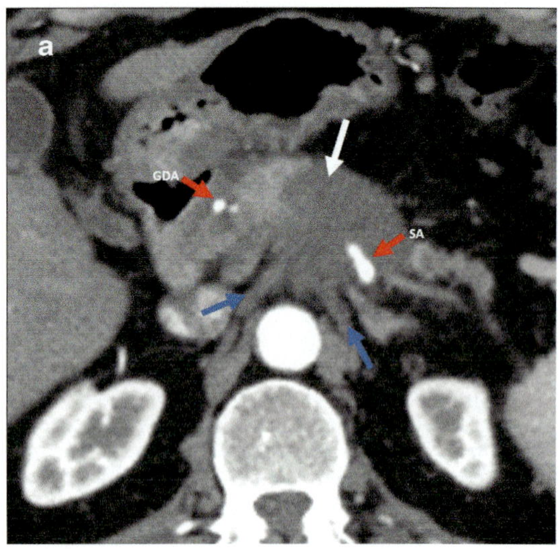

Fig. 2.12 Pancreatic cancer extending to celiac ganglion. (**a**) Pancreatic phase axial MDCT image shows retroperitoneal extension of large pancreatic body mass (white arrow) with involvement of bilateral celiac ganglia (blue arrows) (Celiac ganglia are seen as linear and slender soft tissue which are thickened in this case)

Imaging Findings Significant to Staging

Tumor Location

Most pancreatic cancers (approximately 60–70%) involve the pancreatic head (located to the right of superior mesenteric vein -portal vein (SMV-PV) confluence), about 10–20% are in the body (between the SMV-PV confluence and left lateral margin of the aorta) and 5–10% in the tail (lateral to the aorta) [51]. The location of tumor is important, as it determines the surgical technique for tumor resection; pancreaticoduodenectomy (Whipple procedure) for pancreatic head tumors, distal pancreatectomy for tumors in the body and tail of pancreas, and total pancreatectomy for tumors involving the neck of the pancreas. The location of tumor can also predict the potential route of perineural spread of disease (Fig. 2.12). Perineural invasion is common with head and uncinate process tumor (up to 70% of cases) and can result in positive resection margins at surgery. It can be seen in early stages and even with small tumors (2 cm or less). Perineural spread is seen as soft tissue extending along the gastroduodenal artery, the posterior inferior pancreaticoduodenal artery, and the posterior aspect of portal vein to the celiac/mesenteric ganglion or mesenteric root. Pancreatic cancer can also directly invade adjacent organs (like the stomach, duodenum, adrenal gland, and colon), but if this can be safely removed with pancreatic tumor, the disease is still considered operable [52–55].

Assessment of Vascular Involvement

Once metastatic disease is ruled out, establishing the relationship between the pancreatic cancer and the peripancreatic vessels is the most important anatomic assessment, since the extent of vascular involvement classifies tumor into different categories (resectable, borderline resectable, and locally advanced). Tumor resectability is determined by the degree of vessel involvement, specifically the celiac artery (CA), superior mesenteric artery (SMA), hepatic artery (HA), PV, and SMV, which impacts the potential for R0 resection [11, 20, 56]. Involvement of the gastroduodenal and splenic artery should be mentioned, but this does not directly affect resectability. It is also critical to identify any involvement of aorta and inferior vena cava which may preclude tumor resection. Occasionally, tumor extension to renal veins and renal arteries can be seen, and such findings should be documented to provide information for decisions regarding surgical management. When describing vessel involvement, consistent terminology should be used to give clear information to the referring physician. A vessel is considered free of tumor if it has well-defined fat plane all around and without contour deformity. Arterial involvement should be described as abutment or encasement; abutment refers to <180° contact with the tumor, while encasement is defined as ≥180° circumferential involvement (Fig. 2.13) [11, 20, 49]. This distinction is particularly critical with regards to the celiac axis and superior mesenteric artery, because arterial abutment in these locations is not considered a contraindication to resection, but encasement is generally considered a contraindication. Reporting of these radiographic findings is aimed to maximize specificity so that clinicians are better able to correctly identify the patients with potentially operable disease who may benefit from surgery. Unlike the evaluation and reporting of arterial involvement, the involvement of the PV and SMV is often more descriptive since tumor abutment or encasement-induced narrowing or even short segment occlusion does not preclude resection if a suitable length of proximal and distal segments of vein is available for reconstruction (Fig. 2.14). When the

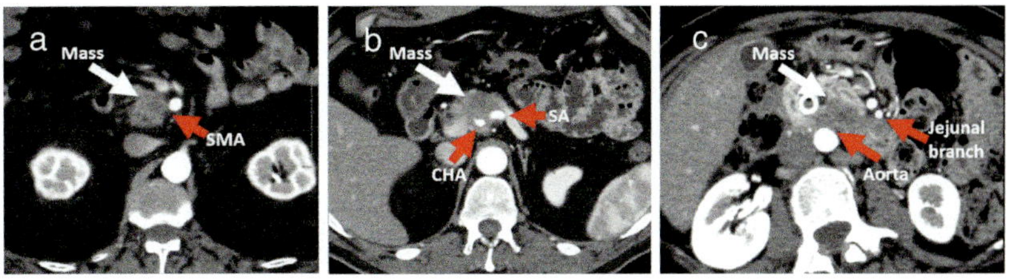

Fig. 2.13 Grading of arterial involvement with pancreatic cancer. Pancreatic phase axial MDCT images from different cases demonstrate spectrum of arterial involvement. (**a**) Pancreatic head mass (white arrow) abutting (<180°) the proximal SMA (red arrow). (**b**) Pancreatic neck mass (white arrow) encases (≥180°) the CHA and SA (red arrows). (**c**) Large pancreatic head mass (white arrow) abutting abdominal aorta and first jejunal branch of SMA (red arrows). (SMA superior mesenteric artery, CHA common hepatic artery, SA splenic artery)

SMV is involved, the caudal extension and proximity to jejunal and/or ileocolic branches should be identified, as such extension could alter surgical technique or preclude the ability to perform venous bypass when multiple branch vessels are involved [11, 20, 57]. It is important to note that pancreatic cancers typically narrow and ultimately occludes veins but rarely invades them. In the setting of PV or SMV invasion, alternate diagnoses, particularly pancreatic neuroendocrine tumors, should be strongly considered [26].

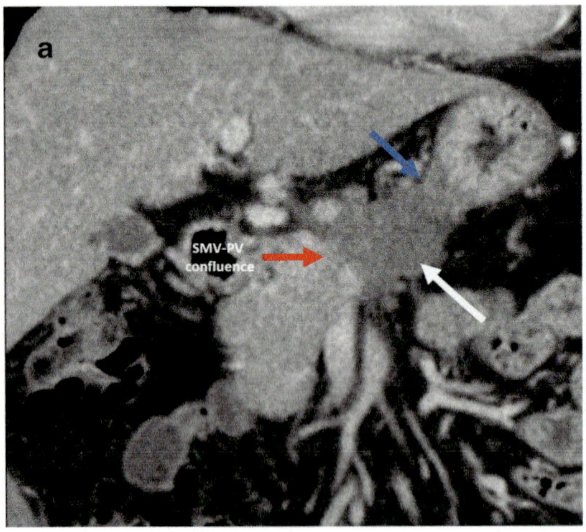

Fig. 2.14 Borderline resectable pancreatic cancer involvement of venous structures. (**a**) Portal venous coronal MDCT image shows encasement and complete occlusion of the SMV-PV confluence (red arrow) by pancreatic body mass (white arrow). Also note direct extension of pancreatic mass to the lesser curvature of stomach (blue arrow). (SMV superior mesenteric vein, PV portal vein)

Subtle degrees of vascular involvement may not be readily visible on axial images. This is particularly true when the tumor involves the undersurface of the CA, HA, or the proximal SMA which can run parallel or oblique to axial source images (Fig. 2.15). A combination of coronal, sagittal, and oblique reformatted images will enhance the characterization of the degree of vascular involvement. For the assessment of veins, concurrent viewing of axial, coronal, and 3-D MIP images provides an excellent view to appreciate the surgical anatomy and the craniocaudal extent of venous involvement [23, 25, 58]. At our institution, multi-planar reformats and 3-D image reconstructions are routinely made available for interpretation.

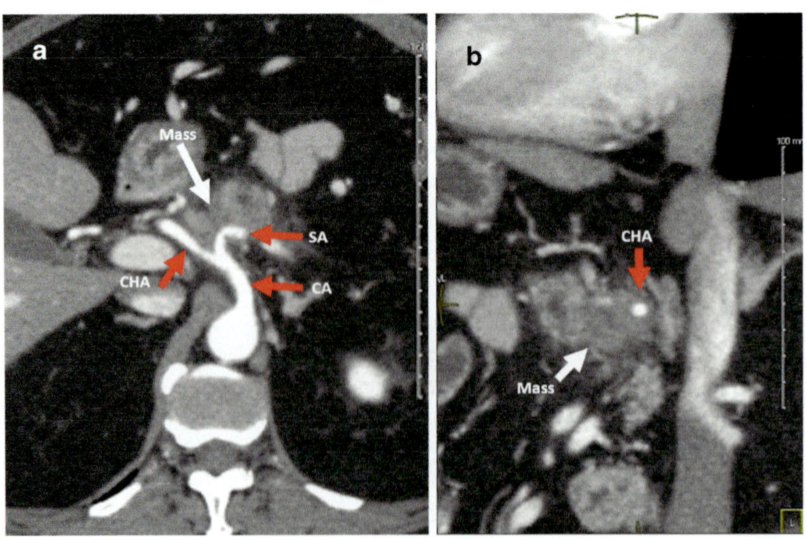

Fig. 2.15 Significance of multiplanar reconstruction for the accurate assessment of arterial involvement. Pancreatic phase axial (**a**) and oblique sagittal (**b**) MDCT images at the level of celiac axis show pancreatic body tumor (white arrow) involving common hepatic artery (CHA) and splenic artery (SA) (red arrow) but difficult to determine the extent of encasement. Oblique sagittal reformatted image (**b**) confirms greater than 180-degree encasement of the CHA by the pancreatic tumor (white arrow)

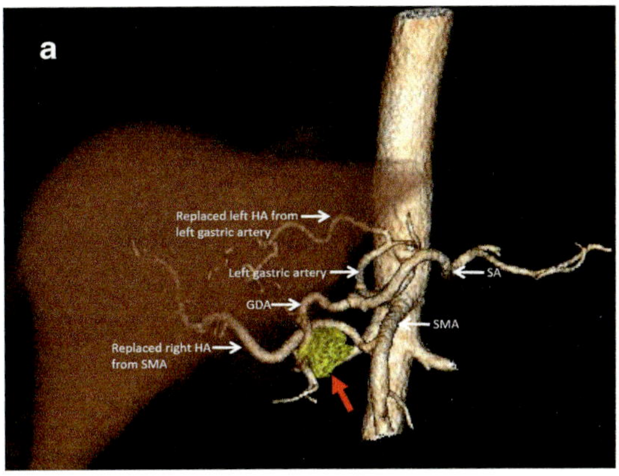

Fig. 2.16 Anatomical variations in mesenteric artery anatomy. (**a**) Coronal volume rendered image shows replaced right hepatic artery (HA) arising from superior mesenteric artery (SMA) and replaced left HA arising from left gastric artery. Pancreatic head cancer surface shaded with fluorescent color (red arrow) abuts gastroduodenal artery (GDA) and replaced right HA. Such variations in mesenteric artery anatomy and their involvement by tumor can alter surgical planning

It is equally important to describe the variants of the CA and SMA anatomy, as their presence can alter surgical planning. The most commonly seen variation is a replaced right HA, or sometimes, even common HA arising from SMA (Fig. 2.16). Other variants are also seen, replaced or accessory left HA arising from the left gastric artery or a common trunk of the CA and SMA. Another consideration that can lead to alteration in surgical planning is celiac artery stenosis, most frequently due to the presence of a median arcuate ligament [21, 59].

Assessment of Metastatic Disease

Pancreatic cancer most commonly spreads to the liver and peritoneum, with the liver being the most common non-nodal site of metastatic disease (Figs. 2.11 and 2.17). Liver metastases are typically hypovascular (with and without rim enhancement)

Fig. 2.17 Metastatic pancreatic cancer involving different organs (red arrows). (**a**) Liver (multiple hypodense lesions), (**b**) peritoneum (thickening and nodularity), (**c**) lymph node (necrotic periportal node), and (**d**) lungs (multiple bilateral pulmonary nodules). Pancreatic tail mass (white arrow) is evident on image (**c**)

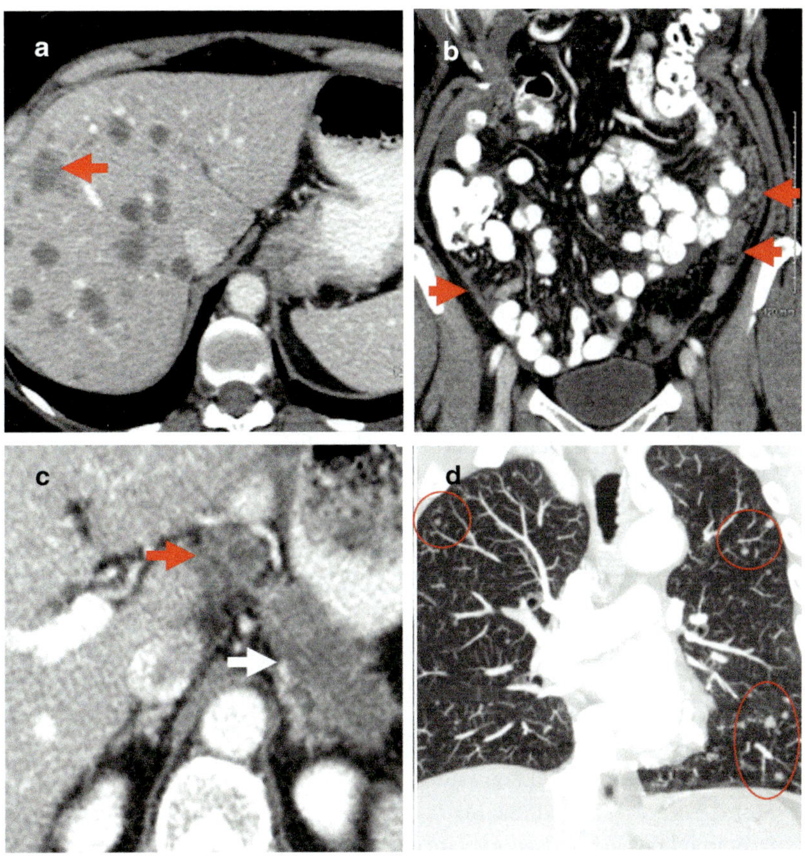

and best evaluated on the portal venous phase. The arterial phase is less useful as small lesions can be easily missed. MRI has better sensitivity and specificity for the detection and characterization of small lesions (<1 cm) which are often indeterminate on MDCT. The performance of MRI is further enhanced by diffusion-weighted imaging (DWI) and new liver-specific contrast agents (Fig. 2.11) [18, 60–63]. In contrast, none of the imaging modalities currently available are sensitive for the detection of early peritoneal disease. Peritoneal disease can have different appearances, including peritoneal thickening and enhancement, micro and macronodular appearance, peritoneal stranding, discrete implants, and frank omental caking (Fig. 2.17). The presence of unexplained ascites is considered suspicious and should prompt careful evaluation of the peritoneal cavity. Peritoneal disease in the subdiaphragmatic spaces, root of the mesentery, hepatic hilum, gallbladder fossa, and serosal surface of the small bowel is particularly difficult to evaluate [64–67]. Other distant sites of disease involvement include the lungs and bones, although bony involvement is usually a late manifestation of this disease. Lung metastases can appear as round or irregular nodules (cavitation can be seen) or have lymphangitic appearance (Fig. 2.17). From a clinical standpoint, chest imaging provides low diagnostic yield and is not usually performed at the initial staging, unless there is a strong clinical suspicion. Nevertheless, chest CT is usually a part of restaging scans [68].

The presence of nodal disease also has important implications on patient prognosis and management; this is particularly influenced by the location of involved lymph nodes (regional vs distant nodes). However, both MDCT and MRI are not particularly sensitive in detecting metastatic lymph nodes. Abnormal lymph nodes are usually defined by size criteria (>1 cm in short axis diameter) and morphology (rounded morphology with cystic/necrotic appearance) (Fig. 2.17). The presence or absence of regional lymph node metastases rarely influences the decision of tumor's resectability, as lymph nodes in this region are almost always resected along with the pancreatic tumor. On the other hand, the involvement of distant lymph nodes (e.g., lymph nodes in infrarenal or retroperitoneal compartment, or to the left of the SMA or within the jejunal mesentery) is classified as distant metastatic disease [69–73].

Reporting of Imaging Findings

Consistent interpretation of a MDCT/MRI study, using a reporting format that is systematic and easily understood by all physicians who are involved in the patient's care, is the next important step. Ambiguous, non-specific reports can lead to miscommunication and could potentially result in repeat imaging, especially when patients move between institutions, or in the worst case, misclassification of disease stage. Standardized reporting using a template with a checklist can ensure that the imaging features described above are consistently included in all radiology reports. Structured reports not only improve the efficiency and accuracy of reporting, they are well accepted and preferred by both radiologists and clinicians. The reporting template should at least include the following information: size and location of the pancreatic tumor, vascular involvement (CA, CHA, SMA, portal vein, and SMV), arterial variants, nodal involvement, and distant metastases. A standardized reporting template for pancreatic cancer published by the Society of Abdominal Radiology (SAR) and the American Pancreatic Association (APA) which highlights various descriptive findings is available [20].

Defining Resectable, Borderline Resectable, and Unresectable Pancreatic Cancer

The multidisciplinary Pancreatic Cancer Program at the Medical College of Wisconsin (MCW) defines resectable disease as localized to the pancreas and without evidence of distant metastases with no abutment of arterial structures (CA, HA, and SMA) and <50% narrowing of the SMV-PV. This definition differs slightly from that of the AHPBA/SSO/SSAT and NCCN guidelines, which similarly require no evidence of arterial abutment but limits tumor contact to $\leq 180°$ contact of the SMV-PV without vein contour irregularity. Patients classified as resectable based on imaging criteria are potential candidates for an R0 resection (possible in 80–90% of patients) (Fig. 2.4) (Table 2.1) [12–14, 16, 74].

The definition of borderline resectable disease is more uniform and includes tumors with arterial abutment and more advanced venous involvement. The arterial abutment can involve the SMA (usually pertinent to tumors of the pancreatic head) or short segment encasement of the CHA (usually pertinent to tumors of the pancreatic head/neck tumor), with or without >50% narrowing of the SMV-PV or short segment SMV-PV occlusion amenable to venous reconstruction. At MCW, borderline resectable disease is defined as tumor abutment of ≤180° of the SMA or celiac axis, short segment tumor abutment/encasement of the hepatic artery (HA) without extension to HA bifurcation or celiac artery or ≥50% narrowing of SMV, PV, SMV-PV, or short segment occlusion with suitable proximal and distal target for reconstruction (Fig. 2.18) (Table 2.1) [7, 9, 13, 16].

Locally advanced disease is defined by >180° involvement of SMA or CA or HA, or SMV-PV occlusion without potential for reconstruction. In contrast to borderline resectable disease, where surgery is a part of planned treatment sequence, locally advanced disease is considered unresectable at the time of initial presentation. At our institution, locally advanced disease is divided into type A and type B based on tumor-vessel relationship (degree of encasement/extent of SMA, CA, and HA involvement) (Fig. 2.19) (Table 2.1). With improvements in response rates to available

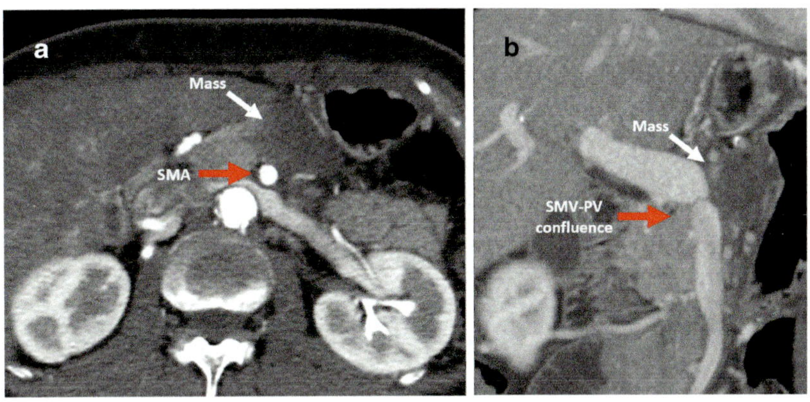

Fig. 2.18 Borderline resectable pancreatic cancer. (**a**, **b**) Axial pancreatic phase (**a**) and coronal portal venous phase (**b**) MDCT images show large pancreatic neck mass abutting SMA (red arrow on **a**) and causing >50% narrowing of SMV and PV confluence (red arrow on **b**). (PV portal vein, SMV superior mesenteric vein, SMA superior mesenteric artery)

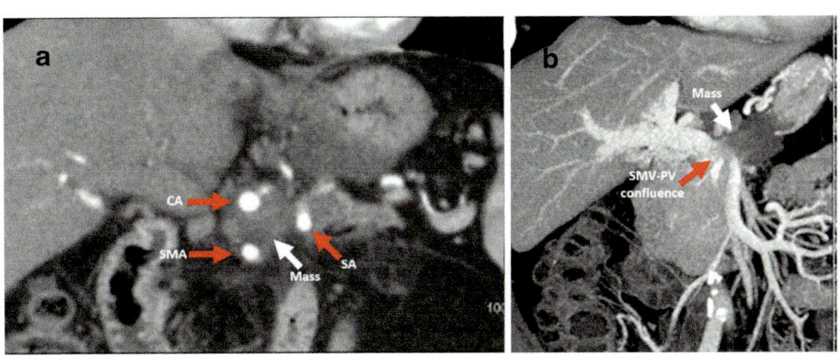

Fig. 2.19 Locally advanced (type B) pancreatic cancer. (**a**, **b**) Coronal pancreatic phase (**a**) and portal venous phase (**b**) MDCT images show a large pancreatic body mass encasing CA, SMA, SA (red arrows on **a**) and completely occluding SMV-PV confluence (red arrow on **b**). (PV portal vein, SMV superior mesenteric vein, SV splenic vein, SA splenic artery, SMA superior mesenteric artery, CA celiac axis)

systemic therapies and established safety of vascular resection and reconstruction employed during pancreatectomy, successful resection of pancreatic cancer may be considered for patients with type A disease but are rarely possible in patients with type B disease [4, 13]. It is important to note that differences in published guidelines are influenced by institutional practice and preferences, expertise of practicing surgeons, and ability to perform arterial and venous resection and reconstruction.

MDCT/MRI Performance in Staging

Local Staging

Dedicated pancreatic MDCT protocol has high sensitivity (89–97%) in detecting pancreatic tumor, although this varies based on tumor size, with low sensitivity of 77% for small tumors (<2 cm). Several studies have shown excellent positive predictive value (PPV) (range 92–100%) of MDCT in defining which tumors are unresectable. However, its performance is inferior in predicting tumor resectability (PPV = 45–79%) [31, 75–77]. This difference is related to diagnostic criteria for vessel invasion (such as vessel encasement and deformity) which are designed to favor specificity in order to minimize patients being denied of a curative resection who indeed have potentially resectable disease [11, 20, 78]. It is important to note that referenced studies were performed on older generation MDCT scanners with lower spatial and temporal resolutions than the current generation of MDCT scanners. It may be possible that the performance of newer scanners is substantially better, although that data are still emerging. Studies comparing MDCT and MRI for the diagnosis and staging of pancreatic cancer have shown comparable performances. However, MDCT overall has a better-established role, is readily available, and better tolerated by patients due to ultrafast scanning which makes it the preferred technique at most institutions. In addition, most radiologists and surgeons have more experience and greater level of comfort with interpreting MDCTs as compared to MRIs. Due to superior image resolution, it is also easier to identify and grade, subtle vascular involvement on MDCT. On the other hand, because of better soft tissue resolution MRI may be preferable in detecting and characterizing small pancreatic lesions (≤2 cm in size) [18, 79].

Unlike radiographic staging at baseline, accurate restaging following preoperative chemoradiation is difficult. Following neoadjuvant therapy, cross-sectional imaging cannot differentiate between treated (nonviable) tumor from residual viable tumor or distinguish perivascular post radiation changes (which manifest as soft tissue stranding) from residual disease. In one study which evaluated the response of borderline resectable tumor to neoadjuvant therapy, only 0.8% of patients were down staged to resectable disease by radiographic indicators, whereas 66% of patients were found to be resectable at surgery. In a consensus statement, the *ISGPS* recommends that following neoadjuvant therapy and in the absence of disease progression (distant metastasis) on subsequent imaging, surgical exploration and resection should be considered [49, 80–82].

Metastases

Lymph nodes are easily seen on MDCT and MR, but irrespective of the modality used, the accuracy for assessing nodal disease is limited, as nodes are considered suspicious primarily based on size; ancillary findings such as change in shape and necrosis are considered when evident. Usually a size threshold of greater than 1 cm (short axis) has been used in identifying metastatic nodes. This approach is non-specific as larger lymph nodes can be reactive and smaller lymph nodes may still harbor micrometastases without being enlarged. In one study, the accuracy of MDCT for the diagnosis of lymph node metastases was only 59.5%. In another study using a size threshold of 1.5 cm, preoperative MDCT identified just 16.7% of patients with nodal disease. Other studies have reported even more inferior performance. In this setting, PET/CT is probably more useful; especially if biopsy is being considered so that most suspicious node is targeted [69, 72, 73].

Regarding identification of liver metastases, MRI is superior to MDCT and is often used as problem-solving tool. A recent study using MDCT showed sensitivity of 48.4% and specificity of 97.9% for liver metastases in pancreatic cancer. In another study comparing MDCT and MRI with gadoxetic acid contrast agent (which is a liver-specific contrast agent), MRI had greater sensitivity than CT (85% vs 69%). The struggle of MDCT is particularly for lesions smaller than 1 cm, both in terms of sensitivity and specificity. However, in cancer patients, benign lesions (such as cyst or hemangioma) are very common and can be followed to ensure stability. Nevertheless, when needed, MRI can characterize majority of the liver lesions that are deemed indeterminate on MDCT. In general, metastases on MRI tend to be T1 hypointense and T2 hyperintense (albeit much less hyperintense than a cyst or hemangioma) and will often show perilesional enhancement around the margins. In addition, MRI also can be useful for identifying liver metastases that are not visible on MDCT, particularly with the inclusion of DWI images, which are significantly more sensitive for small liver metastases as compared to both MDCT and conventional MRI imaging sequences [62, 63, 83].

The diagnosis of peritoneal carcinomatosis, especially low-volume disease, is difficult by any imaging modality. The underperformance of MDCT and MRI is not specific to pancreatic cancer but applicable to any cancer that involves peritoneum. Studies have shown test sensitivity as low as 6% for MDCT when peritoneal implants are 1 cm or smaller. This limitation has led to the approach of using laparoscopy to screen patients for peritoneal disease before performing laparotomy in patients considered for pancreatectomy [64, 67].

Conclusion

There is little doubt that imaging plays an important role in the diagnosis and management of pancreatic cancer. While MDCT is the preferred and most validated imaging modality, MRI plays an important adjunct role. Standardization of imaging protocols and appropriately timed scan acquisition maximizes accurate local and distant staging of pancreatic cancer. A detailed and accurate evaluation of the primary tumor, its locoregional extension (particularly tumor-vessel relationship), and distant metastatic disease is necessary for the accurate classification of disease into resectable (resectable and borderline resectable) and unresectable (locally advanced and metastatic) categories.

References

1. Vincent A, Herman J, Schulick R, Hruban RH, Goggins M. Pancreatic cancer. Lancet. 2011;378(9791):607–20.
2. Ferrone CR, Brennan MF, Gonen M, Coit DG, Fong Y, Chung S, et al. Pancreatic adenocarcinoma: the actual 5-year survivors. J Gastrointest Surg. 2008;12(4):701–6.
3. Siegel RL, Miller KD, Jemal A. Cancer statistics, 2017. CA Cancer J Clin. 2017;67(1):7–30.
4. Li D, Xie K, Wolff R, Abbruzzese JL. Pancreatic cancer. Lancet. 2004;363(9414):1049–57.
5. Oettle H, Neuhaus P, Hochhaus A, Hartmann JT, Gellert K, Ridwelski K, Niedergethmann M, Zülke C, Fahlke J, Arning MB, Sinn M, Hinke A, Riess H. Adjuvant chemotherapy with gemcitabine and long-term outcomes among patients with resected pancreatic cancer: the CONKO-001 randomized trial. JAMA. 2013;310(14):1473–81.
6. Sohn TA, Yeo CJ, Cameron JL, Koniaris L, Kaushal S, Abrams RA, et al. Resected adenocarcinoma of the pancreas-616 patients: results, outcomes, and prognostic indicators. J Gastrointest Surg. 2000;4(6):567–79.
7. Evans DB, Farnell MB, Lillemoe KD, Vollmer C Jr, Strasberg SM, Schulick RD. Surgical treatment of resectable and borderline resectable pancreas cancer: expert consensus statement. Ann Surg Oncol. 2009;16(7):1736–44.
8. Winter JM, Brennan MF, Tang LH, D'Angelica MI, Dematteo RP, Fong Y, et al. Survival after resection of pancreatic adenocarcinoma: results from a single institution over three decades. Ann Surg Oncol. 2012;19(1):169–75.
9. Luberice K, Downs D, Sadowitz B, Ross S, Rosemurgy A. Has survival improved following resection for pancreatic adenocarcinoma? Am J Surg. 2017;214(2):341–6.
10. Varadhachary GR, Tamm EP, Abbruzzese JL, Xiong HQ, Crane CH, Wang H, et al. Borderline resectable pancreatic cancer: definitions, management,

and role of preoperative therapy. Ann Surg Oncol. 2006;13(8):1035–46.
11. NCCN clinical practice guidelines in oncology for pancreatic adenocarcinoma. Version 3.2017-September 11, 2017. Available from: https://www.nccn.org/professionals/physician_gls/pdf/pancreatic.pdf.
12. Callery MP, Chang KJ, Fishman EK, Talamonti MS, William Traverso L, Linehan DC. Pretreatment assessment of resectable and borderline resectable pancreatic cancer: expert consensus statement. Ann Surg Oncol. 2009;16(7):1727–33.
13. Chatzizacharias NA, Tsai S, Griffin M, Tolat P, Ritch P, George B, et al. Locally advanced pancreas cancer: staging and goals of therapy. Surgery. 2018;163:1053–62.
14. Evans DB, George B, Tsai S. Non-metastatic pancreatic cancer: resectable, borderline resectable, and locally advanced-definitions of increasing importance for the optimal delivery of multimodality therapy. Ann Surg Oncol. 2015;22(11):3409–13.
15. Chun YS, Pawlik TM, Vauthey JN. 8th edition of the AJCC cancer staging manual: pancreas and hepatobiliary cancers. Ann Surg Oncol. 2018;25:845–7.
16. Appel BL, Tolat P, Evans DB, Tsai S. Current staging systems for pancreatic cancer. Cancer J. 2012;18(6):539–49.
17. Kinney T. Evidence-based imaging of pancreatic malignancies. Surg Clin North Am. 2010;90(2):235–49.
18. Wong JC, Lu DS. Staging of pancreatic adenocarcinoma by imaging studies. Clin Gastroenterol Hepatol. 2008;6(12):1301–8.
19. Fleischmann D, Kamaya A. Optimal vascular and parenchymal contrast enhancement: the current state of the art. Radiol Clin North Am. 2009;47(1):13–26.
20. Al-Hawary MM, Francis IR, Chari ST, Fishman EK, Hough DM, Lu DS, et al. Pancreatic ductal adenocarcinoma radiology reporting template: consensus statement of the society of abdominal radiology and the american pancreatic association. Gastroenterology. 2014;146(1):291–304.e1.
21. Perez-Johnston R, Lenhart DK, Sahani DV. CT angiography of the hepatic and pancreatic circulation. Radiol Clin North Am. 2010;48(2):311–30, viii.
22. Fletcher JG, Wiersema MJ, Farrell MA, Fidler JL, Burgart LJ, Koyama T, et al. Pancreatic malignancy: value of arterial, pancreatic, and hepatic phase imaging with multi-detector row CT. Radiology. 2003;229(1):81–90.
23. Ichikawa T, Erturk SM, Sou H, Nakajima H, Tsukamoto T, Motosugi U, et al. MDCT of pancreatic adenocarcinoma: optimal imaging phases and multiplanar reformatted imaging. AJR Am J Roentgenol. 2006;187(6):1513–20.
24. Vargas R, Nino-Murcia M, Trueblood W, Jeffrey RB Jr. MDCT in pancreatic adenocarcinoma: prediction of vascular invasion and resectability using a multiphasic technique with curved planar reformations. AJR Am J Roentgenol. 2004;182(2):419–25.
25. Fukushima H, Itoh S, Takada A, Mori Y, Suzuki K, Sawaki A, et al. Diagnostic value of curved multiplanar reformatted images in multislice CT for the detection of resectable pancreatic ductal adenocarcinoma. Eur Radiol. 2006;16(8):1709–18.
26. Raman SP, Chen Y, Fishman EK. Cross-sectional imaging and the role of positron emission tomography in pancreatic cancer evaluation. Semin Oncol. 2015;42(1):40–58.
27. Catalano C, Laghi A, Fraioli F, Pediconi F, Napoli A, Danti M, et al. Pancreatic carcinoma: the role of high-resolution multislice spiral CT in the diagnosis and assessment of resectability. Eur Radiol. 2003;13(1):149–56.
28. Al-Hawary MM, Kaza RK, Wasnik AP, Francis IR. Staging of pancreatic cancer: role of imaging. Semin Roentgenol. 2013;48(3):245–52.
29. Pietryga JA, Morgan DE. Imaging preoperatively for pancreatic adenocarcinoma. J Gastrointest Oncol. 2015;6(4):343–57.
30. Tamm EP, Bhosale PR, Vikram R, de Almeida Marcal LP, Balachandran A. Imaging of pancreatic ductal adenocarcinoma: state of the art. World J Radiol. 2013;5(3):98–105.
31. Bronstein YL, Loyer EM, Kaur H, Choi H, David C, DuBrow RA, et al. Detection of small pancreatic tumors with multiphasic helical CT. AJR Am J Roentgenol. 2004;182(3):619–23.
32. Tamm EP, Loyer EM, Faria SC, Evans DB, Wolff RA, Charnsangavej C. Retrospective analysis of dual-phase MDCT and follow-up EUS/EUS-FNA in the diagnosis of pancreatic cancer. Abdom Imaging. 2007;32(5):660–7.
33. Prokesch RW, Chow LC, Beaulieu CF, Bammer R, Jeffrey RB Jr. Isoattenuating pancreatic adenocarcinoma at multi-detector row CT: secondary signs. Radiology. 2002;224(3):764–8.
34. Morgan DE. Dual-energy CT of the abdomen. Abdom Imaging. 2014;39(1):108–34.
35. Kulkarni NM, Hough DM, Tolat PP, Soloff EV, Kambadakone AR. Pancreatic adenocarcinoma: cross-sectional imaging techniques. Abdom Radiol (NY). 2018;43:253–63.
36. Patel BN, Thomas JV, Lockhart ME, Berland LL, Morgan DE. Single-source dual-energy spectral multidetector CT of pancreatic adenocarcinoma: optimization of energy level viewing significantly increases lesion contrast. Clin Radiol. 2013;68(2):148–54.
37. O'Neill E, Hammond N, Miller FH. MR imaging of the pancreas. Radiol Clin North Am. 2014;52(4):757–77.
38. Chen FM, Ni JM, Zhang ZY, Zhang L, Li B, Jiang CJ. Presurgical evaluation of pancreatic cancer: a comprehensive imaging comparison of CT versus MRI. AJR Am J Roentgenol. 2016;206(3):526–35.
39. Keppke AL, Miller FH. Magnetic resonance imaging of the pancreas: the future is now. Semin Ultrasound CT MR. 2005;26(3):132–52.
40. Tirkes T, Menias CO, Sandrasegaran K. MR imaging techniques for pancreas. Radiol Clin North Am. 2012;50(3):379–93.

41. Jeffrey RB. Pancreatic cancer: radiologic imaging. Gastroenterol Clin North Am. 2012;41(1):159–77.
42. Ly JN, Miller FH. MR imaging of the pancreas: a practical approach. Radiol Clin North Am. 2002;40(6):1289–306.
43. Hammond NA, Miller FH, Day K, Nikolaidis P. Imaging features of the less common pancreatic masses. Abdom Imaging. 2013;38(3):561–72.
44. Miller FH, Rini NJ, Keppke AL. MRI of adenocarcinoma of the pancreas. AJR Am J Roentgenol. 2006;187(4):W365–74.
45. Wang Y, Miller FH, Chen ZE, Merrick L, Mortele KJ, Hoff FL, et al. Diffusion-weighted MR imaging of solid and cystic lesions of the pancreas. Radiographics. 2011;31(3):E47–64.
46. Birchard KR, Semelka RC, Hyslop WB, Brown A, Armao D, Firat Z, et al. Suspected pancreatic cancer: evaluation by dynamic gadolinium-enhanced 3D gradient-echo MRI. AJR Am J Roentgenol. 2005;185(3):700–3.
47. Wang Y, Chen ZE, Nikolaidis P, McCarthy RJ, Merrick L, Sternick LA, et al. Diffusion-weighted magnetic resonance imaging of pancreatic adenocarcinomas: association with histopathology and tumor grade. J Magn Reson Imaging. 2011;33(1):136–42.
48. Park HS, Lee JM, Choi HK, Hong SH, Han JK, Choi BI. Preoperative evaluation of pancreatic cancer: comparison of gadolinium-enhanced dynamic MRI with MR cholangiopancreatography versus MDCT. J Magn Reson Imaging. 2009;30(3):586–95.
49. Bockhorn M, Uzunoglu FG, Adham M, Imrie C, Milicevic M, Sandberg AA, et al. Borderline resectable pancreatic cancer: a consensus statement by the International Study Group of Pancreatic Surgery (ISGPS). Surgery. 2014;155(6):977–88.
50. Bhalla M, Aldakkak M, Kulkarni NM, O'Connor SD, Griffin MO Jr, Christians KK, Evans DB, Tsai S, Tolat PP. Characterizing indeterminate liver lesions in patients with localized pancreatic cancer at the time of diagnosis. Abdom Radiol. 2017; https://doi.org/10.1007/s00261-017-1404-0.
51. de la Santa LG, Retortillo JA, Miguel AC, Klein LM. Radiology of pancreatic neoplasms: an update. World J Gastrointest Oncol. 2014;6(9):330–43.
52. Nakao A, Harada A, Nonami T, Kaneko T, Takagi H. Clinical significance of carcinoma invasion of the extrapancreatic nerve plexus in pancreatic cancer. Pancreas. 1996;12(4):357–61.
53. Tian H, Mori H, Matsumoto S, Yamada Y, Kiyosue H, Ohta M, et al. Extrapancreatic neural plexus invasion by carcinomas of the pancreatic head region: evaluation using thin-section helical CT. Radiat Med. 2007;25(4):141–7.
54. Patel BN, Olcott E, Jeffrey RB. Extrapancreatic perineural invasion in pancreatic adenocarcinoma. Abdom Radiol (NY). 2018;43:323–31.
55. Deshmukh SD, Willmann JK, Jeffrey RB. Pathways of extrapancreatic perineural invasion by pancreatic adenocarcinoma: evaluation with 3D volume-rendered MDCT imaging. AJR Am J Roentgenol. 2010;194(3):668–74.
56. Lu DS, Reber HA, Krasny RM, Kadell BM, Sayre J. Local staging of pancreatic cancer: criteria for unresectability of major vessels as revealed by pancreatic-phase, thin-section helical CT. AJR Am J Roentgenol. 1997;168(6):1439–43.
57. Christians KK, Tsai S, Tolat PP, Evans DB. Critical steps for pancreaticoduodenectomy in the setting of pancreatic adenocarcinoma. J Surg Oncol. 2013;107(1):33–8.
58. Raman SP, Horton KM, Fishman EK. Multimodality imaging of pancreatic cancer-computed tomography, magnetic resonance imaging, and positron emission tomography. Cancer J. 2012;18(6):511–22.
59. Hazirolan T, Metin Y, Karaosmanoglu AD, Canyigit M, Turkbey B, Oguz BS, et al. Mesenteric arterial variations detected at MDCT angiography of abdominal aorta. AJR Am J Roentgenol. 2009;192(4):1097–102.
60. Ward J, Robinson PJ, Guthrie JA, Downing S, Wilson D, Lodge JP, et al. Liver metastases in candidates for hepatic resection: comparison of helical CT and gadolinium- and SPIO-enhanced MR imaging. Radiology. 2005;237(1):170–80.
61. Trede M, Rumstadt B, Wendl K, Gaa J, Tesdal K, Lehmann KJ, et al. Ultrafast magnetic resonance imaging improves the staging of pancreatic tumors. Ann Surg. 1997;226(4):393–405; discussion -7.
62. Ikuta Y, Takamori H, Ikeda O, Tanaka H, Sakamoto Y, Hashimoto D, et al. Detection of liver metastases secondary to pancreatic cancer: utility of combined helical computed tomography during arterial portography with biphasic computed tomography-assisted hepatic arteriography. J Gastroenterol. 2010;45(12):1241–6.
63. Motosugi U, Ichikawa T, Morisaka H, Sou H, Muhi A, Kimura K, et al. Detection of pancreatic carcinoma and liver metastases with gadoxetic acid-enhanced MR imaging: comparison with contrast-enhanced multi-detector row CT. Radiology. 2011;260(2):446–53.
64. Dromain C, Leboulleux S, Auperin A, Goere D, Malka D, Lumbroso J, et al. Staging of peritoneal carcinomatosis: enhanced CT vs. PET/CT. Abdom Imaging. 2008;33(1):87–93.
65. Lim JS, Kim MJ, Yun MJ, Oh YT, Kim JH, Hwang HS, et al. Comparison of CT and 18F-FDG pet for detecting peritoneal metastasis on the preoperative evaluation for gastric carcinoma. Korean J Radiol. 2006;7(4):249–56.
66. Iafrate F, Ciolina M, Sammartino P, Baldassari P, Rengo M, Lucchesi P, et al. Peritoneal carcinomatosis: imaging with 64-MDCT and 3T MRI with diffusion-weighted imaging. Abdom Imaging. 2012;37(4):616–27.
67. Pisters PW, Lee JE, Vauthey JN, Charnsangavej C, Evans DB. Laparoscopy in the staging of pancreatic cancer. Br J Surg. 2001;88(3):325–37.
68. Pappas SG, Christians KK, Tolat PP, Mautz AP, Lal A, McElroy L, et al. Staging chest computed tomography and positron emission tomography in patients

with pancreatic adenocarcinoma: utility or futility? HPB (Oxford). 2014;16(1):70–4.
69. Valls C, Andia E, Sanchez A, Fabregat J, Pozuelo O, Quintero JC, et al. Dual-phase helical CT of pancreatic adenocarcinoma: assessment of resectability before surgery. AJR Am J Roentgenol. 2002;178(4):821–6.
70. Tamm EP, Balachandran A, Bhosale PR, Katz MH, Fleming JB, Lee JH, et al. Imaging of pancreatic adenocarcinoma: update on staging/resectability. Radiol Clin North Am. 2012;50(3):407–28.
71. Nanashima A, Sakamoto I, Hayashi T, Tobinaga S, Araki M, Kunizaki M, et al. Preoperative diagnosis of lymph node metastasis in biliary and pancreatic carcinomas: evaluation of the combination of multidetector CT and serum CA19-9 level. Dig Dis Sci. 2010;55(12):3617–26.
72. Kim JH, Eun HW, Kim KW, Lee JY, Lee JM, Han JK, et al. Diagnostic performance of MDCT for predicting important prognostic factors in pancreatic cancer. Pancreas. 2013;42(8):1316–22.
73. Imai H, Doi R, Kanazawa H, Kamo N, Koizumi M, Masui T, et al. Preoperative assessment of para-aortic lymph node metastasis in patients with pancreatic cancer. Int J Clin Oncol. 2010;15(3):294–300.
74. Vauthey JN, Dixon E. AHPBA/SSO/SSAT consensus conference on resectable and borderline resectable pancreatic cancer: rationale and overview of the conference. Ann Surg Oncol. 2009;16(7):1725–6.
75. Brennan DD, Zamboni GA, Raptopoulos VD, Kruskal JB. Comprehensive preoperative assessment of pancreatic adenocarcinoma with 64-section volumetric CT. Radiographics. 2007;27(6):1653–66.
76. Evans DB, Erickson BA, Ritch P. Borderline resectable pancreatic cancer: definitions and the importance of multimodality therapy. Ann Surg Oncol. 2010;17(11):2803–5.
77. Klauss M, Mohr A, von Tengg-Kobligk H, Friess H, Singer R, Seidensticker P, et al. A new invasion score for determining the resectability of pancreatic carcinomas with contrast-enhanced multidetector computed tomography. Pancreatology. 2008;8(2):204–10.
78. Nakayama Y, Yamashita Y, Kadota M, Takahashi M, Kanemitsu K, Hiraoka T, et al. Vascular encasement by pancreatic cancer: correlation of CT findings with surgical and pathologic results. J Comput Assist Tomogr. 2001;25(3):337–42.
79. Tamm EP, Loyer EM, Faria S, Raut CP, Evans DB, Wolff RA, et al. Staging of pancreatic cancer with multidetector CT in the setting of preoperative chemoradiation therapy. Abdom Imaging. 2006;31(5):568–74.
80. Cloyd JM, Katz MH, Prakash L, Varadhachary GR, Wolff RA, Shroff RT, et al. Preoperative therapy and pancreatoduodenectomy for pancreatic ductal adenocarcinoma: a 25-year single-institution experience. J Gastrointest Surg. 2017;21(1):164–74.
81. Katz MH, Fleming JB, Bhosale P, Varadhachary G, Lee JE, Wolff R, et al. Response of borderline resectable pancreatic cancer to neoadjuvant therapy is not reflected by radiographic indicators. Cancer. 2012;118(23):5749–56.
82. Morgan DE, Waggoner CN, Canon CL, Lockhart ME, Fineberg NS, Posey JA 3rd, et al. Resectability of pancreatic adenocarcinoma in patients with locally advanced disease downstaged by preoperative therapy: a challenge for MDCT. AJR Am J Roentgenol. 2010;194(3):615–22.
83. Bhalla M, Aldakkak M, Kulkarni NM, O'Connor SD, Griffin MO Jr, Christians KK, et al. Characterizing indeterminate liver lesions in patients with localized pancreatic cancer at the time of diagnosis. Abdom Radiol (NY). 2018;43:351–63.

3 Coordination of Endoscopic Ultrasound-Guided FNA and Biliary Drainage in Pancreatic Cancer

Kulwinder S. Dua

Acronyms

ERCP: Endoscopic Retrograde Cholangiopancreatography
EUS: Endoscopic Ultrasound
FNA: Fine Needle Aspiration
FNAB: Fine Needle Aspiration Biopsy
PC: Pancreatic cancer
ROSE: Rapid On-Site Evaluation
SEMS: Self-expanding Metal Stent (Biliary)

Introduction

Over a period of three decades from 1980 to 2000, pancreatic cancer (PC)-related mortality rates have virtually remained unchanged [1]. In an attempt to improve survival outcomes, some of the approaches introduced in the recent past have included giving neoadjuvant therapy even to patients with resectable PCs and using molecular profiling of the cancer to deliver tailored chemotherapy. The rationale behind using neoadjuvant therapy followed by pancreaticoduodenectomy ("delayed surgery") is discussed in other chapters in this book. As against "early surgery" (pancreaticoduodenectomy followed by adjuvant therapy), the approach of using neoadjuvant therapy has had a significant impact on the role and timing of endoscopy in patients with PC, especially with regard to procedures like endoscopic ultrasound (EUS), fine needle aspiration (FNA) or aspiration biopsy (FNAB), and endoscopic retrograde cholangiopancreatography (ERCP). The focus of this chapter will be on the coordination of EUS-FNA/FNAB and ERCP in patients in whom surgery is going to be delayed.

Over 70% of patients with PC present with bile duct obstruction [2]. In majority of these patients, a mass in the head of the pancreas will be identified on a CT scan. It was debated if this radiographic finding alone would suffice for making a diagnosis of PC; especially if associated with significant weight loss and a high carbohydrate antigen (CA 19-9) level and whether tissue diagnosis was necessary. Tessler et al. reviewed 150 patients with jaundice and a mass in the head of the pancreas on CT scan who underwent pancreatoduodenectomy [3]. One hundred two of these patients had no prior tissue diagnosis. The authors found that weight loss of over 20 pounds along with bilirubin greater than 3 mg/dl and CA 19-9 greater than 37 U/ml had a positive predictive value of almost 100% for PC. If any two of these criteria were present, the predictive value dropped to 89.5%. Hence, the need for tissue diagnosis was questioned in

K. S. Dua (✉)
Department of Medicine, Division of Gastroenterology and Hepatology, The Medical College of Wisconsin, Milwaukee, WI, USA
e-mail: kdua@mcw.edu

S. Tsai et al. (eds.), *Management of Localized Pancreatic Cancer*,
https://doi.org/10.1007/978-3-319-98944-0_3

patients going for early surgery who fulfilled these criteria [2]. However, all pancreatic masses may not be PC, and other lesions like neuroendocrine neoplasms, acinar cell carcinoma, lymphomas, and metastasis may also present with a mass in the pancreas. Moreover, benign lesions like focal chronic pancreatitis or autoimmune pancreatitis can also present as a mass. Tissue diagnosis therefore is highly recommended. Since an increasing number of patients with PC nowadays are receiving neoadjuvant therapy for resectable and borderline resectable PC, tissue diagnosis is also essential in these patients. The material obtained for tissue diagnosis by *EUS-guided fine needle aspiration* (*FNA*) or *fine needle biopsy* (*FNAB*) can also be used for molecular profiling of the tumor to tailor the chemotherapy based on the profile. Last, but not the least, on-site tissue diagnosis of cancer can permit the endoscopist to do an *ERCP* and place a self-expanding metal bile duct stent for durable bile duct decompression if surgery is going to be delayed and if the patient is likely to receive neoadjuvant therapy, requires stabilization of comorbidities, or needs to be transferred to a tertiary-care center.

Sequencing of Tests

Staging: Imaging Studies

Currently, contrast-enhanced, multiphasic, multidetector helical computed tomography (CT) scan (*pancreas-protocol CT scan*) is the most commonly accepted imaging modality for the initial evaluation of patients with suspected PC. Besides identifying metastatic disease, it can accurately stage the lesion in relation to the surrounding vessels and is nowadays the cornerstone for staging as compared to EUS [4, 5].

It is highly recommended that a pancreas-protocol CT scan be done on all patients with suspected PC before these patients undergo EUS-FNA and/or ERCP and that the CT scan should be repeated if a previous CT scan was not performed with a dual phase contrast technique. Since both EUS-FNA and ERCP can be associated with complications like pancreatitis and/or bleeding/edema, these complications can alter the CT appearances of the lesion and may not permit accurate staging if the CT scan is done after these procedures. Hence, in the sequencing of tests, a pancreas-protocol scan should be the first order of business.

Tissue Diagnosis: EUS with FNA/FNAB

Following a pancreas-protocol scan, the next procedure should be an EUS with *fine needle aspiration* (FNA) for tissue diagnosis unless the patients have had an ERCP at an outside hospital and the brushing from the bile duct or the pancreatic duct was positive for adenocarcinoma. If the brushings were suspicious, the slides can be reviewed by another pathologist at the tertiary-care center. Either way, EUS-FNA may be required if additional tissue is required for *molecular profiling*. This approach relies on selecting molecular targets from the tissue sample for tailoring chemotherapy appropriate to the molecular targets and is discussed elsewhere in this book.

The linear EUS endoscope is used for FNA. As shown in Fig. 3.1, orientation of the EUS image with the linear endoscope is along the long axis of the US probe. Hence, the echogenic FNA needle is clearly visible, and its path into the mass with to-and-fro movements can be monitored in real time thereby avoiding blood vessels. The needle is moved back and forth several times in various directions (fanning technique) within the mass. The ideal method of tissue acquisition (suction versus no suction; stylet versus no stylet; saline versus stylet aspirations; needle gauge: 25G, 22G, 19G; etc.) has yet to be determined. For lesions of the body and tail of the pancreas, the likelihood of spilling malignant cells into the peritoneum or along the needle track is significantly less with trans-gastric EUS-FNA compared to percutaneous CT-guided biopsy of the mass. Micames et al. reported peritoneal carcinomatosis in 1 of 46 patients (2.2%) who underwent EUS-FNA compared to 7 of 43 patients (16.3%) who had CT-guided FNA of pancreas masses ($p < 0.025$) [6]. As against percutaneous CT-guided FNA, spillage of malignant cells

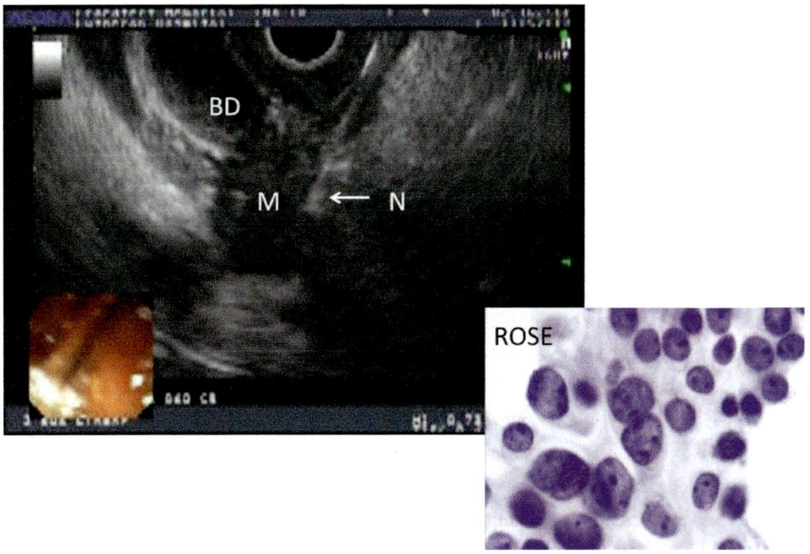

Fig. 3.1 Endoscopic ultrasound with fine needle aspiration. BD, obstructed and dilated common bile duct; M, around 1 cm mass in the head of the pancreas; N, a 25-gauge fine needle used for aspirating cells; ROSE, rapid on-site evaluation showed malignant cells

along the needle track with transduodenal EUS-FNA for pancreas head lesions is not a major issue as it is within the zone of pancreatoduodenectomy.

Several studies have evaluated the sensitivity, specificity, and accuracy of EUS-FNA in diagnosing PC including the observation that better results are obtained from centers performing more than 100 EUS procedures per year [7–11]. In a meta-analysis that included over 3600 patients with solid pancreas masses, the pooled sensitivity and specificity for EUS-FNA for pancreatic cancer were 88.6% [95% CI: 87.2–89.9] and 99.3% (95% CI: 98.7–99.7), respectively [12]. For tissue diagnosis, the presence of an on-site cytopathology faculty for *rapid on-site evaluation* (*ROSE*) was a major determinant of the success of EUS-FNA in making tissue diagnosis [12]. In a study where one faculty performed EUS-FNA at two campuses, one campus with ROSE and other without, there were more unsatisfactory specimen reports from the center without ROSE (9% versus 20%; $p = 0.03$) [13]. This group also showed that more proportion of patients were likely to have a positive or negative tissue diagnosis in the center with an on-site cytopathologist as compared to the other center (79% versus 53%; $p = 0.001$). However, unfortunately, ROSE facility is not available in many centers. To reduce the likelihood of getting an unsatisfactory sample and thereby the need to call the patient back for another attempt, some have advocated training the ultrasonographer GI faculty to perform ROSE themselves [14]. In a study on a group of patients with no ROSE or with ROSE performed by the ultrasonographer, the accuracy of diagnosis increased for 79–95% [15]. Others have advocated the use of *fine needle aspiration biopsy* (*FNAB*) instead of FNA if ROSE is not available. In a recent study, on 333 patients with solid pancreas lesions who underwent FNAB with ROSE ($n = 140$) or without ROSE ($n = 193$), the sensitivity, specificity, and accuracy of EUS-FNA with ROSE were 91%, 100%, and 92%, respectively, compared to those without ROSE (87%, 100%, 88%; $p = 0.2$) [16]. Another recent study showed that more histology material was obtained with the fork-tip FNAB needle compared to a standard FNA needle (59% versus 5%, $p < 0.001$) [17]. Complication rates were similar between the two groups. In a recent prospective, randomized, multicenter study on 408 patients, FNAB was shown to give a better diagnostic yield as compared to FNA (93% versus 83%; $p = 0.001$) [18]. Others have shown no differences in the yield between a standard and a core needle although fewer passes were required with the core needle [19]. Similarly, Aadam et al. showed that the diagnostic yield of FNA was similar to FNAB for pancreatic masses although

FNAB was superior to FNA for non-pancreatic masses [20]. FNAB tissue acquisition is highly recommended when the lesion in the pancreas is suspected to be lymphoma, stromal tumor, or metastasis. Similarly, FNAB is superior to FNA when the mass in the pancreas is suspected to be autoimmune pancreatitis [21].

For fear of higher complication rates with FNAB (pancreatitis, bleeding), many centers tend to initially perform FNA with ROSE, and if the cytology is inconclusive despite several FNA passes, then proceed to use FNAB needle. Although the sensitivity, specificity, and accuracy of FNAB may be similar to with or without ROSE [16], the advantage of getting a diagnosis on-site with ROSE can help in deciding what type of biliary stent can be used for decompressing the bile duct if ERCP is being performed in the same setting immediately after EUS-FNA as described below. Moreover, irrespective of using FNA or FNAB, ROSE is highly recommended if one is collecting material for molecular profiling of the tumor for personalized therapy. In our series of 130 patients, adequate material for profiling was obtained in 94 patients (72%) [22]. Similarly, in a previous large trial, adequate specimen could be obtained in over 85% of patients [23]. Intuitively, similar to better histology material, FNAB may also give better material for profiling, but this has not been formally studied.

For stereotactic radiation therapy, precise location of the lesion is important. This can be obtained with concomitant imaging-guided approach or by placement of *fiducials*. Fiducials are radio-opaque markers that can be placed into the tumor with EUS guidance without fluoroscopy, and the EUS-guided approach is preferred over CT-guided placement. Larger fiducials requiring a 19G FNA needle are being replaced with newer coil design fiducials that can be placed with a 22G FNA needle which is more flexible and hence better for lesions in the head of the pancreas where the EUS endoscope tip is turned at an angle in the duodenum making passage of a 19G needle difficult [24–27].

For those patients who have failed pain management with medications or are having significant side effect from pain medications, *EUS-guided celiac plexus/ganglion block or neurolysis* with bupivacaine/alcohol [28–30] is a more direct approach as compared to the CT-guided approach. The advantage of the EUS over CT for celiac block/neurolysis is that with EUS, one can in real time visualize the celiac ganglion and approach it from the anterior aspect thereby avoiding the retro-crural space. Hence, it is considered to be safer than the CT-guided approach [31, 32]. In a meta-analysis of 8 studies involving over 280 patients, EUS-guided celiac plexus neurolysis was successful in pain control in over 80% of patients [33]. Some have recommended performing early EUS-guided celiac plexus neurolysis as it gave better pain control as compared to those who had the neurolysis done later as a rescue approach [34]. Besides injury to the blood vessels, one of the most dreaded but rare complications of celiac plexus neurolysis is paraplegia secondary to spinal artery spasm.

Although medical and surgical oncologic approaches are currently the mainstay of treatment of resectable, borderline resectable, and locally advanced PC, several *EUS-guided therapies* are emerging [35]. For example, EUS-guided lavage and ablation of cystic neoplasms of the pancreas can be considered as an alternative for those who are not fit for surgery [36–38]. Compared to saline, 80% ethanol resulted in a significant decrease in cyst diameter, and with additional ethanol lavage sessions, complete and durable cyst resolution was observed in 33% of patients [36, 37]. Others have tried combining alcohol or saline with chemotherapeutic agents like paclitaxel or paclitaxel-gemcitabine with variable results [39–43]. Until further data from large-scale prospective randomized studies with long-term follow-up is available, currently EUS-guided ablation of cystic neoplasms of the pancreas should be considered only in those in whom there is a high risk for malignant transformation within the expected life span of the patient who is not fit for surgical removal. For solid tumors of the pancreas, experimental EUS-guided therapy has included brachytherapy by implanting radioactive seeds (iodine-125), [44, 45] irinotecan microspheres, [46] gemcitabine, [47] adenovirus, [48] and immunotherapy [49]. The rationale behind using these approaches is to achieve better tissue penetration as compared to systemic therapy. EUS-guided tissue ablative therapy such as photodynamic therapy and radiofrequency ablation has also been reported [50, 51]. Although initial results from these pilot studies are encouraging, these approaches cannot be recommended at the present time until further large-scale prospective randomized studies are done.

Bile Duct Decompression: ERCP

Although tissue acquisition for diagnosis with brushings and/or cholangioscopic biopsies is possible during ERCP, the sensitivity is poor. Hence EUS-FNA/FNAB is still the method of choice for tissue diagnosis. The primary role of ERCP in the management of patients with PC is biliary decompression.

Majority of the patients with PC of the head of the pancreas present with bile duct obstruction. Decompressing the bile duct is not required in patients going for early pancreaticoduodenectomy. In a meta-analysis of five studies on patients with bile duct obstruction who underwent early pancreaticoduodenectomy, preoperative bile duct decompression gave not additional benefits and was associated with higher perioperative complications [19]. In a subsequent study from Europe on patients with resectable PC with bile duct obstruction going for early pancreaticoduodenectomy, 94 patients underwent surgery without preoperative biliary drainage, and 102 patients had preoperative bile duct decompression. Serious complications were observed in 74% of patients who underwent bile duct decompression as compared to those who went directly for surgery (37%; $p < 0.001$) [52]. In this study, ERCP was successful in draining the bile duct in only 75% of patients which is significantly lower than what one would expect of ERCP compared to national standards in the USA (over 95%). Hence, several patients in this group required percutaneous drainage. Moreover, plastic bile duct stents were used, and several patients did not undergo surgery early enough as one would expect from centers in the USA. These weaknesses of this study could have confounded the results. Nevertheless, preoperative biliary drainage does not offer any significant benefits, especially since patients with malignant bile duct obstruction rarely develop cholangitis unless the bile duct is instrumented. Hence, bile duct drainage is not recommended for patients in whom early pancreatoduodenectomy is planned.

An increasing number of patients nowadays are receiving neoadjuvant therapy for resectable PC. The rationale for this approach is described elsewhere in this book. These patients require tissue diagnosis and then undergo several months of preoperative therapy before surgery is done. Surgery can also be delayed in those who need stabilization of comorbidities or those who are awaiting a date for surgery or awaiting transfer to a tertiary-care center. Durable bile duct drainage is required in these patients, especially since near normalization of liver test is required before chemotherapeutic agents can be given.

Obstructed bile duct can be drained by using either a 10 French (3.3 mm) *plastic stent* or a self-expandable metal stent (*SEMS*). The diameter of SEMS is 10 mm which is equal to around nine plastic stents of 3.3 mm diameter in terms of areas of the circumference. Hence, SEMS offer durable bile duct drainage (patency rates of almost 9–12 months) as compared to plastic stents (patency rates of 6–12 weeks) (Fig. 3.2) [53, 54]. Plastic stents are cheap and can be removed. Hence, they are ideal for short-term drainage and for strictures where the diagnosis is awaiting confirmation. As compared to plastic stents, SEMS are expensive and cannot be removed once deployed across the stricture, especially if they are of the uncovered variety where the crevices of the wire mesh are bare allowing for tissue ingrowth (embedded stent). Hence, these stents should not be placed in patients with benign or indeterminate strictures. SEMS covered with a plastic membrane (covered SEMS) to prevent tissue ingrowth are also available and potentially can be removed (not as yet cleared by the FDA for removable indications) [55]. Higher rates of pancreatitis and cholangitis have been reported with covered SEMS presumably due to occlusion of

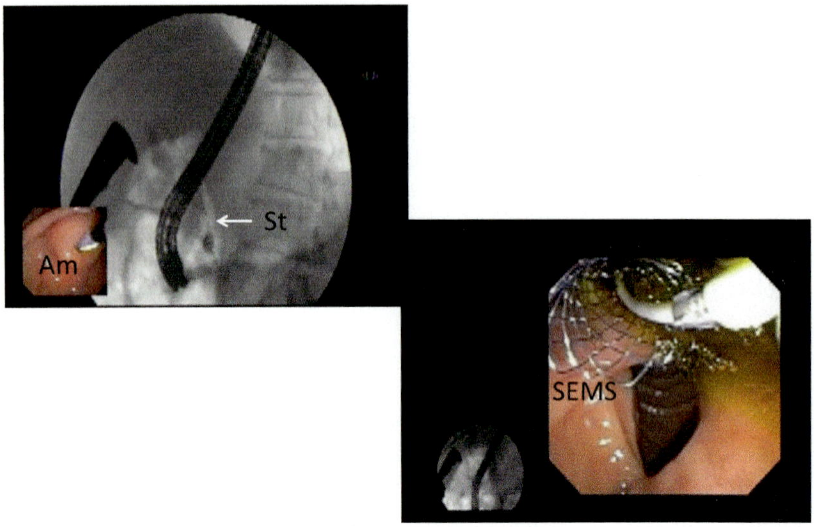

Fig. 3.2 Malignant bile duct stricture with placement of a self-expanding metal stent. Immediately after the EUS-FNA with ROSE showing malignant cells in the patient shown in Fig. 3.1, an ERCP was performed (Am, ampulla was cannulated). Cholangiogram showed a malignant bile duct stricture (white arrow) with placement of a self-expanding metal stent (SEMS)

pancreatic orifice and the cystic duct opening by the plastic membrane. Lack of tissue ingrowth also can lead to higher migration rates [56–58].

Until recently, SEMS were not cleared by the FDA for use in patients with malignant bile duct obstruction in whom there were plans for pancreaticoduodenectomy for fear of causing technical difficulties during surgery. Hence, in those in whose surgery was delayed, plastic stents were placed. This resulted in high complication rates such as cholangitis from frequent stent occlusion that required multiple re-interventions. In a study on 49 patients receiving neoadjuvant therapy for PC in whom 10F plastic stents were placed, 27 (55%) patients presented with stent occlusion-related complication at a median of 83 days (range 14–183 days), cholangitis in 13 patients, and worsening liver tests with jaundice in 14 patients [59]. This resulted in hospitalization for a median of 3 days in 17 patients and interruption of neoadjuvant therapy for a median of 8 days in 13 patients. All these patients required repeat ERCPs. In another recent study on 173 patients receiving neoadjuvant therapy, 35.6% of patients presented with complications secondary to premature occlusion of plastic stents at a median of 53 days [60].

Secondary to the dismal performance of plastic stents, several centers are now placing SEMS in those in whom surgery is delayed such as those who are receiving neoadjuvant therapy. In a prospective, nonrandomized, pilot study on 55 patients with resectable and borderline resectable PC receiving neoadjuvant therapy, SEMS provided durable biliary decompression through the duration of neoadjuvant therapy (neoadjuvant therapy duration: median 104 days; range 70–260 days) [61]. At the median duration point of 104 days, only 12% of SEMS-related adverse events were encountered compared to 35–55% observed with historical control where plastic stents were used. The adverse events noted with SEMS that required re-intervention were cholestasis, cholangitis, and cholecystitis.

The shortest length of SEMS required to bridge the PC-related intrapancreatic bile duct stricture should be used so as to leave at least 1–2 cm of extra-pancreatic bile duct for subsequent surgical anastomosis ("short metal stent"). Hence, it is not necessary to remove the stent prior to surgery. No major technical issues were encountered during surgery using this approach [61–63]. In a retrospective comparative study, surgery time, intraoperative blood loss, and hospital stay were similar between patients who had SEMS in situ at the time of surgery compared to those without SEMS [62]. Based on some of these recent studies, the FDA has now cleared to use SEMS in patients with malignant bile duct obstruction in whom there are intentions for surgery.

One-Stop Shop: EUS-FNA-ROSE-ERCP-SEMS

Since neoadjuvant therapy is increasingly becoming the standard of care for resectable and borderline resectable pancreas adenocarcinoma (delayed surgery), we follow the "one-stop shop" approach (Fig. 3.3). Since EUS and ERCP can be associated with complications like pancreatitis that can alter the accuracy of staging by imaging studies, a pancreas-protocol CT scan should be done or repeated prior to these invasive procedures. After confirming that a pancreas protocol CT scan was done and after reviewing the scan, an EUS-FNA/FNAB with rapid on-site evaluation (ROSE) of the cytology specimen by a cytopathology faculty is performed. If ROSE is inconclusive, additional FNA or FNAB samples should be taken while the patient is still sedated. Additional samples may also be required for molecular profiling. If ROSE is positive for adenocarcinoma, the patient can immediately in the same setting undergo ERCP with placement of a short SEMS if the bile duct is obstructed. Frequently patients are referred to tertiary-care centers with ERCP performed at hospital where they do not have EUS-FNA expertise or capabilities of doing ROSE. These patients have plastic stents placed at these outside hospitals. EUS-FNA with ROSE can still be performed in these patients, and if positive for adenocarcinoma, the plastic stent can be exchanged to a short SEMS in the same procedure. Despite several passes with FNA/FNAB, if ROSE is still inconclusive, then a 10 French plastic bile duct stent can be placed, or one can consider a potentially removable fully covered SEMS (not yet approved by the FDA for this indication). However, unlike plastic stent, the metal stent will cause significant artifacts if one were to consider repeating EUS-FNA.

A recent study evaluated the safety and efficacy of the "one-stop shop" approach focusing on the performance of SEMS during neoadjuvant therapy for PC [63]. In this, one of the largest series of patients (333 patients; 2009–2014) with resectable or borderline resectable PCs as determined by a pancreas-protocol scan, tissue diagnosis was made with EUS-FNA/FNAB and

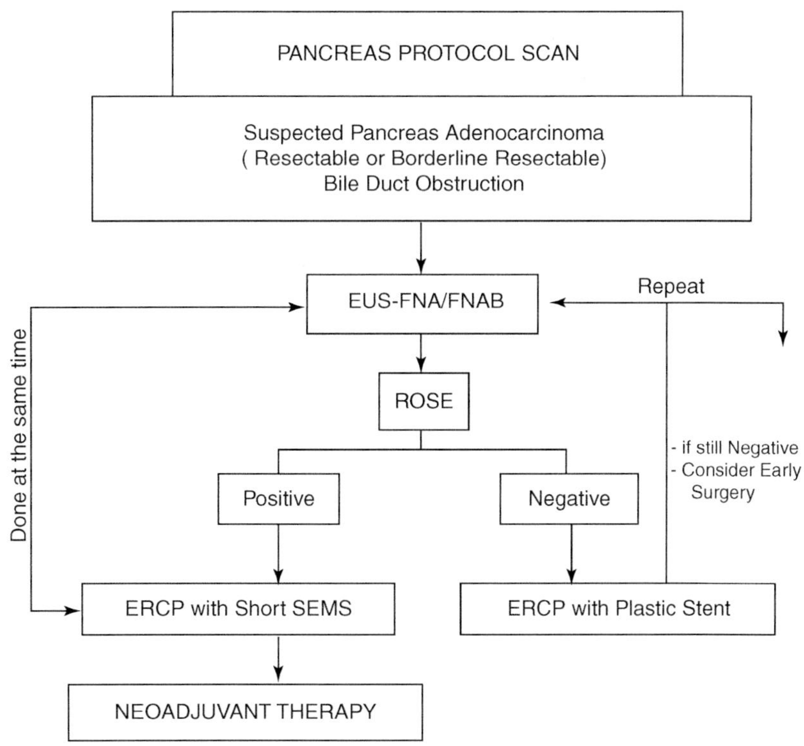

Fig. 3.3 "One-stop shop approach." EUS-FNA/FNB, endoscopic ultrasound with fine needle aspiration/fine needle aspiration biopsy; ROSE, rapid on-site evaluation; ERCP, endoscopic retrograde cholangio-pancreatography; SEMS, self-expanding metal stent (biliary)

ROSE in majority of the patients. Of these, 210 presented with bile duct obstruction. After excluding patients who had already started neoadjuvant therapy prior to placement of SEMS or were lost to follow-up, 142 patients were enrolled. The median duration of neoadjuvant therapy was 111 day (maximum 282 days). SEMS malfunctioned (predominantly occlusion with tissue ingrowth or sludge) in 16 (11%) patients by the median of 111 days (15% by 282 days). On subgroup analysis, no statistical difference in the performance of SEMS was observed between patients with (1) prior plastic stent replaced with SEMS versus up-front SEMS placement, (2) resectable versus borderline resectable PC, (3) chemotherapy alone versus chemoradiation, (4) covered versus uncovered SEMS, and (5) SEMS placed at a community hospital or at a tertiary-care center.

Summary: Resectable and Borderline Resectable Pancreas Adenocarcinoma

Before any invasive endoscopic procedure, a pancreas protocol imaging study should be performed in all patients with suspected PC so as to avoid any procedure-related complications like pancreatitis from confounding accurate staging of the cancer. Since several other malignant and nonmalignant lesions can mimic pancreas adenocarcinoma, it is highly recommended to obtain a tissue diagnosis even if the patient is being considered for early surgery. EUS-FNA or FNAB is the procedure of choice for tissue acquisition. Bile duct decompression does not offer any benefit and can be harmful in those going directly for pancreaticoduodenectomy. However, an increasing number of patients with resectable and borderline resectable pancreas adenocarcinomas are now receiving neoadjuvant therapy. Durable bile duct decompression is essential in these patients. Self-expanding metal stents are better than plastic stent for bile duct drainage but can only be used if the diagnosis of cancer is confirmed. Hence, rapid on-site evaluation of the EUS-FNA/FNAB specimen by a cytology faculty is highly recommended. If positive, additional samples can be taken for molecular profiling, and then, while the patient is still sedated, an ERCP with metal stent placement can be performed immediately after EUS-FNA in the same setting.

References

1. Winter JM, et al. Survival after resection of pancreatic cancer: results from a single institution over three decades. Ann Surg Oncol. 2012;19(1):169–75.
2. Hidalgo M. Pancreatic cancer. N Engl J Med. 2010;362(17):1605–17.
3. Tessler DA, et al. Predictors of cancer in patients with suspected pancreatic malignancy without a tissue diagnosis. Am J Surg. 2006;191(2):191–7.
4. Cassinotto C, et al. Pancreatic cancer: a simple CT score for predicting margin-positive resection in patients with resectable disease. Eur J Radiol. 2017;95:33–8.
5. Glazer ES, et al. Endoscopic ultrasonography complements computed tomography in predicting portal or superior mesenteric vein resection in patients with borderline resectable pancreatic carcinoma. Pancreatology. 2017;17(1):130–4.
6. Micames C, et al. Lower frequency of peritoneal carcinomatosis in patients with pancreatic cancer diagnosed by EUS-guided FNA vs. percutaneous FNA. Gastrointest Endosc. 2003;58(5):690–5.
7. Hewitt MJ, et al. EUS-guided FNA for diagnosis of solid pancreatic neoplasms: a meta-analysis. Gastrointest Endosc. 2012;75(2):319–31.
8. Bang JY, et al. Randomized trial comparing fanning with standard technique for endoscopic ultrasound-guided fine-needle aspiration of solid pancreatic mass lesions. Endoscopy. 2013;45(6):445–50.
9. Puli SR, et al. Diagnostic accuracy of endoscopic ultrasound in pancreatic neuroendocrine tumors: a systematic review and meta analysis. World J Gastroenterol. 2013;19(23):3678–84.
10. Puli SR, et al. How good is endoscopic ultrasound-guided fine-needle aspiration in diagnosing the correct etiology for a solid pancreatic mass?: a meta-analysis and systematic review. Pancreas. 2013;42(1):20–6.
11. Klapman JB, et al. Negative predictive value of endoscopic ultrasound in a large series of patients with a clinical suspicion of pancreatic cancer. Am J Gastroenterol. 2005;100(12):2658–61.
12. Yoon WJ, Seo DW. Endoscopic ultrasound-guided local therapy of pancreatic tumors. Korean J Gastroenterol. 2015;66(3):154–8.
13. Klapman JB, et al. Clinical impact of on-site cytopathology interpretation on endoscopic ultrasound-guided fine needle aspiration. Am J Gastroenterol. 2003;98(6):1289–94.

14. Varadarajulu S, et al. Training endosonographers in cytopathology: improving the results of EUS-guided FNA. Gastrointest Endosc. 2015;81(1):104–10.
15. Ganc RL, et al. Rapid on-site cytopathological examination (ROSE) performed by endosonagraphers and its improvement in the diagnosis of pancreatic solid lesions. Acta Cir Bras. 2015;30(7):503–8.
16. Medioni J, et al. Neoadjuvant dose-dense gemcitabine plus docetaxel and vinorelbine plus epirubicin for operable breast cancer: improved prognosis in triple-negative tumors. Drugs R D. 2011;11(2):147–57.
17. Sun G, et al. Synergistic effects of photodynamic therapy with HPPH and gemcitabine in pancreatic cancer cell lines. Lasers Surg Med. 2012;44(9):755–61.
18. Cheng B, et al. Analysis of fine-needle biopsy versus fine-needle aspiration in diagnosis of pancreatic and abdominal masses: a prospective, multicenter, randomized controlled trial. Clin Gastroenterol Hepatol. 2018;16:1314–21.
19. Sewnath ME, et al. A meta-analysis on the efficacy of preoperative biliary drainage for tumors causing obstructive jaundice. Ann Surg. 2002;236(1):17–27.
20. Aadam AA, et al. A randomized controlled cross-over trial and cost analysis comparing endoscopic ultrasound fine needle aspiration and fine needle biopsy. Endosc Int Open. 2016;4(5):E497–505.
21. Mizuno N, et al. Histological diagnosis of autoimmune pancreatitis using EUS-guided trucut biopsy: a comparison study with EUS-FNA. J Gastroenterol. 2009;44(7):742–50.
22. Tsai S, et al. A phase II clinical trial of molecular profiled neoadjuvant therapy for localized pancreatic ductal adenocarcinoma. Ann Surg. 2018;268:610–9.
23. Chantrill LA, et al. Precision medicine for advanced pancreas cancer: the individualized molecular pancreatic cancer therapy (IMPaCT) trial. Clin Cancer Res. 2015;21(9):2029–37.
24. Choi JH, et al. Fiducial placement for stereotactic body radiation therapy under only endoscopic ultrasonography guidance in pancreatic and hepatic malignancy: practical feasibility and safety. Gut Liver. 2014;8(1):88–93.
25. Park WG, et al. EUS-guided gold fiducial insertion for image-guided radiation therapy of pancreatic cancer: 50 successful cases without fluoroscopy. Gastrointest Endosc. 2010;71(3):513–8.
26. DiMaio CJ, et al. EUS-guided fiducial placement for image-guided radiation therapy in GI malignancies by using a 22-gauge needle (with videos). Gastrointest Endosc. 2010;71(7):1204–10.
27. Khashab MA, et al. Comparative analysis of traditional and coiled fiducials implanted during EUS for pancreatic cancer patients receiving stereotactic body radiation therapy. Gastrointest Endosc. 2012;76(5):962–71.
28. Wyse JM, et al. Practice guidelines for endoscopic ultrasound-guided celiac plexus neurolysis. Endosc Ultrasound. 2017;6(6):369–75.
29. Sahai AV. EUS-guided celiac ganglia neurolysis versus celiac plexus neurolysis: dying to know which is better. Gastrointest Endosc. 2017;86(4):664–5.
30. Sahai AV, et al. Central vs. bilateral endoscopic ultrasound-guided celiac plexus block or neurolysis: a comparative study of short-term effectiveness. Am J Gastroenterol. 2009;104(2):326–9.
31. Doi S, et al. Endoscopic ultrasound-guided celiac ganglia neurolysis vs. celiac plexus neurolysis: a randomized multicenter trial. Endoscopy. 2013;45(5):362–9.
32. Kaufman M, et al. Efficacy of endoscopic ultrasound-guided celiac plexus block and celiac plexus neurolysis for managing abdominal pain associated with chronic pancreatitis and pancreatic cancer. J Clin Gastroenterol. 2010;44(2):127–34.
33. Puli SR, et al. EUS-guided celiac plexus neurolysis for pain due to chronic pancreatitis or pancreatic cancer pain: a meta-analysis and systematic review. Dig Dis Sci. 2009;54(11):2330–7.
34. Wyse JM, et al. Randomized, double-blind, controlled trial of early endoscopic ultrasound-guided celiac plexus neurolysis to prevent pain progression in patients with newly diagnosed, painful, inoperable pancreatic cancer. J Clin Oncol. 2011;29(26):3541–6.
35. Cho CM, Dewitt J, Al-Haddad M. Echo-endoscopy: new therapeutic frontiers. Minerva Gastroenterol Dietol. 2011;57(2):139–58.
36. DeWitt J, DiMaio CJ, Brugge WR. Long-term follow-up of pancreatic cysts that resolve radiologically after EUS-guided ethanol ablation. Gastrointest Endosc. 2010;72(4):862–6.
37. DeWitt J, et al. EUS-guided ethanol versus saline solution lavage for pancreatic cysts: a randomized, double-blind study. Gastrointest Endosc. 2009;70(4):710–23.
38. DiMaio CJ, DeWitt JM, Brugge WR. Ablation of pancreatic cystic lesions: the use of multiple endoscopic ultrasound-guided ethanol lavage sessions. Pancreas. 2011;40(5):664–8.
39. Oh HC, et al. Endoscopic ultrasonography-guided ethanol lavage with paclitaxel injection treats patients with pancreatic cysts. Gastroenterology. 2011;140(1):172–9.
40. Oh HC, Seo DW. Endoscopic ultrasonography-guided pancreatic cyst ablation (with video). J Hepatobiliary Pancreat Sci. 2015;22(1):16–9.
41. Oh HC, et al. Systemic effect of endoscopic ultrasonography-guided pancreatic cyst ablation with ethanol and paclitaxel. Dig Dis Sci. 2014;59(7):1573–7.
42. Moyer MT, et al. The safety and efficacy of an alcohol-free pancreatic cyst ablation protocol. Gastroenterology. 2017;153(5):1295–303.
43. Moyer MT, et al. Is alcohol required for effective pancreatic cyst ablation? The prospective randomized CHARM trial pilot study. Endosc Int Open. 2016;4(5):E603–7.
44. Sun S, et al. Endoscopic ultrasound-guided interstitial brachytherapy of unresectable pancreatic cancer: results of a pilot trial. Endoscopy. 2006;38(4):399–403.

45. Sun S, et al. EUS-guided interstitial brachytherapy of the pancreas: a feasibility study. Gastrointest Endosc. 2005;62(5):775–9.
46. Karaca C, et al. Feasibility of EUS-guided injection of irinotecan-loaded microspheres into the swine pancreas. Gastrointest Endosc. 2011;73(3):603–6.
47. Levy MJ, et al. EUS-guided fine-needle injection of gemcitabine for locally advanced and metastatic pancreatic cancer. Gastrointest Endosc. 2017;86(1):161–9.
48. Hecht JR, et al. A phase I/II trial of intratumoral endoscopic ultrasound injection of ONYX-015 with intravenous gemcitabine in unresectable pancreatic carcinoma. Clin Cancer Res. 2003;9(2):555–61.
49. Chang KJ, et al. Phase I clinical trial of allogeneic mixed lymphocyte culture (cytoimplant) delivered by endoscopic ultrasound-guided fine-needle injection in patients with advanced pancreatic carcinoma. Cancer. 2000;88(6):1325–35.
50. Choi JH, et al. Initial human experience of endoscopic ultrasound-guided photodynamic therapy with a novel photosensitizer and a flexible laser-light catheter. Endoscopy. 2015;47(11):1035–8.
51. Pai M, et al. Endoscopic ultrasound guided radiofrequency ablation, for pancreatic cystic neoplasms and neuroendocrine tumors. World J Gastrointest Surg. 2015;7(4):52–9.
52. van der Gaag NA, et al. Preoperative biliary drainage for cancer of the head of the pancreas. N Engl J Med. 2010;362(2):129–37.
53. Levy MJ, et al. Palliation of malignant extrahepatic biliary obstruction with plastic versus expandable metal stents: an evidence-based approach. Clin Gastroenterol Hepatol. 2004;2(4):273–85.
54. Moss AC, et al. Malignant distal biliary obstruction: a systematic review and meta-analysis of endoscopic and surgical bypass results. Cancer Treat Rev. 2007;33(2):213–21.
55. Isayama H, et al. Polyurethane-covered metal stent for management of distal malignant biliary obstruction. Gastrointest Endosc. 2002;55(3):366–70.
56. Moole H, et al. Covered versus uncovered self-expandable metal stents for malignant biliary strictures: a meta-analysis and systematic review. Indian J Gastroenterol. 2016;35(5):323–30.
57. Almadi MA, Barkun AN, Martel M. No benefit of covered vs uncovered self-expandable metal stents in patients with malignant distal biliary obstruction: a meta-analysis. Clin Gastroenterol Hepatol. 2013;11(1):27–37.e1.
58. Nakai Y, et al. Efficacy and safety of the covered Wallstent in patients with distal malignant biliary obstruction. Gastrointest Endosc. 2005;62(5):742–8.
59. Boulay BR, Gardner TB, Gordon SR. Occlusion rate and complications of plastic biliary stent placement in patients undergoing neoadjuvant chemoradiotherapy for pancreatic cancer with malignant biliary obstruction. J Clin Gastroenterol. 2010;44(6):452–5.
60. Ge PS, et al. Plastic biliary stent patency in patients with locally advanced pancreatic cancer receiving downstaging chemotherapy. Gastrointest Endosc. 2015;81(2):360–6.
61. Aadam AA, et al. Efficacy and safety of self-expandable metal stents for biliary decompression in patients receiving neoadjuvant therapy for pancreatic cancer: a prospective study. Gastrointest Endosc. 2012;76(1):67–75.
62. Mullen JT, et al. Pancreaticoduodenectomy after placement of endobiliary metal stents. J Gastrointest Surg. 2005;9(8):1094–104; discussion 1104–5.
63. Ballard D, et al. Safety and efficacy of self-expanding metal stents for biliary drainage in patients receiving neoadjuvant therapy for pancreatic cancer. Endoscopy International. 2018;6:714–21.

4 Importance of Carbohydrate Antigen 19-9 Monitoring in the Management of Pancreatic Cancer

Ashley N. Krepline, Flavio G. Rocha, and Susan Tsai

Introduction

Although surgical resection is deemed necessary to cure patients with localized pancreatic cancer, surgery alone is associated with a median disease-free survival of 6.7 months in the absence of any additional postoperative (adjuvant) therapy [1]. The high rates of disease recurrence have led to a universal recommendation for adjuvant therapy following surgery, which improves the overall survival from 20 months to 24–28 months and is recommended for all patients with pancreatic cancer, regardless of pathologic stage [1–3]. Recently, the use of multidrug (mFOLFIRINOX) regimens in a highly selected group of patients (with postoperative CA19-9 < 180 U/dL) has been associated with a median overall survival of 54 months, although only 66% of patients completed adjuvant therapy [4]. Unfortunately, post-pancreatectomy complications often prohibit the delivery of adjuvant therapy [5, 6]. In addition, with a surgery-first approach, up to 26% of patients will develop early postoperative disease progression prior to completing adjuvant therapy [7]. As a result, there is a growing interest in preoperative therapy for patients with pancreatic cancer which allows for the early delivery of systemic therapy prior to any potential physiologic surgical perturbation. Among patients who are able to complete neoadjuvant therapy and surgery, the median overall survivals have been reported to be over 40 months, nearly double that of a surgery-first approach [8, 9]. Neoadjuvant therapy is now recommended for all patients with borderline resectable disease and is increasingly being used among patients with resectable disease [3, 8].

Goals of Neoadjuvant Therapy

Although the enthusiasm for neoadjuvant therapy has been rooted in the superior survival of patients who are able to complete all intended therapy and surgery, it is important to note that the neoadjuvant approach was first developed to help identify those patients who would develop early metastatic disease progression in an effort to spare these patients from a surgery which is associated with significant morbidity (Fig. 4.1). As a result, the primary endpoint of neoadjuvant trials has historically focused on the number of patients who are able to com-

A. N. Krepline
Department of Surgery, The Medical College of Wisconsin, Milwaukee, WI, USA

F. G. Rocha
Section of General, Thoracic and Vascular Surgery, Virginia Mason Medical Center, Seattle, WA, USA

S. Tsai (✉)
Department of Surgery, Division of Surgical Oncology, The Medical College of Wisconsin, Milwaukee, WI, USA
e-mail: stsai@mcw.edu

S. Tsai et al. (eds.), *Management of Localized Pancreatic Cancer*,
https://doi.org/10.1007/978-3-319-98944-0_4

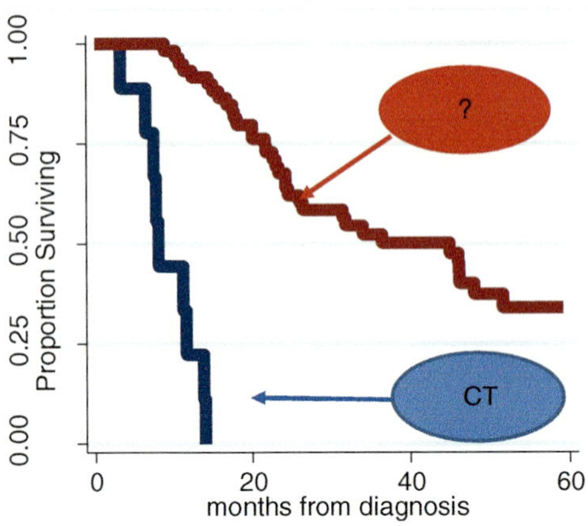

Fig. 4.1 Overall survival of patients who received neoadjuvant therapy for localized pancreatic cancer. Blue curve – patients who are not resected secondary to metastatic disease progression. These patients can be identified by CT or diagnostic laparoscopy. Red curve – patients who complete all intended neoadjuvant therapy and surgery. Currently the selection for surgery is based on the exclusion of patients with metastatic disease progression rather than inclusion of patients who are having a robust response to neoadjuvant therapy. Currently no method is used for positive selection of these patients

plete all neoadjuvant therapy and surgery. In the early experience with neoadjuvant clinical trials, approximately 30% of patients also develop disease progression prior to surgery and experienced a median overall survival of approximately 1 year [10, 11]. In contrast, among patients who are able to complete neoadjuvant therapy and surgery, the median overall survival rates have been reported to range from 33 to 44 months (Fig. 4.1), surpassing that observed with a surgery-first approach [8, 10–13]. This suggests that early systemic therapy may be effective in eradicating radiographically occult metastatic disease in some patients. In the era of increasingly effective systemic regimens, the goal of neoadjuvant therapy may shift to improve the efficacy of neoadjuvant therapy for patients with pancreatic cancer to achieve a greater number of patients who are able to complete all neoadjuvant therapy and surgery.

Assessment of Treatment Response

It is important to note that the current threshold to proceed to surgery is the absence of disease progression rather than the presence of disease response. In fact, a significant radiographic response is seldom observed with neoadjuvant therapy [14, 15]. In general, a radiographic response is rare after neoadjuvant therapy. In a single institutional study of 129 patients, following neoadjuvant therapy, 84 (69%) patients had stable disease, 15 (12%) patients had a partial response, and 23 (19%) patients had disease progression [14]. The inability to accurately discriminate treatment response with disease stabilization is likely responsible for early postoperative recurrences seen in some patients who have received neoadjuvant therapy.

When comparing the patterns of postoperative recurrence following a surgery-first approach as compared with neoadjuvant approach, there are both similarities and differences. With a surgery-first approach, in a study of 636 patients, 531 (77%) of patients developed disease recurrence after surgery at a median of 11.7 months [16]. In contrast, with neoadjuvant therapy, disease recurrence was observed in only 153 (56%) of 272 patients (C. Barnes, in review), suggesting that neoadjuvant therapy was associated with decreased rates of disease recurrence as compared to a surgery-first approach. However, among those patients who developed disease recurrence after neoadjuvant therapy and surgery, the pattern and timing of the disease recurrence was not different from patients who had been treated with a surgery-first approach. This suggests that following neoadjuvant therapy, there are a subset of patients who have radiographically occult metastatic disease which has not been eradicated by neoadjuvant therapy who following surgical resection are at high risk for an early postoperative recurrence. As neoadjuvant strategies evolve, there is an urgent need to develop quantitative assessments of treatment response to improve our understanding of treatment response and better stratify patients for clinical trials.

Carbohydrate Antigen 19-9 (CA19-9)

The limitations of pretreatment radiographic staging in the accurate identification of metastatic disease can be overcome, in part, with the availability of a dynamic biomarker. Carbohydrate antigen 19-9 (CA19-9) is a carbohydrate tumor-associated antigen that was originally isolated from colorectal tumors but has since been shown to have utility as a prognostic biomarker in pancreatic cancer [17, 18]. CA19-9 is a complex carbohydrate formed by the sialyation of the Lewis antigen by a glycosyltransferase. In the setting of a normal total bilirubin level, CA19-9 is typically considered normal if less than 35 U/mL; however the cutoff for a normal value varies slightly by laboratory. It can be falsely elevated in benign conditions such as jaundice, pancreatitis, cholangitis, and cirrhosis. CA19-9 is a Lewis antigen, and among the 5% of patients who are Lewis antigen negative, sialyation cannot occur due to a lack of the required oligosaccharide. These individuals are considered to be CA19-9 nonproducers.

Among patients who are CA19-9 producers, pretreatment CA19-9 levels have been demonstrated to be a highly prognostic biomarker. Patients with high CA19-9 levels prior to treatment were noted to have decreased overall survival and were less likely to be resected [19]. In addition, a decline in CA19-9 in response to neoadjuvant therapy has been associated with improved overall survival and increased rates of surgical resection [20, 21]. Among borderline resectable patients, a decline of >50% in CA19-9 was associated with an improved overall survival (28 vs. 11 months, $p < 0.001$) and was an independent predictor of survival (HR: 0.26, 95% CI: 0.13–0.55). In addition, failure to normalize the CA19-9 level after neoadjuvant therapy and prior to surgery was associated with a 1.37-fold increased risk of death (95% CI:1.08–2.81, $p = 0.02$) [22]. Although previous publications have suggested that CA19-9 may be a valuable predictive biomarker, it remains unclear how to interpret changes in CA19-9 during neoadjuvant therapy. The purpose of this chapter is to help clinicians incorporate CA19-9 monitoring into their practice and provide guidelines for the interpretation of dynamic changes in CA19-9.

Value of Pretreatment CA19-9

A wealth of literature supports the prognostic value of pretreatment CA19-9 levels among patients with pancreatic cancer. Several reports have demonstrated that preoperative CA19-9 is associated with tumor stage, resectability, risk for recurrence, and survival in patients with localized PC treated with a surgery-first approach [18, 19, 23–25]. One of the first studies to describe the prognostic importance of CA19-9 examined 176 patients with localized PC [23]. CA19-9 levels were found to correlate with AJCC pathologic stage, as well as post-resection survival. Of note, patients with preoperative CA19-9 values greater than 1000 U/mL had a median overall survival of only 12 months as compared to 28 months for patients with CA19-9 values less than 1000 U/mL. Similarly, in the largest study examining pretreatment CA19-9 which involved 1626 patients with localized PC, Hartwig et al. observed a strong inverse relationship between preoperative CA19-9 levels and both R0 resection rates and overall survival [19]. In their study, 312 patients had a pretreatment CA19-9 level greater than 1000 U/mL, and in this subgroup, there were no 5-year survivors; the median overall survival after resection was approximately 12 months. As a result, the authors concluded that patients with CA19-9 levels greater than 1000 are at high risk for the development of metastatic disease, and a neoadjuvant treatment approach should be considered.

Although very high levels of CA19-9 have been associated with poor outcome following surgery, there is little available data on exactly how CA19-9 levels should influence treatment sequencing or the decision to proceed to surgery especially in higher-risk patients [18, 26]. We have performed a retrospective analysis of 131 patients who received neoadjuvant therapy for localized pancreatic cancer and performed an initial analysis by quartile of pretreatment CA19-9 levels. We observed that patients with pretreatment CA19-9 in the lowest quartile (<80 U/dL) had the most favorable outcome with a median overall survival of 68 months (Fig. 4.2). The low CA19-9 values in these patients likely represented localized disease with little or no micrometastatic disease burden. Of the remaining 98 patients who had pretx CA19-9 > 80 u/dL, we observed no significant differences in OS following neoadjuvant therapy and surgery among the pretx quartile groups despite a wide range of CA19-9 values (80-6643 U/mL). Our findings support the results from retrospective cohort studies, largely involv-

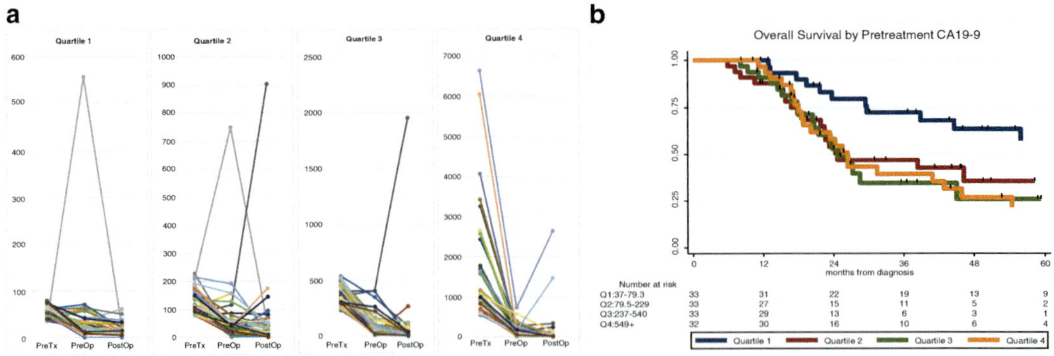

Fig. 4.2 Changes in CA19-9 values during neoadjuvant therapy. Patients are categorized by quartiles of pretreatment CA19-9. (**a**) Longitudinal changes in CA19-9 within quartiles of pretreatment CA19-9 and (**b**) overall survival by quartiles of pretx CA19-9. Note that the lowest quartile of pretreatment CA19-9 has the most favorable overall survival

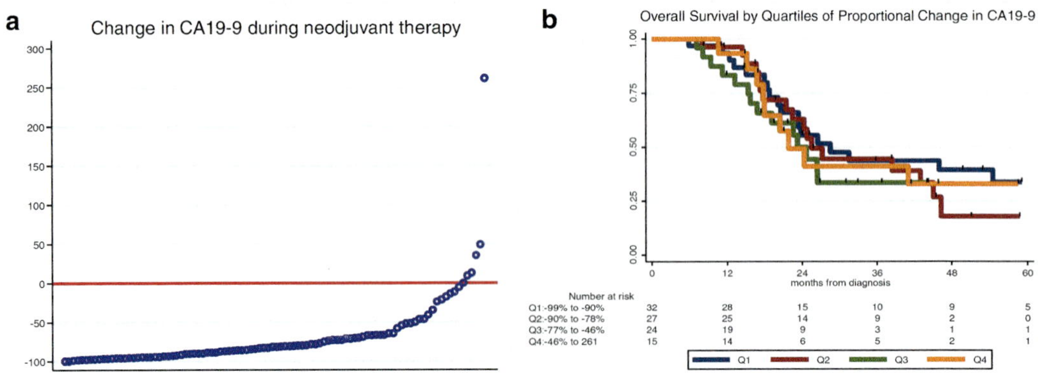

Fig. 4.3 (**a**) Overall survival by normalization of pretx CA19-9 ($n = 98$) (**b**) Overall survival by DCA19-9 (calculated as preop CA19-9-pretreatment CA19-9)/pretreatment CA19-9) after neoadjuvant therapy among patients with pretx CA19-9 > 80 U/mL ($n = 98$). Patients are categorized by quartiles of DCA19-9, with Q1 representing the greatest decline in CA19-9 and Q4 representing the least decline in CA19-9 or increase in CA19-9 after neoadjuvant therapy

ing patients taken directly to surgery, that low pretx CA19-9 (e.g., <80–100 u/dL) is associated with an improved postoperative survival. These patients should be carefully considered during clinical trial allocation to avoid unintended bias.

Changes in CA19-9 with Neoadjuvant Therapy

Among the 98 remaining patients with pretreatment CA19-9 ≥ 80 U/mL, 81 (83%) patients had at least a 50% decline in their CA19-9 level following neoadjuvant therapy, including 30 (94%) of the patients in the highest pretreatment quartile of CA19-9 (Fig. 4.3). However, normalization of preop CA19-9 was achieved in just 29 (30%) of the 98 patients (with a pretreatment CA19-9 ≥ 80 u/dL), and of the remaining 69 patients, an additional 32 (46%) normalized their CA19-9 following surgery. Therefore, dynamic and significant changes in CA19-9 values can occur in response to neoadjuvant therapy, regardless of pretreatment CA19-9 values.

Magnitude of Change of CA19-9 Following Neoadjuvant Therapy

Changes in CA19-9 levels in response to treatment likely represent tumor-specific responses to

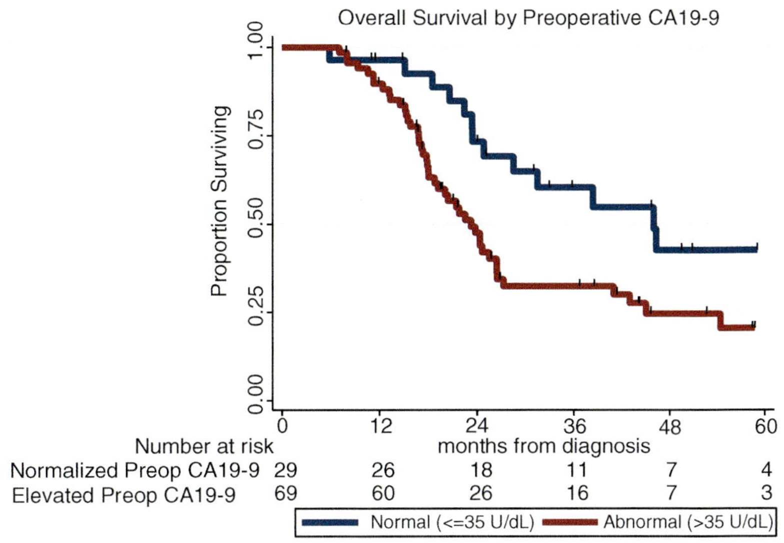

Fig. 4.4 Comparison of patients by perioperative change in CA19-9. CA19-9 was classified as normal or elevated at a cut-point of 35 U/dL. CA19-9 was analyzed at two timepoints: preoperative and postoperative. Perioperative status was classified as: normal/normal, normal/elevated, elevated/normal, elevated/elevated. (**a**) Longitudinal changes in CA19-9 by perioperative CA19-9 status and (**b**) overall survival by perioperative categories of CA19-9

therapy. Among patients with advanced pancreatic cancer, the early decrease in CA19-9 levels was associated with objective changes in radiographic response and survival [27–29]. Similarly, among patients with localized pancreatic cancer, a decrease in CA19-9 in response to neoadjuvant therapy has previously been reported to correlate with overall survival [20, 21]. In a study of 78 patients with localized pancreatic cancer, a 50% reduction in pretreatment CA19-9 after neoadjuvant therapy was associated with improved overall survival (28 vs.11 months, $p < 0.0001$) [20]. In another study of 82 patients with localized pancreatic cancer, a decline in CA19-9 following neoadjuvant therapy was also associated with improved survival (25.7 mo vs. 10.4 mo, $p = 0.01$) [21]. Although prior studies offer a general consensus that a decline in CA19-9 following neoadjuvant therapy is favorable, it may be of modest clinical benefit in the absence of achieving a normal value [20, 21, 30]. In our institutional analysis, the overall survival of patients was compared based on (a) the magnitude of the proportional change in CA19-9 after neoadjuvant therapy and (b) whether a normal CA19-9 value was achieved after neoadjuvant therapy or after surgery. After excluding patients with the lowest quartile pretreatment CA19-9, significant proportional declines in CA19-9 were observed with neoadjuvant therapy; however, the magnitude of the decline was not associated with an improvement in overall survival (Fig. 4.3). In contrast, following the completion of neoadjuvant therapy, patients who normalized their preoperative or postoperative CA19-9 values experienced a doubling in overall survival compared to patients who did not (Fig. 4.4).

Normalization of CA19-9 Following Neoadjuvant Therapy

Having observed that normalization of CA19-9 following neoadjuvant therapy prior to surgery was an important prognostic factor, but could only be achieved in a third of patients, we then examined if postoperative normalization was an important prognostic factor. With regard to perioperative changes of CA19-9, we observed that if the preoperative CA19-9 was normal, it was likely to remain normal after surgery (Fig. 4.5). If the preoperative CA19-9 was elevated, half of patients normalized their postoperative CA19-9. Importantly, the failure to normalize CA19-9 following neoadjuvant therapy and surgery was associated with a 3.18-fold increased risk of death ($p = 0.003$).

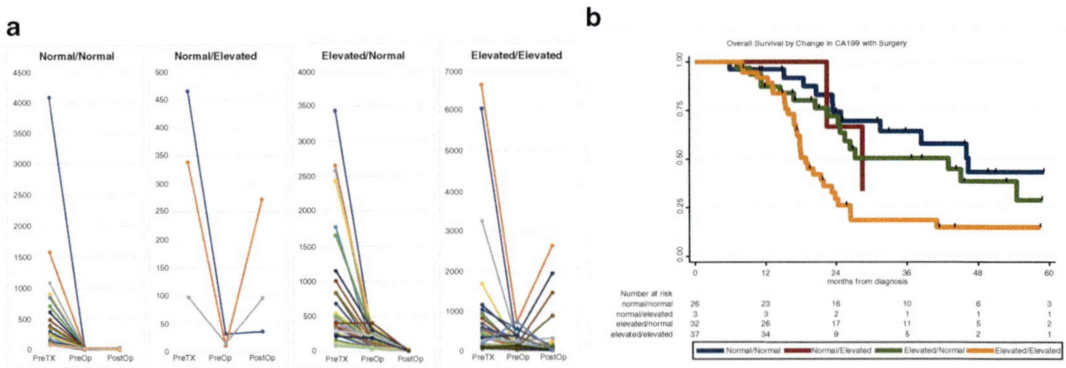

Fig. 4.5 (**a**) Longitudinal changes in CA19-9 among patients who completed all neoadjuvant therapy and surgery, (**b**) Overall survival by perioperative changes in CA19-9 among patients with pretx CA19-9 > 80 U/mL ($n = 98$). Perioperative status (preop and postop) was classified as: normal/normal; normal/elevated; elevated/normal; elevated/elevated

Future Directions

The evolution of treatment for localized pancreatic cancer has evolved from a surgery-first approach to a strategy of neoadjuvant therapy with or without adjuvant therapy. As with many other solid tumor malignancy, there is a growing interest in the delivery of all multimodality therapy (total neoadjuvant therapy) prior to surgery, and thereby diminishing the impact of postoperative complications on the delivery of care. The risk of a total neoadjuvant approach is the potential to deliver inadequate therapy, and therefore the assessment of treatment response is critical. Serial CA19-9 monitoring and treatment adjustments to achieve normalization of CA19-9 will likely be a critical adjunct to radiographic imaging and may help to further guide the design of neoadjuvant trials and the delivery of effective therapies.

Conclusions

In patients with pancreatic cancer who have an elevated CA19-9 at diagnosis, changes in the CA19-9 levels in response to neoadjuvant therapy can be highly prognostic for survival. The normalization of CA19-9 in patients with localized pancreatic cancer may reflect control of systemic micrometastatic disease. Importantly, the CA19-9 response to induction therapy provides a window through which we can begin to understand a complex tumor biology, and the value of extended neoadjuvant therapy to achieve a normalization of CA19-9 should be an area of further study. Additional biomarkers under development will add to the value of posttreatment/preoperative CA19-9 and provide physicians a much more accurate prediction of whether surgery will provide clinically meaningful benefit to an individual patient.

References

1. Oettle H, Neuhaus P, Hochhaus A, et al. Adjuvant chemotherapy with gemcitabine and long-term outcomes among patients with resected pancreatic cancer: the CONKO-001 randomized trial. JAMA. 2013;310(14):1473–81.
2. Neoptolemos JP, Palmer DH, Ghaneh P, et al. Comparison of adjuvant gemcitabine and capecitabine with gemcitabine monotherapy in patients with resected pancreatic cancer (ESPAC-4): a multicentre, open-label, randomised, phase 3 trial. Lancet. 2017;389(10073):1011–1024.
3. Pancreatic Adenocarcinoma. NCCN Clinical Practice Guidelines in Oncology (NCCN Guidelines) 2017; 2015. http://www.nccn.org/professionals/physician_gls/pdf/pancreatic.pdf.
4. Conroy T, Hammel P, Hebbar M, et al. FOLFIRINOX or Gemcitabine as Adjuvant Therapy for Pancreatic Cancer. The New England Journal of Medicine. 2018;379(25):2395–2406.
5. Wu W, He J, Cameron JL, et al. The impact of postoperative complications on the administration of adjuvant therapy following pancreaticoduodenectomy for adenocarcinoma. Ann Surg Oncol. 2014;21(9):2873–81.

6. Mayo SC, Gilson MM, Herman JM, et al. Management of patients with pancreatic adenocarcinoma: national trends in patient selection, operative management, and use of adjuvant therapy. J Am Coll Surg. 2012;214(1):33–45.
7. Tzeng CW, Tran Cao HS, Lee JE, et al. Treatment sequencing for resectable pancreatic cancer: influence of early metastases and surgical complications on multimodality therapy completion and survival. J Gastrointest Surg. 2014;18(1):16–24; discussion 24–15.
8. Christians KK, Heimler JW, George B, et al. Survival of patients with resectable pancreatic cancer who received neoadjuvant therapy. Surgery. 2016;159:893–900.
9. Cloyd JM, Katz MH, Prakash L, et al. Preoperative therapy and pancreatoduodenectomy for pancreatic ductal adenocarcinoma: a 25-year single-institution experience. J Gastrointest Surg. 2017;21(1):164–74.
10. Evans DB, Varadhachary GR, Crane CH, et al. Preoperative gemcitabine-based chemoradiation for patients with resectable adenocarcinoma of the pancreatic head. J Clin Oncol. 2008;26(21):3496–502.
11. Varadhachary GR, Wolff RA, Crane CH, et al. Preoperative gemcitabine and cisplatin followed by gemcitabine-based chemoradiation for resectable adenocarcinoma of the pancreatic head. J Clin Oncol. 2008;26(21):3487–95.
12. Winter JM, Brennan MF, Tang LH, et al. Survival after resection of pancreatic adenocarcinoma: results from a single institution over three decades. Ann Surg Oncol. 2012;19(1):169–75.
13. Winter JM, Cameron JL, Campbell KA, et al. 1423 pancreaticoduodenectomies for pancreatic cancer: a single-institution experience. J Gastrointest Surg. 2006;10(9):1199–210; discussion 1210–1191.
14. Katz MH, Fleming JB, Bhosale P, et al. Response of borderline resectable pancreatic cancer to neoadjuvant therapy is not reflected by radiographic indicators. Cancer. 2012;118(23):5749–56.
15. Ferrone CR, Marchegiani G, Hong TS, Ryan DP, Deshpande V, McDonnell EI, Sabbatino F, Santos DD, Allen JN, Blaszkowsky LS, Clark JW, Faris JE, Goyal L, Kwak EL, Murphy JE, Ting DT, Wo JY, Zhu AX, Warshaw AL, Lillemoe KD, Fernadez-del Castillo C. Radiological and surgical implications of neoadjuvant treatment with FOLFIRINOX for locally advanced and borderline resectable pancreatic cancer. Ann Surg. 2015; 261(1):12–17
16. Groot VP, Rezaee N, Wu W, et al. Patterns, timing, and predictors of recurrence following pancreatectomy for pancreatic ductal adenocarcinoma. Ann Surg. 2018;267:936–45.
17. Koprowski H, Steplewski Z, Mitchell K, Herlyn M, Herlyn D, Fuhrer P. Colorectal carcinoma antigens detected by hybridoma antibodies. Somatic Cell Genet. 1979;5(6):957–71.
18. Humphris JL, Chang DK, Johns AL, et al. The prognostic and predictive value of serum CA19.9 in pancreatic cancer. Ann Oncol. 2012;23(7):1713–22.
19. Hartwig W, Strobel O, Hinz U, et al. CA19-9 in potentially resectable pancreatic cancer: perspective to adjust surgical and perioperative therapy. Ann Surg Oncol. 2013;20(7):2188–96.
20. Boone BA, Steve J, Zenati MS, et al. Serum CA 19-9 response to neoadjuvant therapy is associated with outcome in pancreatic adenocarcinoma. Ann Surg Oncol. 2014;21(13):4351–8.
21. Katz MH, Varadhachary GR, Fleming JB, et al. Serum CA 19-9 as a marker of resectability and survival in patients with potentially resectable pancreatic cancer treated with neoadjuvant chemoradiation. Ann Surg Oncol. 2010;17(7):1794–801.
22. Aldakkak M, Christians KK, Krepline AN, et al. Pretreatment carbohydrate antigen 19-9 does not predict the response to neoadjuvant therapy in patients with localized pancreatic cancer. HPB. 2015;17(10):942–52.
23. Ferrone CR, Finkelstein DM, Thayer SP, Muzikansky A, Fernandez-delCastillo C, Warshaw AL. Perioperative CA19-9 levels can predict stage and survival in patients with resectable pancreatic adenocarcinoma. J Clin Oncol. 2006;24(18):2897–902.
24. Barton JG, Bois JP, Sarr MG, et al. Predictive and prognostic value of CA 19-9 in resected pancreatic adenocarcinoma. J Gastrointest Surg. 2009;13(11):2050–8.
25. Turrini O, Schmidt CM, Moreno J, et al. Very high serum CA 19-9 levels: a contraindication to pancreaticoduodenectomy? J Gastrointest Surg. 2009;13(10):1791–7.
26. Karachristos A, Scarmeas N, Hoffman JP. CA 19-9 levels predict results of staging laparoscopy in pancreatic cancer. J Gastrointest Surg. 2005;9(9):1286–92.
27. Reni M, Cereda S, Balzano G, et al. Carbohydrate antigen 19-9 change during chemotherapy for advanced pancreatic adenocarcinoma. Cancer. 2009;115(12):2630–9.
28. Wong D, Ko AH, Hwang J, Venook AP, Bergsland EK, Tempero MA. Serum CA19-9 decline compared to radiographic response as a surrogate for clinical outcomes in patients with metastatic pancreatic cancer receiving chemotherapy. Pancreas. 2008;37(3):269–74.
29. Hess V, Glimelius B, Grawe P, et al. CA 19-9 tumour-marker response to chemotherapy in patients with advanced pancreatic cancer enrolled in a randomised controlled trial. Lancet Oncol. 2008;9(2):132–8.
30. Xia BT, Fu B, Wang J, et al. Does radiologic response correlate to pathologic response in patients undergoing neoadjuvant therapy for borderline resectable pancreatic malignancy? J Surg Oncol. 2017;115(4):376–83.

5 Treatment Sequencing for Resectable Disease

Mariana I. Chavez

Introduction

Pancreatic cancer (PC) is a rising public health threat and is anticipated to account for over 48,000 cancer-related deaths by 2020 and 63,000 by 2030—being only surpassed by lung cancer [1]. In an era when oncologic treatments of many solid organ cancers have made significant advances, it is sobering that the survival of patients with PC remains largely unchanged [2]. In fact, death rates have been stable over 2005–2014.

Staging of PC is usually done with triphasic pancreatic-protocol computed tomography scan of chest, abdomen, and pelvis. Based upon imaging, the tumor can be classified as resectable, borderline resectable, locally advanced types A or B, and metastatic. Resectable or localized disease is present when there is no arterial tumor contact [with either celiac axis (CA), superior mesenteric artery (SMA), or common hepatic artery (CHA)] and there is no tumor contact with the superior mesenteric vein (SMV) or portal vein (PV) or ≤180-degrees contact without vein contour irregularity on imaging study.

Decades of surgical experience have demonstrated that even among patients with localized PC who were managed with immediate surgery (surgery-first approach), addition of adjuvant therapy provides an improved but still limited survival benefit with median survival rates, at best, of only 24 months [3]. With most patients developing systemic recurrence even after margin-negative (R0) resections, it is suggested that PC is a systemic disease, even in the absence of radiographic evidence of distant metastases [4–6].

Currently, the National Comprehensive Cancer Network (NCCN) practice guidelines recommend a surgery-first approach for resectable PC [7]. An alternative approach is to administer early systemic therapy prior to surgery (neoadjuvant therapy) for the management of systemic disease that is suspected but not radiographically confirmed. This way, patients who have aggressive tumor biology and develop disease progression during neoadjuvant therapy can be spared an operative intervention with limited oncologic benefit. This chapter details the rationale of treatment sequencing for resectable PC and provides specific recommendations for staging and treatment sequencing for patients with resectable pancreatic disease.

Rationale for Neoadjuvant Treatment

Large randomized controlled clinical trials have demonstrated the benefit of adjuvant therapy in PC. Such is the case of CONKO-001

M. I. Chavez (✉)
Department of General Surgery,
The Surgical Clinic,
Nashville, TN, USA

S. Tsai et al. (eds.), *Management of Localized Pancreatic Cancer*,
https://doi.org/10.1007/978-3-319-98944-0_5

(Charité Onkologie 001) and ESPAC4 (European Study Group for Pancreatic Cancer 4) which demonstrated an increase in median overall survival when comparing surgery alone vs either additional of single-agent gemcitabine or gemcitabine and capecitabine [8, 9]. More recent clinical trials, such as the GI PRODIGE 24/CCTG PA.6, have abandoned an observation arm in recognition of the importance of adjuvant therapy [37 38]. Until recently the median overall survival benefit of adjvuant therapy has been modest. However, the recent report of the GI PRODIGE 24/CCTG PA.6 demonstrated a median overal survival of 54 months among patients who received modified fluorouracil, irinotecan, and oxaliplatin (mFOLFIRINOX) as compared to patients receiving gemcitabine [38]. This marks a major advancement in overall survival among patients who undergo upfront surgical resection. However, these findings should be interpreted with caution as the outstanding observed survival benefit may be explained by rigorous selection alone. As compared to the seminal report of adjuvant gemcitabine in the CONKO-001 trial, the median overall survival of patients on the control arm of the GI PRODIGE 24/CCTG PA.6 who received gemcitabine was 35 months as compared to 23 months. It is important to note, that mFOLFIRINOX is recognized to be a challenging regimen to administer, and this may have influenced the selection of patients for the trial. The GI PRODIGE 24/CCCTG PA.6 trial was conducted at 77 centers over 4 years to accrue 493 patients. In total, each center enrolled an average of 6.4 patients over a 4 year period (average 1.6 patients/year). It is likely that the low accrual rate per center, reflects a selection bias which may account for the tremendous survival advancement observed in this trial.

Although universally recommended, the feasibility of delivering adjuvant therapy to patients with PC in the postoperative setting remains problematic. Even at experienced high-volume institutions, almost half of patients will fail to receive any adjuvant therapy following pancreatectomy because of complications, delayed recovery, or failure to return to an adequate baseline performance status acceptable for systemic therapy [10, 11]. In the GI PRODIGE24/CCTG PA.6 trial, 32% of patients who were assigned to mFOLFIRINOX discontinued treatment and only 66% of patients recieved all planned cycles of chemotherapy [37].

To address these limitations, a growing interest has emerged in an alternative treatment sequencing. Preoperative treatment was proposed since 1992 with the premise of avoiding resection in patients with rapidly progressive disease, as well as ensuring completion of multimodality therapy and allowing radiation therapy to be delivered to well-oxygenated cells before surgical devascularization [12].

Since neoadjuvant therapy offers an "induction" phase lasting approximately 2–4 months, individuals with unfavorable tumor biology who develop early metastatic disease are identified prior to surgery. Detecting these patients prior to surgery will spare a major procedure with limited oncologic benefit.

The addition of radiation has important pathologic implications with several series reporting decreased rates of positive margins, either R1 or R2, and node-positive disease [13–15]. This effect could be attributed to the presence of oxygenated environment which improves the efficacy of radiation and decreases the toxicity to adjacent normal tissue [12, 16].

When neoadjuvant therapy was first introduced as an alternative to a surgery-first approach, several concerns were raised by the surgical community pertaining to its safety and feasibility. Foremost was the concern that patients with localized PC may develop local disease progression which would prevent a potentially curative surgical resection; the so-called window of opportunity for surgery could be lost. Over the last decade as the experience with neoadjuvant therapy has matured, concerns regarding local disease progression have not been realized. In the largest combined experience with neoadjuvant therapy for patients with resectable PC, less than 1% of eligible patients were found to have isolated local disease progression at the time of restaging after neoadjuvant therapy and before planned surgery [17, 18].

When disease progression occurs during neoadjuvant therapy, it is usually distant metastatic disease involving the liver or peritoneum. In addition, theoretical concerns over the toxicity of neoadjuvant therapy and the impact of treatment-related side effects on operative morbidity and mortality were also not observed [17–19]. In fact, the incidence of pancreatic fistula—the most frequent serious complication associated with pancreatectomy—has been demonstrated to be reduced after neoadjuvant therapy, probably because the treated pancreas becomes more fibrotic with a decrease in enzyme production [13–15].

With regard to overall complications, a recent analysis of the National Surgical Quality Improvement Program (NSQIP) database demonstrated no differences in 30-day mortality and postoperative morbidity rates among patients treated with neoadjuvant therapy as compared to patients who received surgery-first approach [20].

Multidisciplinary care is the cornerstone of successful administration of neoadjuvant therapy. See Table 5.1 for advantages and disadvantages of neoadjuvant therapy. The scope of the multidisciplinary team is vast and includes medical and surgical oncologists, pathologists, radiation oncologists, diagnostic radiologists, advanced endoscopists, genetic counselors, dietitians, and trained nursing staff. Before embarking on a neoadjuvant approach, all patients should have the benefit of having their case reviewed in a multidisciplinary conference where the optimal treatment plan can be established and the course of treatment outlined prior to the initiation of any therapy.

Table 5.1 Advantages and disadvantages of neoadjuvant therapy

Advantages of neoadjuvant therapy
Usually well tolerated
Ensures the receipt of systemic therapy by all patients
Identification of patients with aggressive tumor biology, manifested as disease progression
Increased efficacy of radiation therapy due to a well-oxygenated environment
Decreased radiation-induced toxicity to adjacent normal tissue as the radiated field is resected at the time of pancreatectomy
Decreased rate of pancreatic fistula formation when radiation is used
Potential for lessening the size of tumors to facilitate surgical resection
Decreased rate of positive resection margins
Disadvantages of neoadjuvant therapy
Potential for complications from pretreatment endoscopic procedures
Biliary stent-related morbidity: cholangitis, cholecystitis
Disease progression obviating resectability
Possibility to increase morbidity and mortality due to side effects of selected pretreatment
Requires involvement and good communication of multidisciplinary physician team

Impact of Treatment Sequencing on Overall Survival

Until recently, the evidence favoring a neoadjuvant approach for localized PC is limited to retrospective and single-arm prospective studies. Multiple investigators have reported results after treating localized PC with neoadjuvant therapy [17, 18, 21, 22] or compared neoadjuvant vs up-front surgery followed by adjuvant therapy [23–25]. Attempts at the prospective comparison of neoadjuvant therapy with a surgery-first approach have been unsuccessful due to poor recruitment [26, 27]. Overall, direct comparisons of single-institutional series are complicated by variability in the staging definitions, chemotherapeutic agents, and radiation therapy plans.

Using the National Cancer Database (NCDB), a study retrospectively compared patients resected within clinical stages I and II who were preceded by neoadjuvant therapy. Neoadjuvant therapy was associated with a 5-month improvement in median survival compared with up-front surgery, from 21 to 26 months. Also, the up-front surgery group was found to have worse pathologic stage, higher positivity of lymph nodes, and positive margin resections [23].

A Markov decision analysis supported the use of neoadjuvant chemotherapy that provided longer overall survival (32 months vs 27 months) and quality-adjusted life expectancy (25 months vs 21 months) in comparison to surgery followed by adjuvant chemotherapy. Sensitivity analysis of the model showed that if the probability of surgical resection after neoadjuvant therapy was lower than 57%, up-front surgery was the best treatment option [25].

Another group compared the efficacy of neoadjuvant chemotherapy with adjuvant treatment with an intention-to-treat analysis using a two-arm Markov model. In the neoadjuvant group, patients were treated with an average of 3 months of neoadjuvant therapy followed by surgery. After surgery, patients who received preoperative chemotherapy did not receive any adjuvant treatment. On the other hand, patients who underwent surgery first underwent chemotherapy after they recovered from their operations. In this model, the median overall survival was longer for the neoadjuvant cohort (22 months) in comparison to the adjuvant group (20 months), and the cumulative quality-adjusted survival for patients who underwent the neoadjuvant strategy was 19.8 months compared to 18.4 months for patients who had adjuvant therapy. One-way sensitivity analysis showed that the surgery-first approach provided higher-quality-adjusted survival rates if more than 44% of patients treated with neoadjuvant therapy experienced progression of their disease and failed to undergo surgical resection [24].

All these models provided evidence that neoadjuvant therapies have better overall survival and quality of life in comparison to surgery-first approach, although the differences were clinically modest.

Single-institutional series have shown among patients who are able to complete all intended neoadjuvant therapy and surgery, median overall survival is improved by almost 12 months compared with a surgery-first approach (34–45 months vs 22–26 months) [3, 17, 18, 22]. This is a remarkable finding, considering that the survival benefit is not attributable to the addition of novel therapies but rather a change in treatment sequencing.

The results of the PREOPANC study, which was a randomized controlled trial of surgery-first versus neoadjuvant therapy with gemcitabine-based chemoradiation, were reported at the 2018 American Society of Clinical Oncology (ASCO). The patients were randomly assigned to receive immediate surgery or chemoradiotherapy for 10 weeks followed by surgery. Both treatment groups also received chemotherapy after surgery, with an equal total amount of chemotherapy given in both groups. The intention-to-treat analysis of 246 patients demonstrated a median overall survival of 13.1 vs 17.1 months with a surgery-first versus neoadjuvant approach (HR 0.74, $p = 0.07$). There was a significant decrease in time to distant metastases as well as locoregional recurrences (9.9 vs 7.9 months) (HR: 0.73, 0.013; HR 0.55, $p = 0.002$). In a subset analysis of patients who underwent resection, the median overall survival was 16.8 months and 42.2 months for patients who underwent surgery-first versus neoadjuvant therapy ($p < 0.001$). Surgical resection was completed in 72% of patients in the surgery-first group and 62% in the neoadjuvant therapy group. Among patients who had a resection, R0 resection was achieved in a greater proportion of patients who received preoperative treatment (63% vs 31%). The results of this trial have provided the first prospective randomized controlled trial evidence that a neoadjuvant approach is superior to a surgery-first approach.

Table 5.2 summarizes details of selected phase I and II trials reporting the outcomes of patients treated with neoadjuvant chemotherapy or chemoradiation for localized PC [28].

Future Directions

The results from PREOPANC-1 trial brings hope to patients, clinicians and researchers of early stage PC and it seems logical next steps include to study even more effective preoperative treatments. Recent chemotherapy regimens, such as FOLFIRINOX [folinic acid (leucovorin)/5-FU/irinotecan/oxaliplatin], have already demonstrated promising results in a small group of patients with borderline resectable tumors [28]. Given this finding, there are multiple phase III trials undergoing recruitment phase which will help to clarify the role of neoadjuvant therapy, single vs multi-agent therapy, and the addition of radiation in neoadjuvant protocols in the treatment of localized PC (NCT01314027, NCT01900327, NCT02172976, NCT02047513, NCT01150630, NCT02305186, and NCT02775695) [29].

Some examples include NEOPAC trial (NCT01314027) (adjuvant vs neoadjuvant plus adjuvant chemotherapy in resectable PC) which will compare neoadjuvant gemcitabine and oxaliplatin plus adjuvant gemcitabine vs adjuvant gemcitabine alone. NEONAX trial (NCT02047513) will assess the effects of neoadjuvant plus adjuvant nab-paclitaxel plus gem-

Table 5.2 Selected published neoadjuvant phase II trials in resectable PC

Trial/published reference/year	No. of patients	Clinical stage/duration treatment	Study design	Treatment regimen	Resection rate (%)	R0 (%)	Median overall survival (months)
Pisters et al. (2002) [33]	35	Resectable/1.8 months	Phase II Prospective	Paclitaxel (60 mg/m^2) weekly, RT (30 Gy)	57	68	19 with surgery, 10 without surgery
Palmer et al. (2007) [34]	26	Resectable/4 months	Phase II Prospective	Gemcitabine (1000 mg/m^2 weekly) + cisplatin (25 mg/m^2)	70	75	28.4 with surgery
Heinrich et al. (2008) [35]	28	Resectable/2 months	Phase II Prospective	Gemcitabine (1000 mg/m^2 twice weekly) + cisplatin (50 mg/m^2)	89	80	19.1 with surgery
Evans et al. (2008) [17]	80	Resectable/3 months	Phase II Prospective	Gemcitabine (400 mg/m^2 weekly) + RT (30 Gy)	85	82	34 with surgery, 7 without surgery
Varadhachary et al. (2008) [18]	90	Resectable/4 months	Phase II Prospective	Gemcitabine (750 mg/m^2 weekly) + cisplatin (30 mg/m^2) every 2 weeks + RT (30 Gy)	58	96	31 with surgery, 10.5 without surgery
O'Reilly et al. (2014) [36]	38	Resectable	Phase II Prospective	Gemcitabine (1000 mg/m^2) + oxaliplatin (80 mg/m^2) every 2 weeks	77	74	27.2 for the entire cohort, 22-month progression-free survival with surgery
Golcher et al. (2015) [27]	66 A: 33 CRT + surgery B: 33 only surgery	Resectable	Phase II Prospective randomized trial	Gemcitabine (300 mg/m^2) + cisplatin (30 mg/m^2) + RT (50.4 Gy). Only for Arm A	A: 69 B: 57	A: 48 B: 51	A: 18.9 months B: 25 months

citabine vs adjuvant only nab-paclitaxel plus gemcitabine. Other ongoing trials are the multicenter German randomized trial investigating adjuvant gemcitabine compared with neoadjuvant and adjuvant FOLFIRINOX (NCT02172976) and a single-arm nonrandomized trial evaluating preoperative and postoperative FOLFIRINOX in patients with resectable disease (NCT01660711). Other clinical trial development for patients with resectable PC has emphasized molecular profiling of the fine-needle aspiration specimen as a guide to the choice of systemic therapy given before operation (NCT01726582) [29].

In the case of borderline resectable pancreatic cancer (BRPC), the ALLIANCE Trial A021501 will help define standard preoperative treatment regimens for BRPC. In this study, patients with criteria for BRPC will be randomized to receive either eight cycles of modified FOLFIRINOX or to seven cycles of modified FOLFIRINOX followed by stereotactic body radiation therapy. Patients without evidence of disease progression following preoperative therapy will undergo pancreatectomy and will subsequently receive postoperative modified FOLFOX6. The primary endpoint is 18-month overall survival [30].

Emerging clinical trials will answer if systemic therapy followed by chemoradiation, in an effort to deliver all intended nonsurgical therapy before operation in patients with resectable and BRPC, is superior than current practice.

Proposed Treatment Sequencing

Outside of a clinical trial, neoadjuvant treatment of resectable PC may consist of chemotherapy alone or chemoradiation. It is important to consider the patient's response based on three main elements: clinical evaluation, tumor markers trends (Ca 19-9), and radiographic response.

If chemoradiation is used, gemcitabine combined with external-beam radiation therapy is favored. This regimen is a modification of the neoadjuvant treatment schema reported by Evans et al. [18] and includes a standard fractionation course of radiation therapy (1.8 Gy/day, M-F, 28 fractions) to a total dose of 50.4 Gy, with concurrent weekly gemcitabine given on day 1 (day −2 to +1) at a dose of 400 mg/m^{2}at fixed dose rate over 40 minutes. This program resulted in a median survival of almost 3 years in those patients who completed all therapy to include surgery [17]. Restaging with pancreatic-protocol CT imaging is completed 4 weeks after the last radiation treatment, and, in the absence of disease progression, patients are then brought to surgery. The recent reports of both FOLFIRINOX and gemcitabine/nab-paclitaxel, which demonstrated efficacy in patients with advanced disease [31, 32], have generated enthusiasm for their use in patients with localized disease. Acknowledging that the use of chemoradiation remains controversial, neoadjuvant FOLFIRINOX or gemcitabine/nab-paclitaxel delivered over approximately 2 months also represents a logical treatment alternative for patients with resectable disease.

Summary

PC is a systemic disease. With such a premise, multimodality therapy should be considered for localized PC. In contrast to a surgery-first approach, neoadjuvant treatment sequencing will ensure the receipt of systemic therapy by all patients and improve the discrimination between patients who will and who will not benefit from surgery. Currently, regimens are not unified and vary among institutions. There is growing acceptance for this modality, and is expected to incorporate novel investigational drug therapies and evolving techniques and fractionation schemes for the delivery of radiation therapy.

References

1. Rahib L, Smith BD, Aizenberg R, et al. Projecting cancer incidence and deaths to 2030: the unexpected burden of thyroid, liver, and pancreas cancers in the United States. Cancer Res. 2014;74:2913–21.
2. Stat Fact Sheet: Pancreas Cancer [10/30/2013]. Available online: http://seer.cancer.gov/statfacts/html/pancreas.html.
3. Winter JM, Brennan MF, Tang LH, et al. Survival after resection of pancreatic adenocarcinoma: results from a single institution over three decades. Ann Surg Oncol. 2012;19:169–75.
4. Sohal DP, Walsh RM, Ramanathan RK, et al. Pancreatic adenocarcinoma: treating a systemic disease with systemic therapy. J Natl Cancer Inst. 2014;106:dju011.
5. Iacobuzio-Donahue CA, Fu B, Yachida S, et al. DPC4 gene status of the primary carcinoma correlates with patterns of failure in patients with pancreatic cancer. J Clin Oncol. 2009;27:1806–13.
6. Gnerlich JL, Luka SR, Deshpande AD, et al. Microscopic margins and patterns of treatment failure in resected pancreatic adenocarcinoma. Arch Surg. 2012;147:753–60.
7. Tempero MA, Arnoletti JP, Behrman S, et al. Pancreatic adenocarcinoma. J Natl Compr Cancer Netw. 2010;8:972–1017.
8. Oettle H, Post S, Neuhaus P, et al. Adjuvant chemotherapy with gemcitabine vs observation in patients undergoing curative-intent resection of pancreatic cancer: a randomized controlled trial. JAMA. 2007;297:267–77.
9. Neoptolemos JP, Palmer DH, Ghaneh P, et al. Comparison of adjuvant gemcitabine and capecitabine with gemcitabine monotherapy in patients with resected pancreatic cancer (ESPAC-4): a multicentre, open-label, randomised, phase 3 trial. Lancet. 2017;389(10073):1011–1024.
10. Mayo SC, Gilson MM, Herman JM, et al. Management of patients with pancreatic adenocarcinoma: national trends in patient selection, operative management, and use of adjuvant therapy. J Am Coll Surg. 2012;214:33–45.
11. Wu W, He J, Cameron JL, et al. The impact of postoperative complications on the administration of adjuvant therapy following pancreaticoduodenectomy for adenocarcinoma. Ann Surg Oncol. 2014;21:2873–81.
12. Evans DB, et al. Preoperative chemoradiation and pancreaticoduodenectomy for adenocarcinoma of the pancreas. Arch Surg. 1992;127:1335–9.
13. Takahashi H, Ogawa H, Ohigashi H, et al. Preoperative chemoradiation reduces the risk of pancreatic fistula

after distal pancreatectomy for pancreatic adenocarcinoma. Surgery. 2011;150:547–56.
14. Raut CP, Evans DB, Crane CH, et al. Neoadjuvant therapy for resectable pancreatic cancer. Surg Oncol Clin N Am. 2004;13:639–61, ix.
15. Willett CG, Lewandrowski K, Warshaw AL, et al. Resection margins in carcinoma of the head of the pancreas. Implications for radiation therapy. Ann Surg. 1993;217:144–8.
16. Pilepich MV, Miller HH. Preoperative irradiation in carcinoma of the pancreas. Cancer. 1980;46:1945–9.
17. Evans DB, Varadhachary GR, Crane CH, et al. Preoperative gemcitabine-based chemoradiation for patients with resectable adenocarcinoma of the pancreatic head. J Clin Oncol. 2008;26:3496–502.
18. Varadhachary GR, Wolff RA, Crane CH, et al. Preoperative gemcitabine and cisplatin followed by gemcitabine-based chemoradiation for resectable adenocarcinoma of the pancreatic head. J Clin Oncol. 2008;26:3487–95.
19. Christians KK, Tsai S, Mahmoud A, et al. Neoadjuvant FOLFIRINOX for borderline resectable pancreas cancer: a new treatment paradigm? Oncologist. 2014;19:266–74.
20. Cooper AB, Parmar AD, Riall TS, et al. Does the use of neoadjuvant therapy for pancreatic adenocarcinoma increase postoperative morbidity and mortality rates? J Gastrointest Surg. 2015;19:80–6; discussion 86–7.
21. Takahashi H, Ohigashi H, Gotoh K, et al. Preoperative gemcitabine-based chemoradiation therapy for resectable and borderline resectable pancreatic cancer. Ann Surg. 2013;258:1040–50.
22. Christians KK, Heimler JW, George B, et al. Survival of patients with resectable pancreatic cancer who received neoadjuvant therapy. Surgery. 2016;159:893–900.
23. Mokdad AA, Minter RM, Zhu H, et al. Neoadjuvant therapy followed by resection versus upfront resection for resectable pancreatic cancer: a propensity score matched analysis. J Clin Oncol. 2016;35:515–22.
24. Sharma G, Whang EE, Ruan D, et al. Efficacy of neoadjuvant versus adjuvant therapy for resectable pancreatic adenocarcinoma: a decision analysis. Ann Surg Oncol. 2015;22:S1229–37.
25. de Geus SWL, Eskander MF, Tseng JF, et al. Neoadjuvant therapy versus upfront surgery for resected pancreatic adenocarcinoma: a nationwide propensity score matched analysis. Surgery. 2016;161:592–601.
26. Casadei R, Di Marco M, Ricci C, et al. Neoadjuvant chemoradiotherapy and surgery vs surgery alone in resectable pancreatic cancer:a single-center prospective, randomized, controlled trial which failed to achieve accrual targets. J Gastrointest Surg. 2015;19(10):1802–12.
27. Golcher H, Brunner TB, Witzigmann H, et al. Neoadjuvant chemoradiation therapy with gemcitabine/cisplatin and surgery versus immediate surgery in resectable pancreatic cancer: results of the first prospective randomized phase II trial. Strahlenther Onkol. 2015;191(1):7–16.
28. Rahman SH, Urquhart R, Molinari M. Neoadjuvant therapy for resectable pancreatic cancer. World J Gastrointest Oncol. 2017;9(12):457–65.
29. ClinicalTrials.gov [Internet]. Bethesda (MD): National Library of Medicine (US). Identifiers NCT01314027, NCT02047513, NCT02172976, NCT01660711 and NCT01726582. Available from: https://clinicaltrials.gov/
30. Katz MH, et al. Alliance for clinical trials in oncology (ALLIANCE) trial A021501: preoperative extended chemotherapy vs. chemotherapy plus hypofractionated radiation therapy for borderline resectable adenocarcinoma of the head of the pancreas. BMC Cancer. 2017;17:505.
31. Von Hoff DD, Goldstein D, Renschler MF. Albumin-bound paclitaxel plus gemcitabine in pancreatic cancer. N Engl J Med. 2014;370:479–80.
32. Conroy T, Desseigne F, Ychou M, et al. FOLFIRINOX versus gemcitabine for metastatic pancreatic cancer. N Engl J Med. 2011;364:1817–25.
33. Pisters PW, Wolff RA, Janjan NA, et al. Preoperative paclitaxel and concurrent rapid-fractionation radiation for resectable pancreatic adenocarcinoma: toxicities, histologic response rates, and event-free outcome. J Clin Oncol. 2002;20(10):2537–44.
34. Palmer DH, Stocken DD, Hewitt H, et al. A randomized phase 2 trial of neoadjuvant chemotherapy in resectable pancreatic cancer: gemcitabine alone versus gemcitabine combined with cisplatin. Ann Surg Oncol. 2007;14(7):2088–96. Epub 2007 Apr 24.
35. Heinrich S, Pestalozzi BC, Schäfer M, et al. Prospective phase II trial of neoadjuvant chemotherapy with gemcitabine and cisplatin for resectable adenocarcinoma of the pancreatic head. J Clin Oncol. 2008;26(15):2526–31.
36. O'Reilly EM, Perelshteyn A, Jarnagin WR, et al. A single-arm, nonrandomized phase II trial of neoadjuvant gemcitabine and oxaliplatin in patients with resectable pancreas adenocarcinoma. Ann Surg. 2014;260(1):142–8.
37. Van Tienhoven G, Versteijne E, Suker M, Groothuis KBX, Busch OR, Bonsing BA. Preoperative chemoradiotherapy versus immediate surgery for resectable and borderline resectable pancreatic cancer (PREOPANC-1): a randomized, controlled, multicenter phase III trial. J Clin Oncol. 2018;36(18_suppl) https://doi.org/10.1200/JCO.2018.36.18_suppl.LBA4002.
38. Conroy T, Hammel P, Hebbar M, Ben Abdelghani M, Wei AC, Raoul J-L, Choné L, Francois E, Artru P, Biagi JJ, Lecomte T, Assenat E, Faroux R, Ychou M, Volet J, Sauvanet A, Breysacher G, Di Fiore F, Cripps C, Kavan P, Texereau P, Bouhier-Leporrier K, Khemissa-Akouz F, Legoux J-L, Juzyna B, Gourgou S, O'Callaghan CJ, Jouffroy-Zeller C, Rat P, Malka D, Castan F, Bachet J-B. FOLFIRINOX or Gemcitabine as adjuvant therapy for pancreatic cancer. New Eng J Med. 2018;379(25):2395–406.

6 Treatment Sequencing for Borderline Resectable Pancreatic Cancer

Callisia N. Clarke

Introduction

Over 55,000 people will be diagnosed with pancreatic cancer in the United States this year. Traditionally approximately 50% of patients will present with metastatic disease, 20–25% will present with locally advanced disease as determined by tumor involvement of adjacent vascular structures, traditionally considered unresectable, and only 20% will be considered resectable [1]. Patients with unresectable localized pancreatic cancer, when treated with chemotherapy in the setting of good performance status, fair only slightly better than their metastatic counterparts with a median overall survival of up to 16.5 months, compared to 11.1 months [2–4]. Given the continuum of tumor-vasculature interface, it soon became clear that dichotomization of pancreatic patients without metastatic disease into locally advanced and resectable pancreatic cancer was imprecise and excluded patients who could derive benefit from complete resection. A subset of patients with limited vascular involvement responding to neoadjuvant multimodality treatment, as determined by imaging response and a decrease in serum biomarkers, was able to undergo curative pancreatectomy with a high likelihood of achieving a margin-negative (R0) resection and significant oncologic benefit [5, 6]. This new subset of operable patients was termed borderline resectable pancreatic cancer. The distinction between resectable and borderline resectable pancreatic cancer is a critical one, with significant therapeutic and prognostic implications. Patients with borderline resectable are at higher risk of having occult metastatic disease at diagnosis. They may require more complex surgical resections with a need for vascular reconstruction and have a higher rate of margin-positive resection when compared to resectable pancreatic cancer. For these reasons, we believe a period of induction therapy with effective chemotherapy and chemoradiation should be utilized to identify patients who will develop early distant failure, potentially sparing them the morbidity of a noncurative surgery, and to increase the rate of achieving R0 resection due to tumor downsizing and margin sterilization.

Improvements in systemic therapies for pancreatic cancer, in particular, the use of fluorouracil, irinotecan, and oxaliplatin (FOLFIRINOX) and gemcitabine plus nanoparticle albumin-bound paclitaxel, have resulted in improved response rates and survival outcomes across all stages of disease. When used in the neoadjuvant setting, these therapies have dramatically increased the number of patients eligible for surgical resection [3, 4, 7]. For this reason, there is renewed interest in precise clinical staging of localized pancreatic cancer and

C. N. Clarke (✉)
Division of Surgical Oncology, Department of Surgery, The Medical College of Wisconsin, Milwaukee, WI, USA
e-mail: cnclarke@mcw.edu

S. Tsai et al. (eds.), *Management of Localized Pancreatic Cancer*,
https://doi.org/10.1007/978-3-319-98944-0_6

objective early stratification for surgical resectability. In this chapter, we will discuss current clinical staging paradigms and treatment strategies employed in the management of borderline resectable pancreatic cancer with an emphasis on multimodality management and treatment sequencing of local and systemic therapies.

Clinical Staging of Pancreatic Cancer

Helical computed tomography (CT) is the most important and commonly used diagnostic and staging modality in pancreatic cancer. Multidetector-row CT imaging with thin sections and dual-phase contrast (pancreatic and portovenous phases) allows for high-resolution imaging of the primary tumor and its vascular relationship, as well as detection of the lungs, liver, and nodal metastasis [8–10]. Furthermore, advanced image processing, such as volume-rendered, three-dimensional reconstruction, can be used to give additional vascular detail. With high-quality pancreas protocol CT imaging, the correlation between preoperative vascular CT and surgical findings is greater than 90% [11–13]. High-resolution pancreas protocol CT imaging should be obtained prior to any invasive intervention, including biopsy or endoscopic retrograde cholangiopancreatography (ERCP), as these procedures may result in bleeding or inflammation that can obscure tissue planes and impede the ability to determine the relationship of the tumor to critical vasculature and, hence, the accurate clinical stage.

Contemporary pancreatic cancer clinical staging stratifies patients into four categories based on objective CT radiologic determination of disease extent: resectable, borderline resectable, locally advanced, and metastatic (Table 6.1). These classifications simply serve to preopera-

Table 6.1 Classification of resectable, borderline resectable, and locally advanced pancreatic cancer as determined by the Multidisciplinary Pancreatic Cancer Working Group at the Medical College of Wisconsin

		Resectable	Borderline resectable	Locally advanced A	Locally advanced B
Tumor-arterial interface	SMA	None	≤180° abutment	>180° but ≤270° encasement	>270°
	CA	None	≤180° abutment	>180° without extension to aorta with possibility for celiac resection with or without reconstruction	>180° encasement with extension to aorta
	HA	None	Short segment abutment or encasement without extension to CA or HA bifurcation	>180° with extension to CA but not HA bifurcation and amenable to reconstruction	>180° encasement with extension beyond HA bifurcation
Tumor-venous interface	PV-SMV	None	Tumor-induced narrowing >50% of the SMV, PV, or portal confluence with suitable targets above (PV) and below (SMV) for reconstruction	Occlusion of PV/SMV confluence with no targets for reconstruction	
Likely candidate for surgical resection after neoadjuvant therapy		Yes	Yes	Yes	No
Probability of surgical resection after neoadjuvant therapy			63–67% [14, 15]	62% [16]	24% [16]

SMA superior mesenteric artery, *CA* celiac artery, *HA* hepatic artery, *PV* portal vein
Modified from Tsai et al. [17]

tively risk stratification of patients by the likelihood of achieving an R0 (margin-negative) resection at the time of surgery while maintaining critical visceral blood flow. The impact of margin resection in pancreatic cancer is well known. Patients undergoing R0 resection have improved outcomes when compared to patients with R1 (microscopically positive margin) resection with overall survivals of 18–23 months compared to 11–15 months, respectively, in surgery-first cohorts [18–20]. More significantly, patients undergoing R2 resection with gross positive margins have similar outcomes as patients undergoing nonoperative treatment for localized unresectable disease or metastatic disease [18, 20, 21]. For this reason, there is no role for "debulking" in pancreatic cancer, and surgical intervention should only be undertaken with the intent for complete tumor extirpation with regional lymphadenectomy or to palliate symptoms.

As tumor-vascular interface increases, the incidence of margin-negative resection following surgery decreases [22]. While resection of venous involvement/occlusion of the superior mesenteric vein (SMV), portal vein (PV), or portal confluence has been associated with high R0 margin rates and acceptable outcomes [23–25], the same cannot be said for arterial involvement. Unlike veins, the superior mesenteric artery (SMA) and celiac artery are surrounded by a sheath of autonomic neural tissue that is believed to act as a conduit for microscopic tumor extension from the site of the primary tumor along the involved vessel [26]. For this reason, tumors with arterial involvement if not subjected to a pretreatment prior to surgery will often have microscopically positive arterial margins, even away from the gross tumor. As the tumor-artery interface increases from abutment to encasement, the probability of achieving an R0 resection decreases. These clinicopathologic findings and outcomes are central in clinical pancreatic cancer clinical staging and are reflected in the conventional dichotomization to operable (resectable and borderline resectable) and nonoperable (locally advanced and metastatic) pancreatic cancer.

The distinction between borderline resectable and locally advanced disease is also an important one that warrants careful examination of the interface between the tumor and arterial vasculature (SMA, celiac axis, aorta, hepatic arteries) to determine abutment (defined as $\leq 180°$ tumor contact) versus encasement (defined as $>180°$ tumor contact). Additionally, attention must be given to the assessment of tumor-related narrowing or occlusion of the SMV or PV with specific emphasis on a proximal and distal target for reconstruction. At the Medical College of Wisconsin, the borderline resectable disease is limited to tumor abutment at the SMA or celiac axis or short segment encasement of the hepatic artery. Tumor-induced narrowing >50% of the SMV, PV or portal confluence, or occlusion with suitable proximal and distal targets for vascular reconstruction is also defined as borderline resectable (Table 6.1). Locally advanced disease is defined by (1) encasement of the SMA, celiac artery or hepatic artery with extension to the bifurcation or celiac artery, and/or (2) SMV-PV occlusion without an option for venous reconstruction.

In order for borderline resectable pancreatic cancer patients to derive maximal benefit from complex surgical resection, a thoughtful neoadjuvant treatment plan incorporating multimodal sequenced therapies, patient conditioning and selection with the goal of achieving margin-negative resection is paramount. Contemporary studies have shown that with this approach, the majority of borderline resectable patients will undergo curative resection. Katz et al. [6] described their experience with 160 consecutive patients with borderline resectable pancreatic cancer treated at a single high-volume tertiary cancer center over a seven-year period. All patients were treated neoadjuvantly with chemotherapy, chemoradiation, or both. Systemic therapy consisted of single-agent gemcitabine or gemcitabine in combination. Chemotherapy consisted of radiosensitizing doses of 5-fluorouracil (FU), paclitaxel, gemcitabine, or capecitabine given concomitantly with external beam radiation most commonly to 50.4 Gy over 28 fractions. One hundred twenty-five patients (78%) completed neoadjuvant therapy and 66 (41%) proceeded to pancreatectomy with a 94% R0 resection rate. Patients who completed all intended therapy, including pancreatectomy, had a median overall survival of 40 months compared to 13 months in patients who did not undergo resection ($p < 0.001$).

Modern chemotherapy regimens continue to improve rates of resectability in this patient population. Christians et al. [14] describe their early experience in 18 patients with borderline resectable pancreatic cancer treated preoperatively with FOLIFIRINOX followed by gemcitabine- or capecitabine-based chemoradiation. No patient had disease progression on FOLIRINOX at restaging prior to starting chemoradiation. Six patients had progressive disease precluding resection; the remaining 12 (67%) underwent pancreatectomy, with all patients achieving R0 margins and all tumors having a partial pathologic response with >50% nonviable tumor. Ten (83%) patients required vascular (portal vein) resection/reconstruction. Only two (17%) patients were found to have node-positive disease. Median survival was not reached in the pancreatectomy group. At a median follow-up of 22 months, seven (58%) were alive and five (42%) with no evidence of disease. Median survival in patients who progressed precluding resection was 12.5 months.

Treatment Sequencing in Borderline Pancreatic Cancer

In order to maximize survival and clinical outcomes in borderline resectable cancer, a comprehensive treatment plan with consideration of surgical resection in patients with favorable anatomy and good performance status must be made at the time of diagnosis. This approach minimizes suboptimal surgical timing due to prolonged time between chemotherapy and/or chemoradiation, resulting in scarring and fibrosis that may be prohibitive. Initial therapeutic plans are best made in the setting of a multidisciplinary pancreatic cancer conference where input from experienced surgeons, gastroenterologists, medical oncologists, and radiation oncologists is taken into consideration. Additionally, suitability for surgery must be reassessed at each staging evaluation. A total neoadjuvant approach ensures the delivery of all intended therapies in patients undergoing curative pancreatectomy and allows for tumor downsizing and identification of patients with poor tumor biology who develop distant disease or progress locally. These patients are thereby spared the morbidity of a surgery that would offer no survival benefit. In an effort to streamline this assessment and clarify goals of treatment at the time of diagnosis, the Multidisciplinary Pancreatic Cancer Working Group at the author's institution has proposed a neoadjuvant treatment algorithm outlined in Fig. 6.1 based on our experience with borderline resectable pancreatic cancer. Rationales to support each component are detailed below.

Tissue Diagnosis

Multimodal treatment is the cornerstone of management of borderline resectable pancreatic cancer. For this reason, tissue confirmation of malignancy is necessary in order to initiate therapy. Once high-quality cross-sectional imaging has been obtained to determine clinical staging, a biopsy should be performed. Endoscopic ultrasonography (EUS) is often performed in conjunction with endoscopic retrograde cholangiopancreatography (ERCP). In addition to facilitating tissue biopsies, EUS gives additional information regarding the tumor relationship to surrounding vessels and regional nodal status, while ERCP allows for therapeutic stenting of the common bile duct if obstructed [27]. This approach mitigates the potential risk of peritoneal seeding associated with CT-guided biopsies.

Serum Tumor Markers

In addition to routine laboratory studies, serum carbohydrate antigen (CA19-9) can be informative in most patients with pancreatic cancer and

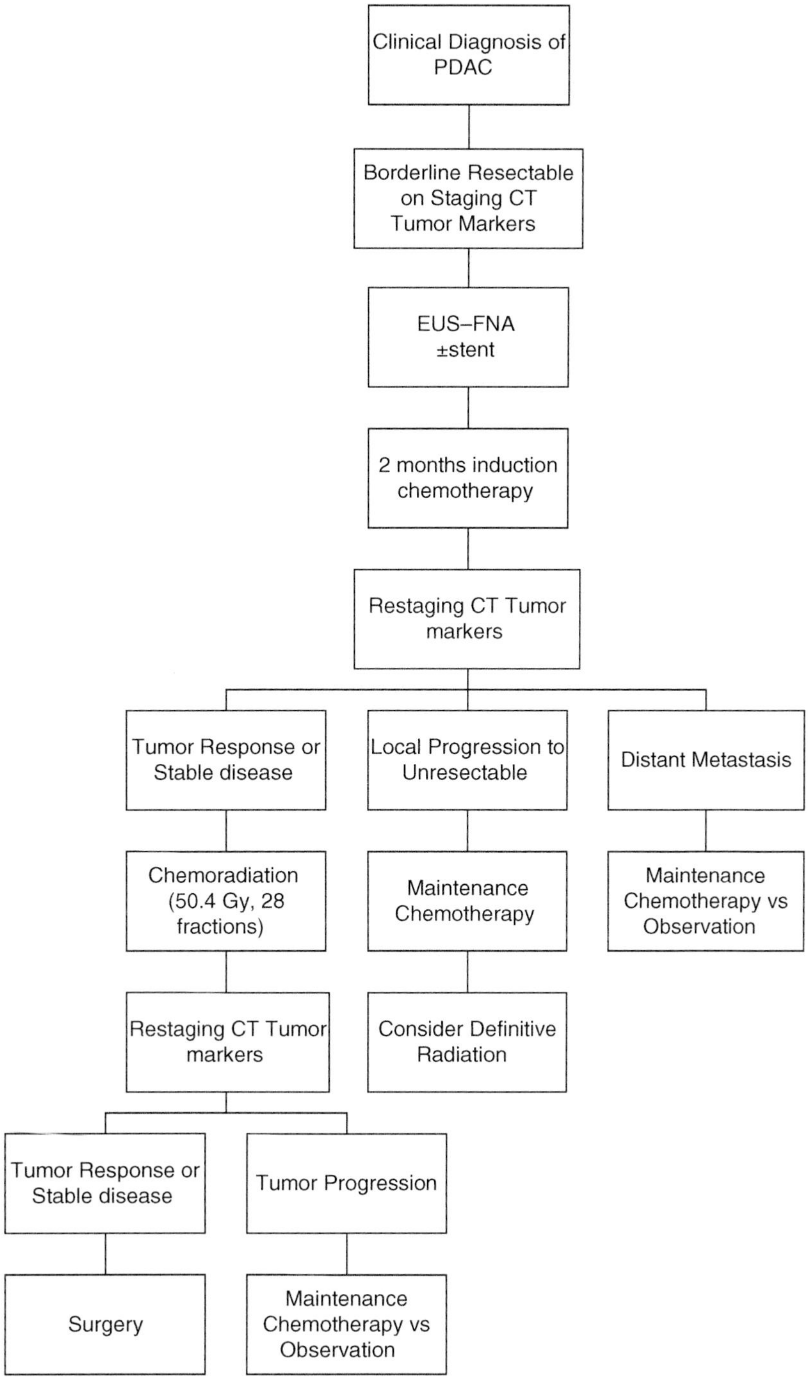

Fig. 6.1 Proposed neoadjuvant treatment sequencing for patients with borderline resectable pancreatic cancer. These patients have a reasonable likelihood of proceeding to curative resection after neoadjuvant therapy. Treatment response is reassessed at each restaging by change in primary tumor radiographic size, serum cancer antigen 19-9 levels, and patient functional status. Surgical resection is offered only to patients with excellent tumor response after receipt of all intended neoadjuvant therapy and with favorable tumor-vasculature anatomy

should be measured prior to initiation of therapy once serum bilirubin has normalized. CA 19-9 is the most widely studied and validated biomarker in pancreatic cancer . While its utility as a screening test is limited due to tissue nonspecificity, elevated CA 19-9 in the setting of a known diagnosis of pancreatic cancer confers valuable information regarding overall disease burden, the potential for R0 resection, response to therapy, and overall survival [28]. Approximately 10% of the patients lack the enzyme required to produce the antigen so that a normal CA 19-9 in the setting of pancreatic cancer can be frequently encountered and offers no additional information. In patients that produce CA 19-9, serum levels can be trended to assess tumor response, especially since the radiographic response is often limited even with highly effective systemic treatments. Following neoadjuvant therapy, a decrease or normalization of CA 19-9 is associated with an increased rate of complete surgical resection and improved overall survival [29]. Additionally, after curative resection, normalization of CA19-9 (<37 U/ml) is associated with improved overall survival [30], while sustained elevations of CA 19-9 are associated with tumor recurrence that often precedes clinical or radiographic evidence by up to 6 months [30–33]. Therefore, it is now widely accepted that immediate or delayed postoperative elevations in CA 19-9 represent persistent disease or tumor recurrence and portend unfavorable outcomes.

Systemic Chemotherapy

Borderline resectable cancer is associated with a high incidence of micrometastatic disease at diagnosis. Given this, systemic chemotherapy is an integral component in the treatment of the disease, and in the multimodality therapy plan, induction chemotherapy is given precedence.

Contemporary chemotherapeutic regimens have significantly improved prognosis in advanced pancreatic cancer with the median survival in unresectable patients approaching 1 year [3]. Combination therapy with 5-FU/leucovorin, oxaliplatin, and irinotecan (FOLFIRINOX) was studied in phase III clinical trial of advanced pancreatic cancer by Conroy et al. [3]. Patients treated on the FOLFIRINOX arm had improved overall survival (OS) (11.1 months vs. 6.8 months, $p < 0.001$) and improved progression-free survival (PFS) (6.4 months vs. 3.3 months, $p < 0.001$) compared to gemcitabine alone.

Nanoparticle albumin-bound (nab)-paclitaxel was developed to increase the solubility and pharmacokinetics of paclitaxel. Von Hoff et al. [4] investigated the clinical efficacy of gemcitabine in combination with nab-paclitaxel in the Metastatic Pancreatic Adenocarcinoma Clinical Trial (MPACT). Combination therapy was associated with improved OS (8.5 months vs. 6.7 months $p < 0.001$), PFS (5.5 months vs. 3.7 months, $p < 0.001$), and response rates (23% vs. 7%, $p < 0.001$). Both of these regimens have been adapted to use in the neoadjuvant therapy for borderline resectable pancreatic cancer.

Chemoradiation

The role of chemoradiation in pancreatic cancer was first investigated in the adjuvant setting to address to the high risk of locoregional recurrence, ranging from 20 to 60% even after R0 pancreatectomy [34–37]. However, subsequent European studies have failed to reproduce these findings, concluding that adjuvant chemoradiation provided no survival benefit and, on the contrary, caused significant harm fueling debate and primarily excluding its use as standard therapy in Europe [38, 39]. While adjuvant chemoradiation has still not been universally adopted, expert consensus agrees that a subset of resected patients with a high risk for locoregional disease recurrence is likely to benefit from the addition of chemoradiation [40].

The benefits of chemoradiation in the neoadjuvant setting prior to pancreatectomy for borderline resectable, however, are slightly less controversial. In the case of borderline resectable pancreatic cancer, the primary goal of chemoradiation is, as an adjunct to systemic chemotherapy, to induce tumor reduction and increase the rate of margin-negative resection in patients proceeding to surgery.

As tumor-vascular interface increases so does the rate of margin-positive resection. The addition of conventional preoperative chemoradiation (typically 50.4 Gy over 28 fractions) has been shown to increase the rate of R0 resection and improve survival in patients with borderline resectable and locally advanced pancreatic cancer [6, 15, 16, 41, 42]. Neoadjuvant chemoradiation is also associated with sterilization of regional lymph nodes with a 73% pathologic node negative (pN0) rate compared to 14% in upfront surgery patients ($p < 0.001$) with a benefit in survival seen in pN0 [41]. Conventional chemoradiation alone has not been associated with significant tumor reduction; however, when used in sequence with effective chemotherapy regimens such as FOLFIRINOX, approximately one-third of patients with unresectable locally advanced pancreatic cancer can be downstaged to resectable, with an associated increase in median overall survival of 10–15 months [7, 43, 44].

Recently, there has been significant interest in treatment abbreviation and the exploration of stereotactic body radiation therapy (SBRT) in this patient cohort. SBRT administers higher doses of radiation per fraction over a shorter period of time. The use of SBRT in the neoadjuvant treatment of localized pancreatic cancer appears to result in comparable local control and margin-negative resection rates as conventional fractionation [45–47]. Rajagopalan et al. [47] applied SBRT in 12 patients with borderline resectable and locally advanced pancreatic cancer, 11 of whom also received prior induction chemotherapy. Seven patients received 36 Gy over three fractions, while five patients received single-fraction radiation therapy to 24 Gy with a median time to surgery of 3.3 months. Eleven patients (92%) achieved R0 resection with three patients (25%) having a complete pathology response and two patients (17%) having <10% tumor viability [47]. The median progression-free survival was 27.4 months with 92% survival at 1 year and 51% at 3 years. Similarly, Chuong et al. [45] reported high rates of local control in borderline resectable and locally advanced pancreatic cancer after SBRT. Seventy-three patients received radiation to 35 Gy at the tumor-vascular interface and 25 Gy to remainder of the tumor over five consecutive fractions. Thirty-two patients underwent curative pancreatectomy with 97% R0 margin resection with a median OS of 19.3 months and a local control rate at 1 year of 81% in locally advanced unresected disease [45]. The rate of node sterilization, however, was lower than reported in conventional fractionation studies with only 20 patients (65%) having pN0 disease. While SBRT is well tolerated in the acute setting, concern for delayed complications associated with SBRT has hampered its widespread adoption. In particular, high rates of gastrointestinal toxicity, postoperative wound complications, and vascular injuries have been reported with at least one resulting death in these small studies [45, 47]. Clinical trials are ongoing to further characterize these toxicities and refine the ideal fractionation in preoperative pancreatic cancer therapy.

Curative Pancreatectomy

The surgeries required to facilitate complete tumor removal in patients with borderline pancreatic cancer carry a significant risk of morbidity and mortality because of the potential need for complex vascular resection and reconstruction. These risks are considerably lower at high-volume pancreatectomy centers presumably due to surgeon expertise as well as institutional resources for "rescue" in the setting of complications [48]. The median age at diagnosis of pancreatic cancer is 70 years [1]; as such, these procedures are often performed in older patients at high risk for deconditioning after heavy pre-treatment. These facts support the need for multidisciplinary patient management with surgical evaluation at each phase of multimodal treatment, at a minimum: (1) at/near diagnosis, (2) at the end of induction chemotherapy, and (3) at the end of chemoradiation. Frequent patient assessment of surgical suitability allows for early identification and intervention of potentially reversible functional loss or sarcopenia, which may render patients unresectable. At the author's institution, surgical resectability of localized disease after multimodal neoadjuvant therapy is based on maintenance of good performance status, improved or stable imaging findings with anatomy favoring R0 resection, and decrease or normalization of serum biomarkers when informative [49]. At many high-volume pancreatic surgery centers, providers have taken advantage of the lengthy period of induction therapy to implement Enhanced Recovery After

Surgery (ERAS) protocols with preoperative or "prehabilitation" interventions aimed at patient education, nutritional optimization, and physical conditioning prior to pancreatectomy. The Enhanced Recovery After Surgery (ERAS®) Society summarized their evidence-based guidelines for perioperative care of patients undergoing pancreaticoduodenectomy, to attenuate loss of function preoperatively and minimize postoperative morbidity [50]. Adaptation of ERAS protocols for patients undergoing pancreatectomy has demonstrated safety without compromising oncologic surgical outcomes in a variety of studies and has been associated with decreased hospital length of stay and postoperative morbidity [51, 52].

Preoperative planning for borderline resectable pancreatic cancer, with special attention to vascular anatomy and tumor-vessel encasement, is critical to good oncologic outcomes, low morbidity and mortality. Unanticipated need for vascular resection may result in vascular injury, major blood loss, or death. High-quality preoperative CT imaging with three-dimensional vascular reconstructions can be particularly helpful when creating a detailed operative plan for vascular resection and reconstruction. A significant portion of borderline resectable patients (10–13%) will have distant metastasis not detected by cross-sectional imaging at the time of surgery, and so diagnostic laparoscopy should precede open exploration in this high-risk patient population [7, 16].

Venous Resection and Reconstruction

There is growing experience with PV and SMV resection/reconstruction in borderline pancreatic cancer. The involved occluded PV-SMV confluence may be resected provided that adequate inflow and outflow targets for reconstruction are present and R0 resection is anticipated. Prior to resection and reconstruction, the venous anatomy must be clearly understood. The SMV arises from the convergence of the jejunal and ileal first-order branches that carry blood away from the proximal and distal small bowel, respectively. The first jejunal branch courses behind the SMA to enter the SMV posterolaterally, while the ileal branch travels along the midline in the mesenteric root. The SMV and splenic vein (SV) coalesce to form the PV, which runs posterior to the pancreatic neck. The inferior mesenteric vein (IMV) typically drains into the SV but may also drain directly into the SMV just inferior to or at the SMV-CV confluence [53]. Given the variation in patient anatomy, resection of the PV-SMV confluence in the setting of locally advanced pancreatic cancer must be well planned and individualized. If the IMV drains into the splenic vein, then the splenic vein can be ligated with impunity at the PV-SMV confluence as the IMV provides sufficient collateral drainage from the spleen into the systemic venous circulation. If the IMV drains into the SMV or at the confluence, then division of the SV leaves only the short gastric veins of the stomach to decompress the spleen. This leads to sinistral hypertension that may later manifest as upper gastrointestinal bleeding. With this venous anatomy, we recommend performing an end-to-side splenorenal shunt [54]. Christians et al. [54] described their initial experience with temporary mesocaval shunting to facilitate safe portal dissection in patients with cavernous transformation of the PV due to tumor occlusion. Interestingly, this technique also nicely exposes the SMA and root of mesentery and has since been expanded to locally advanced patients with PV/SMV occlusion as well as SMA involvement to ease arterial dissection [54, 55].

Arterial Resection and Reconstruction

Early studies of arterial resection for pancreatic cancer demonstrated high morbidity and poor survival outcomes related to incomplete resection and lack of effective systemic therapies [56]. However, advances in multimodal therapy, surgical techniques, and more effective systemic chemotherapeutics have renewed interest in identifying select patients who may benefit from pancreatectomy with arterial resection. Christians et al. [55] demonstrated safe and effective arterial resection with pancreatectomy in a small cohort of patients after extensive multimodal therapy. In this study, 13 locally advanced patients underwent curative pancreatectomy (10 with arterial resection) with 85% margin-negative rate, with acceptable morbidity (20%) and no perioperative deaths [55]. At a median follow-up of 21 months, eight patients (62%) were alive with no evidence of disease, and the median time to development of recurrent (in all five cases metastatic) disease was 33 months. Subsequent larger studies have demonstrated similar outcomes and survival benefit in well-selected locally advanced pancreatic cancer patients undergoing pancreatectomy with arterial resection after extensive neoadjuvant treatment at high-volume pancreas surgery centers [7, 16]. A central tenet in each of these studies is that the intent to treat surgically was determined at diagnosis and reassessed at multiple time points through neoadjuvant therapy.

Assessing tumor-vessel interface sterilization after neoadjuvant therapy can be challenging and further complicates the preoperative planning in localized tumors. Ferrone et al. [7] critically identified discordance between CT imaging findings and pathologic findings after neoadjuvant therapy in patients with borderline resectable and locally advanced pancreatic cancer. Their group noted that even in patients with a good serologic response as evidenced by decreased CA19-9, there was rarely corresponding separation of the tumor from critical vessels on restaging CT imaging after neoadjuvant therapy in patients receiving either FOLFIRINOX or FOLFIRINOX plus chemoradiation. However, intraoperative pathologic assessment of the tumor-vascular interface was most likely to demonstrate fibrosis with no viable cells. For this reason, Ferrone et al. [7] advocate exploration with attempted resection in patients with localized pancreatic cancer, even with persistent imaging evidence of arterial vascular involvement after neoadjuvant FOLFIRINOX-based therapy with intraoperative pathologic assessment. They support proceeding with pancreatectomy in patients with no viable tumor at the vessel interface and aborting the procedure if the arterial perivascular tissue is positive for malignancy. While we agree these findings are provocative, at the author's institution we do not advocate surgical exploration after neoadjuvant therapy without clear intent for curative resection with planned vascular resection as needed. We believe the risks of vascular complication, delay in reinitiation of systemic therapy, and the unmeasurable effect on tumor immunology from a negative laparotomy are too high to justify this approach.

Conclusions

Effective systemic chemotherapy and multimodality treatment strategies have increased the proportion of borderline resectable pancreatic cancer patients undergoing curative pancreatectomy with a significant survival benefit. Clinical staging should be aimed at the identification of these patients at diagnosis in order to facilitate ideal multimodal therapy. Early surgical consideration based on clinical staging and thoughtful neoadjuvant treatment sequencing results in optimal surgical outcomes and survival benefits. Complete surgical resection may mandate complex vascular resection and reconstruction and should only be undertaken at high-volume pancreas surgery centers to mitigate the associated morbidity and mortality.

References

1. NooneAM, Howlader N, Krapcho M, Miller D, Brest A, Yu M, Ruhl J, Tatalovich Z, Mariotto A, Lewis DR, Chen HS, Feuer EJ, Cronin KA,editors. SEER cancer statistics review, 1975–2015. Bethesda: National Cancer Institute; 2018.https://seer.cancer.gov/csr/1975_2015/, based on November 2017 SEER data submission, posted to the SEER website, April 2018. Accessed 2 May 2018.
2. Hammel P, et al. Effect of chemoradiotherapy vs chemotherapy on survival in patients with locally advanced pancreatic cancer controlled after 4 months of gemcitabine with or without erlotinib: the LAP07 randomized clinical trial. JAMA. 2016;315(17):1844–53.
3. Conroy T, et al. FOLFIRINOX versus gemcitabine for metastatic pancreatic cancer. N Engl J Med. 2011;364(19):1817–25.
4. Von Hoff DD, et al. Increased survival in pancreatic cancer with nab-paclitaxel plus gemcitabine. N Engl J Med. 2013;369(18):1691–703.
5. Varadhachary GR, et al. Borderline resectable pancreatic cancer. Curr Treat Options Gastroenterol. 2005;8(5):377–84.
6. Katz MH, et al. Borderline resectable pancreatic cancer: the importance of this emerging stage of disease.

J Am Coll Surg. 2008;206(5):833–46; discussion 846–8.
7. Ferrone CR, et al. Radiological and surgical implications of neoadjuvant treatment with FOLFIRINOX for locally advanced and borderline resectable pancreatic cancer. Ann Surg. 2015;261(1):12–7.
8. Brennan DD, et al. Comprehensive preoperative assessment of pancreatic adenocarcinoma with 64-section volumetric CT. Radiographics. 2007;27(6):1653–66.
9. Balachandran A, et al. Imaging of pancreatic neoplasms. Surg Oncol Clin N Am. 2014;23(4):751–88.
10. Lee ES, Lee JM. Imaging diagnosis of pancreatic cancer: a state-of-the-art review. World J Gastroenterol. 2014;20(24):7864–77.
11. Lee JK, et al. Prediction of vascular involvement and resectability by multidetector-row CT versus MR imaging with MR angiography in patients who underwent surgery for resection of pancreatic ductal adenocarcinoma. Eur J Radiol. 2010;73(2):310–6.
12. Lu DS, et al. Local staging of pancreatic cancer: criteria for unresectability of major vessels as revealed by pancreatic-phase, thin-section helical CT. AJR Am J Roentgenol. 1997;168(6):1439–43.
13. Tamm EP, et al. Staging of pancreatic cancer with multidetector CT in the setting of preoperative chemoradiation therapy. Abdom Imaging. 2006;31(5):568–74.
14. Christians KK, et al. Neoadjuvant FOLFIRINOX for borderline resectable pancreas cancer: a new treatment paradigm? Oncologist. 2014;19(3):266–74.
15. Kharofa J, et al. Neoadjuvant chemoradiation with IMRT in resectable and borderline resectable pancreatic cancer. Radiother Oncol. 2014;113(1):41–6.
16. Chatzizacharias NA, et al. Locally advanced pancreas cancer: staging and goals of therapy. Surgery. 2018;163:1053.
17. Tsai S, et al. Multimodality therapy in patients with borderline resectable or locally advanced pancreatic cancer: importance of locoregional therapies for a systemic disease. J Oncol Pract. 2016;12(10):915–23.
18. Winter JM, et al. 1423 pancreaticoduodenectomies for pancreatic cancer: a single-institution experience. J Gastrointest Surg. 2006;10(9):1199–210; discussion 1210–1.
19. Fatima J, et al. Pancreatoduodenectomy for ductal adenocarcinoma: implications of positive margin on survival. Arch Surg. 2010;145(2):167–72.
20. Neoptolemos JP, et al. Influence of resection margins on survival for patients with pancreatic cancer treated by adjuvant chemoradiation and/or chemotherapy in the ESPAC-1 randomized controlled trial. Ann Surg. 2001;234(6):758–68.
21. Bilimoria KY, et al. Effect of hospital volume on margin status after pancreaticoduodenectomy for cancer. J Am Coll Surg. 2008;207(4):510–9.
22. Katz MH, et al. Borderline resectable pancreatic cancer: need for standardization and methods for optimal clinical trial design. Ann Surg Oncol. 2013;20(8):2787–95.
23. Tran Cao HS, et al. Radiographic tumor-vein interface as a predictor of intraoperative, pathologic, and oncologic outcomes in resectable and borderline resectable pancreatic cancer. J Gastrointest Surg. 2014;18(2):269–78; discussion 278.
24. Leach SD, et al. Survival following pancreaticoduodenectomy with resection of the superior mesenteric-portal vein confluence for adenocarcinoma of the pancreatic head. Br J Surg. 1998;85(5):611–7.
25. Tseng JF, et al. Pancreaticoduodenectomy with vascular resection: margin status and survival duration. J Gastrointest Surg. 2004;8(8):935–49; discussion 949–50.
26. Nagakawa T, et al. Patterns of neural and plexus invasion of human pancreatic cancer and experimental cancer. Int J Pancreatol. 1991;10(2):113–9.
27. Brugge WR, Van Dam J. Pancreatic and biliary endoscopy. N Engl J Med. 1999;341(24):1808–16.
28. Ballehaninna UK, Chamberlain RS. The clinical utility of serum CA 19-9 in the diagnosis, prognosis and management of pancreatic adenocarcinoma: an evidence based appraisal. J Gastrointest Oncol. 2012;3(2):105–19.
29. Aldakkak M, Christians KK, Krepline AN, George B, Ritch PS, Erickson BA, Johnston FM, Evans DB, Tsai S. Pre-treatment carbohydrate antigen 19-9 does not predict the response to neoadjuvant therapy in patients with localized pancreatic cancer. HPB. 2015;17(10):942–52. https://doi.org/10.1111/hpb.12448.
30. Tian F, et al. Prognostic value of serum CA 19-9 levels in pancreatic adenocarcinoma. Ann Surg. 1992;215(4):350–5.
31. Hernandez JM, et al. CA 19-9 velocity predicts disease-free survival and overall survival after pancreatectomy of curative intent. J Gastrointest Surg. 2009;13(2):349–53.
32. Hata S, et al. Prognostic impact of postoperative serum CA 19-9 levels in patients with resectable pancreatic cancer. Ann Surg Oncol. 2012;19(2):636–41.
33. Montgomery RC, et al. Prediction of recurrence and survival by post-resection CA 19-9 values in patients with adenocarcinoma of the pancreas. Ann Surg Oncol. 1997;4(7):551–6.
34. Khawaja MR, et al. Adjuvant gemcitabine and gemcitabine-based chemoradiotherapy versus gemcitabine alone after pancreatic cancer resection: the Indiana University experience. Am J Clin Oncol. 2017;40(1):42–6.
35. Sohn TA, et al. Resected adenocarcinoma of the pancreas-616 patients: results, outcomes, and prognostic indicators. J Gastrointest Surg. 2000;4(6):567–79.
36. Hishinuma S, et al. Patterns of recurrence after curative resection of pancreatic cancer, based on autopsy findings. J Gastrointest Surg. 2006;10(4):511–8.
37. Smeenk HG, et al. Long-term survival and metastatic pattern of pancreatic and periampullary cancer after adjuvant chemoradiation or observation: long-term results of EORTC trial 40891. Ann Surg. 2007;246(5):734–40.

38. Klinkenbijl JH, et al. Adjuvant radiotherapy and 5-fluorouracil after curative resection of cancer of the pancreas and periampullary region: phase III trial of the EORTC gastrointestinal tract cancer cooperative group. Ann Surg. 1999;230(6):776–82; discussion 782–4.
39. Neoptolemos JP, et al. A randomized trial of chemoradiotherapy and chemotherapy after resection of pancreatic cancer. N Engl J Med. 2004;350(12):1200–10.
40. Abrams RA, et al. Combined modality treatment of resectable and borderline resectable pancreas cancer: expert consensus statement. Ann Surg Oncol. 2009;16(7):1751–6.
41. Chun YS, et al. Defining venous involvement in borderline resectable pancreatic cancer. Ann Surg Oncol. 2010;17(11):2832–8.
42. Takahashi H, et al. Preoperative chemoradiation reduces the risk of pancreatic fistula after distal pancreatectomy for pancreatic adenocarcinoma. Surgery. 2011;150(3):547–56.
43. Sadot E, et al. FOLFIRINOX induction therapy for stage 3 pancreatic adenocarcinoma. Ann Surg Oncol. 2015;22(11):3512–21.
44. Gillen S, et al. Preoperative/neoadjuvant therapy in pancreatic cancer: a systematic review and meta-analysis of response and resection percentages. PLoS Med. 2010;7(4):e1000267.
45. Chuong MD, et al. Stereotactic body radiation therapy for locally advanced and borderline resectable pancreatic cancer is effective and well tolerated. Int J Radiat Oncol Biol Phys. 2013;86(3):516–22.
46. Mahadevan A, et al. Stereotactic body radiotherapy and gemcitabine for locally advanced pancreatic cancer. Int J Radiat Oncol Biol Phys. 2010;78(3):735–42.
47. Rajagopalan MS, et al. Pathologic response with neoadjuvant chemotherapy and stereotactic body radiotherapy for borderline resectable and locally-advanced pancreatic cancer. Radiat Oncol. 2013;8:254.
48. Finks JF, Osborne NH, Birkmeyer JD. Trends in hospital volume and operative mortality for high-risk surgery. N Engl J Med. 2011;364(22):2128–37.
49. Evans DB, George B, Tsai S. Non-metastatic pancreatic cancer: resectable, borderline resectable, and locally advanced-definitions of increasing importance for the optimal delivery of multimodality therapy. Ann Surg Oncol. 2015;22(11):3409–13.
50. Lassen K, et al. Guidelines for perioperative care for pancreaticoduodenectomy: Enhanced Recovery After Surgery (ERAS(R)) Society recommendations. World J Surg. 2013;37(2):240–58.
51. Takagi K, et al. Effect of an enhanced recovery after surgery protocol in patients undergoing pancreaticoduodenectomy: a randomized controlled trial. Clin Nutr. 2019;38:174–81.
52. Xiong J, et al. Enhanced recovery after surgery program in patients undergoing pancreaticoduodenectomy: a PRISMA-compliant systematic review and meta-analysis. Medicine (Baltimore). 2016;95(18):e3497.
53. Katz MH, et al. Anatomy of the superior mesenteric vein with special reference to the surgical management of first-order branch involvement at pancreaticoduodenectomy. Ann Surg. 2008;248(6):1098–102.
54. Pilgrim CH, et al. Mesocaval shunting: a novel technique to facilitate venous resection and reconstruction and enhance exposure of the superior mesenteric and celiac arteries during pancreaticoduodenectomy. J Am Coll Surg. 2013;217(3):e17–20.
55. Christians KK, et al. Arterial resection at the time of pancreatectomy for cancer. Surgery. 2014;155(5):919–26.
56. Fortner JG. Regional resection of cancer of the pancreas: a new surgical approach. Surgery. 1973;73(2):307–20.

Delivery of Neoadjuvant Versus Adjuvant Therapy in Localized Pancreatic Cancer

7

Ben George and Paul S. Ritch

Introduction

Cancer of the exocrine pancreas is a highly lethal malignancy. Approximately 53,670 people develop exocrine pancreatic cancer each year in the United States, and almost all are expected to die from the disease [1]. Worldwide, pancreatic cancer is the eighth leading cause of cancer deaths in men (138,100 deaths annually) and the ninth in women (127,900 deaths annually) [2]. It is the third leading cause of cancer-related death in the United States after recently eclipsing breast cancer-related mortality and is expected to become the second leading cause of cancer-related mortality in the United States in the next decade, second only to lung cancer [1].

More than 90% of these tumors are adenocarcinomas arising from the ductal epithelium. This chapter will be dealing exclusively with adenocarcinoma of the exocrine pancreas and will use the terms pancreatic cancer (PC) and pancreatic ductal adenocarcinoma (PDAC) interchangeably. Surgical resection is the only potentially curative treatment. Unfortunately, because of the late presentation, only 15–20% of patients are candidates for pancreatectomy. Prognosis is poor, even after a complete resection; 5-year survival after margin-negative (R0) pancreaticoduodenectomy is approximately 30% for node-negative and 10% for node-positive disease [3].

B. George
Pancreatic Cancer Program, Division of Hematology and Oncology, Department of Medicine, Phase 1 Clinical Trials Program, Froedtert and Medical College of Wisconsin, Milwaukee, WI, USA

P. S. Ritch (✉)
Pancreatic Cancer Program, Division of Hematology and Oncology, Department of Medicine, Froedtert and Medical College of Wisconsin, Clinical Cancer Center, Milwaukee, WI, USA
e-mail: pritch@mcw.edu

Pancreatic Ductal Adenocarcinoma Staging

Accurate staging is important because it impacts both prognostication and clinical decision-making. Staging for PDAC can be both pathologic and clinical. The pathologic staging system is applied to patients who undergo a surgery-first approach, while the clinical staging system, based on computed tomography (CT) scan/magnetic resonance imaging (MRI) and/or endoscopic ultrasound (EUS), is applied to patients who are evaluated for neoadjuvant therapy.

The preferred pathologic staging system for PDAC is the tumor, node, and metastasis (TNM) system of the combined American Joint Committee on Cancer (AJCC)/Union for International Cancer Control (UICC) [4]. The pathologic staging system in PDAC evolved due to the importance of surgical resection in curative intent treatment of this disease. However, with

S. Tsai et al. (eds.), *Management of Localized Pancreatic Cancer*,
https://doi.org/10.1007/978-3-319-98944-0_7

the recognition that PDAC is a systemic disease and surgery for localized PDAC is necessary but not sufficient for cure, multimodality therapy (chemotherapy, chemoradiation, and surgery) has assumed an increasingly important role in the management of this disease. Effective utilization and sequencing of multimodality therapy in the contemporary management of localized PDAC require a robust and reliable clinical staging system. Clinical staging classifies PDAC into resectable, borderline resectable, locally advanced, and metastatic disease. Patients with resectable and borderline resectable disease are considered operable, whereas patients with locally advanced and metastatic disease are largely considered inoperable [5, 6]. Throughout this chapter, we will be referencing both clinical and pathologic staging based on the context in which multimodality therapy is discussed (neoadjuvant versus adjuvant therapy).

Adjuvant Therapy for Resected Pancreatic Cancer

The goal of adjuvant therapy in PDAC is to eliminate microscopic (occult) disease and thus potentially facilitate a cure. Multimodality therapy – chemotherapy, concurrent chemoradiation or a combination of the two – has been utilized to minimize both systemic and local relapse. The chemotherapy regimen of choice, the optimal radiotherapy dose and fractionation schedules, as well radiosensitizing chemotherapy continue to evolve. The contemporary adjuvant therapy strategies that have been employed over the past few decades are summarized below.

Adjuvant Chemotherapy

The practice defining randomized phase III adjuvant chemotherapy trials have been summarized in Table 7.1.

ESPAC-1 The European Study for Pancreatic Cancer (ESPAC)-1 trial initially randomized patients to a 2×2 factorial design to ascertain the benefit of adjuvant chemotherapy, chemoradiotherapy, or chemoradiotherapy followed by chemotherapy compared with observation alone. Fear of poor accrual led to a modification in trial design where clinicians were allowed to choose from three randomization schemes – (i) adjuvant chemoradiotherapy versus no chemoradiotherapy, (ii) adjuvant chemotherapy versus no chemotherapy, and (iii) a 2×2 factorial design trial with four groups: chemoradiotherapy, chemotherapy, both, or observation. The primary endpoint was overall survival (OS), and results were published separately [7, 8]. In the initial report of the pooled analysis, there was a significant survival benefit for adjuvant chemotherapy alone when the patients ($N = 238$) who received it were compared with the patients ($N = 235$) who did not (19.7 months versus 14 months; HR 0.66; 95% CI 0.52–0.83; $p = 0.005$). Analysis of the ESPAC-1 results was criticized due to concerns about selection biases compromising the validity of the results since (i) patients and clinicians were allowed to select which trial to enter; (ii) comparisons of treatment groups were pooled together by treatment actually received, rather than "intent-to-treat" analysis; and (iii) clinicians were allowed, according to their own preferences, to deliver "background" chemoradiation or chemotherapy in addition to protocol-directed therapy.

CONKO-001 The multinational European Charité Onkologie (CONKO)-001 trial randomized 368 patients with grossly complete (R0 or R1) surgical resection and a preoperative carbohydrate antigen 19–9 (CA 19–9) level < 2.5 times the upper limit of normal to gemcitabine (1000 mg/m^2 days 1, 8, and 15 every 4 weeks for 6 months) or observation after surgery [9]. The primary endpoint was disease-free survival (DFS). Patients were stratified by surgical margin status (R1–17%) tumor (T) stage and nodal (N1–74%) status. Patients who received adjuvant gemcitabine had a statistically significant improvement in both DFS (13.4 months vs. 6.7 months, HR 0.55; 95% CI 0.44–0.69; $p < 0.001$) and OS (22.8 months vs. 20.2 months;

Table 7.1 Selected adjuvant chemotherapy trials

Trial	Number of patients	Primary endpoint	Randomization	R0 status (%)	Node positive (%)	Local recurrence rate (%)	DFS (months)	OS (months)
ESPAC-1	473	OS	Bolus 5-FU vs. observation	81%	53%	–	–	19.7 vs. 14.0 (HR 0.66; 95% CI 0.52–0.83; $p = 0.005$)
CONKO-001	368	DFS	Gemcitabine vs. observation	82.3%	74.4%	34% vs. 41%	13.4 vs. 6.7 (HR 0.55; 95% CI 0.44–0.69; $p < 0.001$)	22.8 vs. 20.2 (HR 0.76; 95% CI 0.61–0.95; $p = 0.01$)
JSAP-02	119	OS	Gemcitabine vs. observation	84%	69%	23% vs. 32%	11.4 vs. 5.0 (HR 0.6; 95% CI 0.40–0.89; $p = 0.01$)	22.3 vs. 18.4 (HR 0.77; 95% CI 0.51–1.14; $p = 0.19$)
ESPAC-3	1088	OS	Gemcitabine vs. bolus 5-FU/LV	65%	72%	–	14.3 vs. 14.1 (HR 0.96; 95% CI 0.84–1.10; $p = 0.53$)	23.6 vs. 23.0 (HR 0.94; 95% CI 0.81–1.08; $p = 0.39$)
ESPAC-4	732	OS	Gemcitabine + capecitabine vs. gemcitabine	40%	80%	46% vs. 53%	–	28.0 vs. 25.5 (HR 0.82; 95% CI 0.68–0.98; $p = 0.032$)
PRODIGE-24	493	DFS	Modified-FOLFIRINOX vs. gemcitabine	57.2%	76.5%	–	21.6 vs. 12.8 (HR 0.58; 95% CI 0.46–0.73, $P < 0.001$)	54.4 vs. 35.0 (HR 0.64; 95% CI 0.48–0.86; $p = 0.003$)
APACT	866	DFS	Nab-paclitaxel + gemcitabine vs. gemcitabine	76%	72%	–	19.4 vs. 18.8 (HR 0.88; 95% CI 0.729–1.063; $p = 0.1824$)	40.5 vs. 36.2 (HR 0.82; 95% CI 0.680–0.996; $p = 0.045$)

HR 0.76; 95% CI 0.61–0.95; $p = 0.01$). Final updated long-term results of the CONKO-001 trial demonstrated that adjuvant treatment with gemcitabine for 6 months in patients with R0/R1 resection of pancreatic ductal adenocarcinoma leads to a 24% improvement in overall survival, with a statistically significant 10.3% improvement in the absolute 5-year OS (20.7% vs. 10.4%) and a 4.5% improvement in the 10-year OS (12.2% vs. 7.7%), compared with observation alone [10].

JSAP-02 *This multicenter* phase III Japanese trial randomized patients who underwent macroscopically curative resection of invasive ductal carcinoma of the pancreas to adjuvant chemotherapy with gemcitabine (1000 mg/m^2 days 1, 8, and 15 for 3 months only) or observation [11]. The primary endpoint was OS. Patients were stratified by resection status (R0 versus R1), pathological stage (I–II versus III–IV), and enrollment center; a total of 119 patients were enrolled. Patients who received adjuvant gemcitabine experienced a significant improvement in median DFS (11.4 months vs. 5 months; HR 0.6; 95% CI 0.40–0.89; $p = 0.01$), but the difference in OS (22.3 months vs. 18.4 months; HR 0.77; 95% CI 0.51–1.14; $p = 0.19$) was not statistically significant.

ESPAC-3 The multicenter European Study for Pancreatic Cancer (ESPAC)-3 trial randomly allocated 1088 patients with resected exocrine pancreatic cancer to 6 months of postoperative adjuvant treatment with either gemcitabine (1000 mg/m^2 weekly for three of every 4 weeks) or leucovorin-modulated bolus 5-FU (leucovorin 20 mg/m^2 followed by 5-FU 425 mg/m^2 intravenous [IV] bolus days 1 through 5 every 28 days) [12]. Patients were stratified at randomization by country and resection margin status (R0 vs. R1), and the primary outcome measure was OS. After a median of follow-up of 34.2 months (interquartile range, 27.1–43.4), median OS in patients treated with 5-FU plus folinic acid (23.0 months) was similar to those treated with gemcitabine (23.6 months) (HR 0.94; 95% CI 0.81–1.08; $p = 0.39$). However, the patients assigned to FU/leucovorin had more grade 3 to 4 treatment-related toxicity, including stomatitis (10 versus 0%), diarrhea (13 versus 2%), and more treatment-related hospitalizations. An extended subgroup analyses from the study explored the optimal duration of adjuvant therapy and the ideal window after surgery to initiate such therapy [13], leading to some interesting observations. Overall survival favored patients who completed the full 6 months of therapy versus those who did not (median OS 28 versus 15 months, HR 0.51, 95% CI 0.44–0.60). Further, there was no survival disadvantage from delaying the start of adjuvant chemotherapy for up to 12 weeks after surgery; conversely, there was no survival advantage for starting early treatment, within 8 weeks of surgery. In fact, initiating chemotherapy within 8 weeks of surgery versus later was an important survival factor only for the subgroup of patients who did not complete all 6 months of therapy (in this group, survival favored later initiation of therapy).

ESPAC-4 In this phase III, two-group, open-label, multicenter, randomized clinical trial, 732 patients with macroscopically resected (R0/R1) pancreatic ductal adenocarcinoma were randomly assigned to 6 months of gemcitabine alone (1000 mg/m^2 on days 1, 8, and 15 of each 28-day cycle) or the same dose of gemcitabine plus capecitabine (1660 mg/m^2 per day, divided twice daily on day 1 through 21 of each 28-day cycle) [14]. Majority of patients in both arms had an R1 resection (60%) and involved lymph nodes (80%). The primary endpoint was OS. The median overall survival for patients in the gemcitabine plus capecitabine group was 28.0 months compared to 25.5 months in the gemcitabine group (HR 0.82; 95% CI 0.68–0.98; $p = 0.032$). The estimated 5-year overall survival in the gemcitabine plus capecitabine-treated group was 28.8% (22.9–35.2) compared with 16.3% (10.2–23.7) in the gemcitabine group. Of the grade 3 or 4 adverse effects, diarrhea (5 versus 2%), hand foot syndrome (7 versus 0%), and neutropenia (38 versus 24%) were significantly more common with combined therapy, although there were no significant differences in the rates of treatment-related serious adverse events. The results of the ESPAC-4 trial reinforced the efficacy of combination cytotoxic chemotherapy in pancreatic cancer that was previously appreciated in the metastatic setting.

PRODIGE-24 The multicenter PRODIGE-24 trial randomly assigned 493 patients with histologically proven pancreatic ductal adenocarcinomas who underwent an R0 or R1 resection to 6 months of gemcitabine alone (28-day cycles of gemcitabine 1000 mg/m^2 on days 1, 8, and 15) or modified-FOLFIRINOX (oxaliplatin [85 mg per square meter of body surface area], irinotecan [180 mg per square meter, reduced to 150 mg per square meter after a protocol-specified safety analysis], leucovorin [400 mg per square meter], and fluorouracil [2400 mg per square meter] every 2 weeks) [15]. Majority of the patients had an R0 resection (57.2%) and positive lymph nodes (76.5%). The primary end point was DFS. The median DFS was 21.6 months in the modified-FOLFIRINOX arm and 12.8 months in the gemcitabine arm (HR 0.58; 95% CI 0.46–0.73; $p < 0.001$). The DFS rate at 3 years was 39.7% in the modified-FOLFIRINOX arm and 21.4% in the gemcitabine arm. The median overall survival was 54.4 months in the modified-FOLFIRINOX arm and 35.0 months in the gemcitabine arm (HR 0.64; 95% CI 0.48–0.86; $p = 0.003$). Grade 3 or 4 adverse effects occurred more frequently in the modified-FOLFIRINOX group compared to the gemcitabine group (75.9% vs. 52.9%). These data suggest that modified-FOLFIRINOX should be the new standard for adjuvant therapy in patients with resected PDAC. Further, these results should be the benchmark for evaluating the results of future adjuvant therapy trials.

APACT Preliminary results of APACT, a phase III, multicenter, international, open-label, randomized trial that compared adjuvant therapy with nab-paclitaxel + gemcitabine versus single agent gemcitabine was reported at the American Society of Clinical Oncology (ASCO) annual meeting (2019). The study randomized 866 patients with histologically proven pancreatic ductal adenocarcinoma who underwent an R0 or R1 resection to 6 months of gemcitabine alone (gemcitabine 1000 mg/m^2 on days 1, 8, and 15 of a 28 day cycle) or nab-paclitaxel along with gemcitabine (nab-paclitaxel 125 mg/m^2 and gemcitabine 1000 mg/m^2 on days 1.8,15 of a 28-day cycle). Majority of the patients had an R0 resection (76%) and positive lymph nodes (72%). The primary end point was DFS. The median DFS was 19.4 months in the nab-paclitaxel + gemcitabine arm compared to 18.8 months in the gemcitabine arm (HR 0.88; 95% CI 0.729–1.063; $p = 0.1824$) suggesting a lack of benefit with the combination arm. The median overall survival was 40.5 months in the nab-paclitaxel + gemcitabine arm compared to 36.2 months in the gemcitabine arm (HR 0.82; 95% CI 0.680–0.996; $p = 0.045$). The reason for the lack of improved efficacy with the combination arm in the adjuvant setting, contrary to the data in the metastatic setting, is not clear. Final publication of the data is awaited.

Chemoradiation

The pivotal adjuvant chemoradiation trials have been summarized in Table 7.2.

GITSG study In this study conducted by the Gastrointestinal Tumor Study Group (GITSG), patients with resected pancreatic cancer were randomly assigned to either observation or EBRT (40 Gy) plus concurrent bolus fluorouracil (FU 500 mg/m^2 per day on the first 3 and last 3 days of RT), followed by maintenance chemotherapy (FU 500 mg/m^2 per day for 3 days monthly) for 2 years or until disease progression [16]. The study was terminated after 8 years due to poor patient accrual ($N = 43$). While these data need to be interpreted with caution, it is notable that patients who received postoperative chemoradiotherapy had significantly longer median DFS (11 versus

Table 7.2 Selected adjuvant chemoradiation trials

Trial	Number of patients	Primary endpoint	Randomization	R0 (%)	N1 (%)	RT dose/chemo	Chemotherapy	LR (%)	DFS (months)	OS (months)
GITSG	43	OS & DFS	CCRT → bolus 5-FU vs. observation	–	28%	40Gy/5-FU	Bolus 5-FU	–	11 vs. 9	20 vs. 11
EORTC	218	OS	CCRT vs. observation	81%	47%	40 Gy/5-FU	–	15% vs. 15%	17.4 vs. 16	24.5 vs. 19.0 $p = 0.208$
ESPAC-1	353	OS	CCRT vs. observation	82.4%	55.6%	20 Gy/5-FU	Bolus 5-FU	–	–	15.5 vs. 16.1 (HR 1.18; 95% CI 0.90–1.55; $p = 0.24$)
RTOG-9704	451	OS	Gemcitabine vs. 5-FU	41.7%	66.3%	50.4 Gy/5-FU	Gemcitabine vs. 5-FU	25% vs. 30%		20.5 vs. 16.9 (pancreatic head tumors (HR 0.82; 95% CI 0.65–1.03; $p = 0.09$)

LR local recurrence, *RT* radiotherapy

9 months) and median overall survival (20 versus 11 months) with a doubling of the 2-year survival rate (20% versus 10%) compared to patients in the observation arm.

EORTC study The European Organisation for Research and Treatment of Cancer (EORTC) conducted a randomized study that assigned 218 resected pancreatic cancer patients (1987–1995) to postoperative concurrent FU (25 mg/kg per day by continuous infusion) plus EBRT (40 Gy in split courses) or observation [17]. The primary endpoint was OS. Patients were stratified for institution and tumor localization (pancreatic head vs. periampullary). In the treatment arm, 21 patients (20%) received no treatment because of postoperative complications or patient refusal. The median duration of survival was 19.0 months for the observation group and 24.5 months in the treatment group (log rank, $p = 0.208$). In patients with cancer of the head of the pancreas, a larger difference was found; the median duration of survival was 17.1 months in the treatment group and 12.6 months in the observation group, suggesting a trend in favor for adjuvant treatment ($p = 0.099$). The 2-year survival estimates were 41% and 51%, respectively. No reduction in locoregional recurrence was seen with combined modality therapy. Similar to the GITSG study, there were several criticisms raised against this study, including the split course RT, suboptimal RT dose, and the lack of prospective assessment of surgical margins.

ESPAC-1 The design of ESAPC-1 has already been described in the section under adjuvant chemotherapy [7, 8]. The final results were presented in two separate publications, one that pooled the results from the three parallel randomized trials [7] and a later report that focused on the 289 patients randomized to the four-arm study [8].

In the initial report of the pooled analysis, overall results showed no benefit for adjuvant chemoradiotherapy with a median survival of 15.5 months in the 175 patients with chemoradiotherapy vs. 16.1 months in 178 patients without (HR 1.18; 95% CI 0.90–1.55; $p = 0.24$). In a subsequent report that included only the 289 patients randomized to the four-arm study [8], there was no significant benefit for chemoradiotherapy in the two groups that received it; in fact, the data suggested a trend toward worse survival for this group. The estimated 5-year survival rate was 10% among patients assigned to receive chemoradiotherapy and 20% among patients who did not receive chemoradiotherapy ($p = 0.05$). There were no significant imbalances for known prognostic factors (nodal positivity, resection margin status, histologic grade) in the two arms that could have contributed to these results. Local recurrence rates were similar in both groups, but there were more recurrences overall (84 versus 74) in the chemoradiotherapy group and a shorter recurrence-free interval (10.7 versus 15.2 months, respectively). There were several limitations associated with this study including the lack of an "intent-to-treat" analysis, split course RT, the nonuniform dose of RT (ranging from 40 to 60 Gy), and the "background" chemoradiation or chemotherapy administered according to clinician discretion. Although the trial was underpowered to perform formal statistical comparisons among the four individual treatment groups, patients in both chemoradiotherapy groups had an inferior median overall survival (13.9 months for chemoradiotherapy alone and 14.2 months for chemoradiotherapy plus chemotherapy) as compared with those undergoing observation alone (16.9 months), suggesting that treatment-related toxicity may have accounted for some of these results.

RTOG 9704 The US Intergroup Study (Radiation Therapy Oncology Group [RTOG] 9704) addressed the role of systemic therapy with adjuvant gemcitabine versus 5-fluorouracil over and beyond concomitant FU-based chemoradiotherapy in patients with resected PDAC [18]. This phase III trial enrolled 451 patients who had undergone gross total resections for T1–4, N0–1 PDAC (taking in at least 1500 calories daily postoperatively) and randomized them to one of the following two treatment arms: (a) 5-FU arm, 3 weeks of continuous infusion 5-FU

(250 mg/m^2 daily) followed by chemoradiotherapy (50.4 Gy in 1.8 Gy daily fractions for 5.5 weeks with concurrent infusional 5-FU 250 mg/m^2 daily) and, starting 3–5 weeks later, two 4-week courses of continuous infusion 5-FU (250 mg/m^2 daily, with a 2-week rest in between courses), or (b) gemcitabine arm, three weekly doses of gemcitabine alone (1000 mg/m^2 per week) followed by the same chemoradiotherapy protocol as for the conventional chemoradiotherapy arm and, starting 3–5 weeks later, 3 months of single-agent gemcitabine (1000 mg/m^2 weekly for three of every 4 weeks). The primary endpoints were survival for all patients and survival for patients with pancreatic head tumors. Patients were stratified by nodal status (uninvolved vs. involved), tumor diameter (<3 cm vs. ≥3 cm), and surgical margin status (negative vs. positive vs. unknown). Overall, the addition of gemcitabine to adjuvant fluorouracil-based chemoradiation was associated with a survival benefit for patients with resected pancreatic cancer, but this improvement was not statistically significant. Patients with pancreatic head tumors (n = 388) had a median OS of 20.5 months and a 3-year survival of 31% in the gemcitabine group vs. a median OS of 16.9 months and a 3-year survival of 22% in the fluorouracil group (HR 0.82; 95% CI 0.65–1.03; p = 0.09); this effect was strengthened on multivariate analysis (HR 0.80; 95% CI 0.63–1.00; p = 0.05), suggesting a trend toward survival benefit. In the updated analysis, there were no significant differences in 5-year overall survival or DFS between the two groups [19].

In summary, the authors feel that it is safe to draw the following conclusions from the various adjuvant therapy trials that have been conducted thus far.

1. Local relapse occurs in a substantial number of patients with resected PDAC, but distant relapse appears to be the primary mode of failure.
2. There is clear evidence to support the role of adjuvant systemic therapy in patients with resected PDAC. Combination cytotoxic chemotherapy appears to provide incremental benefit compared to single-agent cytotoxic therapy in the adjuvant setting, as evidenced by the results of ESPAC-4 and PRODIGE-24 trials, respectively.
3. The robust data from PRODIGE-24 suggests that modified-FOLFIRINOX should be the new standard for adjuvant therapy in eligible patients with resected PDAC.
4. While there are no clear randomized data to support the role of adjuvant chemoradiation over and beyond systemic chemotherapy, the low local recurrence rates noted in RTOG 9704, where central QA was employed, suggests an important role for this modality.
5. The currently available adjuvant therapy data does not shed adequate light on the number of patients who undergo curative intent resection and never undergo adjuvant therapy due to either early relapse or inadequate postoperative recovery.

Neoadjuvant Therapy for PDAC

Any discussion regarding the role of neoadjuvant therapy in the treatment of PDAC needs to be placed in the context of accurate clinical staging of PDAC. Improvements in imaging modalities, specifically, contrast-enhanced multiplanar computed tomography, provide highly accurate assessments of tumor-vessel associations which can be used to reproducibly define the clinical stage of PDAC. Although cross-sectional imaging studies are extremely accurate at defining the extent of the primary tumor, the detection of metastatic disease continues to be challenging. More than 76% of patients who undergo surgical resection of the primary tumor will develop distant metastatic disease as the first evidence of disease recurrence [20, 21]. Furthermore, within 6 months of successful surgery, up to 60% of patients with PDAC experience disease relapse, as reported in the CONKO-001 study [9]. Thus, it is clear that one of the greatest challenges in treating patients with localized PDAC is the treatment of clinically/radiographically occult metastases which are present but unappreciated in most patients who are eligible for surgical resection.

In this chapter, we have reviewed results of multiple randomized clinical trials that have consistently demonstrated an overall improvement in median survival with adjuvant therapy (median overall survival, approximately 24 months) as compared with surgery alone. However, there are similar limitations to this approach. First, adjuvant trials have an inherent selection bias in that they do not provide accurate information on the true denominator that undergoes curative intent pancreatic resection and the proportion of patients that never makes it to adjuvant therapy due to either early relapse or postoperative complications. Prolonged postoperative recovery can prevent the delivery of adjuvant therapy in approximately 25% of patients even in a highly specialized academic setting and up to 50% in some series [22]. Analysis of the Surveillance, Epidemiology, and End Results Program database suggests that only 51% of eligible patients received adjuvant therapy following major pancreatic resection for cancer [23] indicative of "real-world" trends. Therefore, the survival durations reported in adjuvant trials following pancreatectomy apply only to a subset of all patients who underwent surgery with curative intent and are superior to what can be achieved in general practice. Second, completion of adjuvant therapy can be challenging even when successfully initiated in the postoperative setting. In the CONKO-001 trial, 90% of patients (168/186) received a single dose of therapy, 87% (138/161) received one cycle of therapy, and only 62% of patients (111/179) were able to complete all six cycles of gemcitabine [10]. Third, neoadjuvant therapy affords a window in which patients with unfavorable tumor biology (10–30%), who are at risk for developing distant metastatic disease progression early, can be identified prior to surgery, thus avoiding unnecessary operative intervention and delay in exposure to alternative systemic therapy.

Initial concerns regarding the safety and feasibility of neoadjuvant therapy have been largely unfounded. Foremost was the concern that patients with potentially resectable PDAC may develop local progression, thus losing the "window of opportunity" for a potentially curative surgery. Data from two prospective, phase II, neoadjuvant trials (N = 176) showed that less than 1% of eligible patients were found to have isolated local disease progression at the time of preoperative restaging (after neoadjuvant therapy) [24, 25]. In a contemporary experience from our institution, only 4 of 246 patients (1.6%) were found to have local disease progression after neoadjuvant therapy; all 4 patients were assessed as having BLR disease at the time of diagnosis [26]. Further, concerns over the toxicity of neoadjuvant therapy and the effect of treatment-related adverse effects on operative morbidity and mortality have not been observed [24, 25, 27]. The incidence of pancreatic fistula, the most frequent serious complication associated with pancreatectomy, is actually reduced after neoadjuvant therapy as the treated pancreas becomes more firm in response to chemoradiation [28–30]. An analysis of the National Surgical Quality Improvement Program database demonstrated no differences in 30-day mortality and morbidity rates among patients treated with neoadjuvant therapy as compared with patients who received surgery first [31]. Furthermore, the addition of radiation may have important implications as several series have reported decreased rates of positive margins (R1 or R2) and node-positive disease following neoadjuvant therapy [29, 30]. Most importantly, among patients who are able to complete all intended neoadjuvant therapy and surgery, median overall survival is improved by almost 12 months (34–45 months vs. 22–26 months) as compared with a surgery-first approach [24, 25, 32, 33].

A summary of selected large series of neoadjuvant trials in patients with localized (resectable and borderline resectable) PDAC is provided in Tables 7.3 and 7.4. At least three meta-analyses have addressed the benefit of neoadjuvant therapy in patients with initially potentially resectable pancreatic cancer [34–36]. The largest analysis of 111 studies [36], including 56 phase I/II trials and with 96% of the patients receiving chemotherapy and 94% RT, concluded that, among patients with initially resectable disease, 35% had an objective response to neoadjuvant therapy, while 21% had progressive disease.

Table 7.3 Selected neoadjuvant studies in patients with resectable PDAC

Author	*N*	Neoadjuvant regimen	Resected (%)	R0 (%)	Survival
Evans DB, 1992 [40]	28	CCRT (5-FU)	61%	82%	–
Staley, 1996 [41]	39	CCRT (5-FU)	100%	54%	19 months
Pisters PW, 1998 [42]	35	CCRT(5-FU) + EB-IORT	74%	88%	3-yr survival 23%
Hoffman JP, 1998 [43]	53	CCRT (5-FU and mitomycin)	45%	71%	9.7 months
White RR, 2001 [44]	53	CCRT (5-FU)	53%	72%	–
Pisters PW, 2002 [45]	35	CCRT (paclitaxel) + EB-IORT	57%	68%	3-yr survival, 28%
Moutardier V, 2004 [46]	61	CCRT (5-FU and cisplatin)	65%	92.5%	13 months
Talamonti MS, 2006 [47]	20	CCRT (gemcitabine)	85%	94%	26 months for resected patients
Palmer DH, 2007 [48]	50	Gemcitabine vs. gemcitabine + cisplatin	Gemcitabine −38% Gemcitabine + cisplatin −70%	Gemcitabine −75% Gemcitabine + cisplatin −75%	1-yr survival Gemcitabine −42% Gemcitabine + cisplatin −62%
Heinrich S, 2008 [49]	28	Gemcitabine + cisplatin	93%	80%	26.5 months
Evans DB, 2008 [24]	86	CCRT (gemcitabine)	74%	89%	34 months (resected patients)
Varadachary, GR, 2008 [25]	90	Gemcitabine +cisplatin → CCRT (gemcitabine)	66%	96%	31 months (resected patients)
Le Scodan R, 2009 [50]	41	CCRT (5-FU and cisplatin)	63%	81%	2-yr survival, 32%
O'Reilly, EM, 2014 [51]	38	Gemcitabine +oxaliplatin	71%	74%	27.2 months
Christians, KK, 2016 [32]	69	Chemotherapy (various) and chemoradiation	87%	97%	31.5 months

CCRT concurrent chemoradiation, *EB-IORT* electron beam intraoperative radiotherapy

Table 7.4 Selected neoadjuvant studies in patients with borderline resectable PDAC

Author	*N*	Neoadjuvant regimen	Number resected (%)	R0 resection (%)	Survival
Kim S, 2016 [52]	26	FOLFIRINOX ($n = 26$) then RT ($n = 4$)	26 (100)	22 (92)	Median survival not reached at median follow-up 27.6 months
Katz M, 2016 [53]	22	FOLFIRINOX then CRT	15 (68)	14 (93)	Median 21.7 months
Takahashi H, 2013 [54]	80	Gem-RT	43 (54)	42 (98)	5-year: 34%
Kim E, 2013 [55]	39	GEMOX-RT	24 (62)	NR	Median 18.4 months
Kang C, 2012 [56]	32	Gem with or without Cis-RT	32 (100)	28 (88)	NR
Barugola G, 2012 [57]	27	Various	27 (100)	NR	NR
Stokes J, 2011 [58]	40	Cape-RT	16 (40)	12 (75)	NR
Chun Y, 2010 [59]	74	Various	74 (100)	44 (60	Median 21 months
McClaine R, 2010 [60]	29	Various	12 (41)	8 (75)	NR

Resectability rates were 74% (95% CI 65.9–80.6%). Such data needs to be interpreted with caution due to the heterogeneity of the trials involved in the analysis.

Attempts at prospective comparison of neoadjuvant therapy with a surgery-first approach have been unsuccessful [37, 38]. It is not surprising that such clinical trials have failed to meet accrual targets as many patients and referring physicians are unwilling to participate in clinical trials (phase II or III) that involve randomization to two drastically different treatment arms.

The National Cancer Database (NCDB) was used to identify on 15,237 patients who underwent a potentially curative resection for early stage PDAC (clinical stage I or II according to the 2010 TNM classification) from 2006 to 2012 [39]. Patients who underwent neoadjuvant therapy followed by curative-intent resection were matched by propensity score with patients whose tumors were resected upfront. Overall survival was compared by using a Cox proportional hazards regression model. The conditional probability of receiving neoadjuvant therapy (the propensity score) was estimated based upon age, gender, race, ethnicity, year of diagnosis, income, insurance type, area of residence, comorbidity, facility type, clinical stage, and type of surgery. From the group receiving neoadjuvant therapy (47% multiagent, 43% single agent, 10% unspecified), 2005 patients were propensity score matched to 6015 patients who had upfront resection. The neoadjuvant therapy group demonstrated an improved survival compared with the upfront surgery group (median OS, 26 months vs. 21 months, HR 0.72; 95% CI, 0.68–0.78; $p < 0.01$). Patients in the upfront resection group had higher pathologic T stage (pT3 and T4: 86% vs. 73%; $P < 0.01$), higher positive lymph nodes (73% vs. 48%; $P < 0.01$), and higher positive resection margin (24% vs. 17%; $P < 0.01$). Compared with a subset of upfront surgery patients who received adjuvant therapy, patients who received neoadjuvant therapy had a better median OS (26 vs. 23 months; HR 0.83; 95% CI 0.73–0.89; $p < 0.01$). Rates of 3- and 5-year survival were also modestly higher in the neoadjuvant therapy group (35% and 21% versus 29% and 18%, respectively). This difference was smaller when patients receiving neoadjuvant therapy were compared with the subset of patients undergoing upfront surgery who also received adjuvant therapy (3- and 5-year survival rates 35% and 21% versus 31% and 18%, respectively). Clearly, such data need to be interpreted with caution due to inherent limitations of retrospective analyses of data from large databases and the fact that patients in the neoadjuvant therapy group represented only those who tolerated neoadjuvant therapy and successfully underwent resection.

In a similar approach, 593 patients were identified from the NCDB-377 (63.6%) in the neoadjuvant cohort, wherein 104 (27.6%) experienced preoperative attrition, and 216 (36.4%) in the surgery-first cohort, of whom 30 (13.9%) failed to receive intended adjuvant chemotherapy. Intention-to-treat Kaplan-Meier analysis demonstrated superior median OS for the neoadjuvant cohort compared to the surgery-first cohort (20.7 months vs. 13.7 months, $p < 0.001$). Intention-to-treat, multivariable regression analysis revealed a decreased mortality hazard (HR 0.68, 95% CI 0.53–0.86, $p = 0.0012$) for the neoadjuvant cohort compared to the surgery-first cohort. Again, these data need to be interpreted with caution, keeping in mind the limitations associated with analysis of retrospective data from a large database, including, but not limited to, the heterogeneity of patient characteristics, differences in stage definitions/evaluations, diversity in chemotherapy regimens administered, and different doses/techniques in delivery of radiotherapy.

Value of Biomarkers in Guiding Neoadjuvant Therapy

Serum carbohydrate antigen 19–9 (CA 19–9), or sialyl Lewis (a) antigen, is a biomarker that was initially discovered in the serum of patients with advanced colorectal, gastric, and pancreatic cancers; the assay was originally developed using a colorectal cancer cell line [61, 62]. Although this biomarker does not have value as a screening assay, it is used as an adjunct tool in the diagnosis of PDAC, to monitor response to therapy and for prognostic purposes [63–66]. Individuals who are Lewis antigen negative (up to 10% of the population) lack the enzyme fucosyltransferase needed for CA 19–9 production; these patients do not express CA 19–9 and are considered nonsecretors [67, 68]. CA 19–9 is also secreted by normal biliary epithelium, contributing to its lack of specificity [69]. Significant elevated levels of CA19–9 in the setting of benign or malignant biliary obstruction have been well described and may obfuscate interpretation, particularly in the context of a known PDAC [70, 71].

There has been considerable debate about the prognostic impact of CA 19–9 production, its absolute levels, and the relevance of normalization with therapy. Previous reports have suggested that CA 19–9 nonsecretors have a better prognosis compared with secretors [72, 73].

A large study utilizing the NCDB commented on the prognostic impact of CA19–9 in patients with PDAC [74]. Among a total of 113,145 patients queried, 28,074 (24.8%) patients had CA 19–9 measured and reported. Survival was worse in all stages in patients with CA 19–9 elevation; this survival effect was greatest in the early stage patients (median OS 22.3 vs. 11.3 months, $p < 0.001$). Nonsecretors had survival similar to that of patients with normal CA19–9 levels. Early stage patients with elevated CA 19–9 had decreased survival at 1, 2, and 3 years (56% vs. 68%, 30% vs. 42%, 15% vs. 25%, all $p < 0.001$) compared to patients with normal levels; this was confirmed by adjusted modeling (HR 1.26, 95% CI 1.20–1.32, $p < 0.001$). To investigate the possible effect of CA 19–9 elevation on OS among patients receiving equivalent therapy, unadjusted Kaplan-Meier analysis was performed on early stage patients who received curative intent surgical therapy either alone or in conjunction with either adjuvant systemic chemotherapy or neoadjuvant systemic chemotherapy followed by curative intent surgery. Neoadjuvant systemic chemotherapy followed by curative intent surgery was the only treatment sequence that completely eliminated the observed negative effect on survival due to CA 19–9 elevation; results were confirmed by repetition of a stage- and therapy-specific Cox proportional hazards survival model ($p = 0.11$). A similar study performed using the NCDB found that pretreatment CA 19–9 levels >800 was associated with advanced disease and negatively associated with long-term survival, while levels ≤800 had no significant association with survival [75].

At our institution, we have analyzed the significance of pretreatment CA19–9 level in predicting response to neoadjuvant therapy [76]. In a retrospective evaluation of 235 patients, we categorized pretreatment CA19–9 levels (with concomitant normal bilirubin level) in patients with localized PC as normal (≤35), low (36–200), moderate (201–1000), or high (>1000). Posttreatment CA19–9 levels were measured after neoadjuvant therapy, prior to surgery. Of the 235 patients, 168 (71%) completed all planned therapy including a pancreatectomy: 44 (73%), 62 (79%), 46 (67%), and 16 (57%) of the normal, low, moderate, and high groups ($p = 0.10$). Among these 168 patients, the median overall survival was 43.6, 44.7, 27.2, and 26.4 months for normal, low, moderate, and high CA19–9 groups (log rank $p = 0.72$). Thus, in our experience, in patients completing all planned therapy including surgery, an elevated pretreatment CA19–9 was of little prognostic value; instead, it was the CA19–9 response to neoadjuvant therapy that was prognostic (HR 1.80, $p = 0.02$).

The significance of CA 19–9 normalization with neoadjuvant therapy and its oncologic impact is gaining some attention. A single institution retrospective series that evaluated the impact of "duration of neoadjuvant therapy" found that the most favorable median OS was noted in the group patients whose CA19–9 level normalized, regardless of the duration of therapy [77]. In our institutional experience (unpublished data), the median OS for the 98 patients who did (29, 30%) or did not (69) normalize their preoperative CA19–9 with neoadjuvant therapy was 46 and 23 months, respectively ($p = 0.02$). Following surgery, 32 (46%) of the 69 patients with an elevated preoperative CA19–9 normalized their postoperative CA19–9. Failure to normalize preop or postop CA19–9 was associated with a 2.77-fold increased risk of death ($p < 0.003$).

In summary, the limited body of available evidence suggests that the absolute CA 19–9 level at diagnosis (in the context of a normal bilirubin) may have a prognostic impact. More importantly, normalization of CA19–9 levels with preoperative therapy or at minimum postoperatively in patients who have received neoadjuvant therapy appears to have highly significant, favorable prognostic implications.

Current Clinical Trials

There are several large clinical trials evaluating the use of more modern chemotherapy regimens in the adjuvant setting and as neoadjuvant treatment for resectable and borderline resectable pancreatic cancer. Many protocols include perioperative treatment that includes both neoadjuvant and adjuvant therapy, and many incorporate preoperative radiation therapy in addition to systemic chemotherapy. Some trials have met the accrual goal or are nearing completion of enrollment. Many additional smaller studies include new cytotoxic drugs, targeted agents, and, increasingly, immunotherapy approaches. The results of these protocols may eventually provide practice-changing information and influence the next generation of clinical trials in pancreatic cancer. Those trials including approximately 100 patients or more are described below and listed in Table 7.5.

Adjuvant Chemotherapy

Preliminary results of the APACT trial (NCT01964430) – a randomized phase III comparison of nab-paclitaxel plus gemcitabine (standard dose and schedule) versus gemcitabine alone in 866 patients following macroscopic complete resection (R0/R1) of PDAC that was surgically staged T1–3, N0–1, and M0 with good performance status and able to start treatment by 12 weeks after surgery – were reported at ASCO (2019) and summarized in the section on adjuvant chemotherapy. Final publication of the results in manuscript format is awaited.

Neoadjuvant Chemotherapy

Several ongoing clinical trials examine administration of chemotherapy prior to surgery, and many deliver perioperative chemotherapy both before and after surgery. The NEOPAC trial (NCT01314027) is a randomized phase III trial comparing neoadjuvant GEMOX every 2 weeks × four cycles (days 1, 15, 29, 43) over 8 weeks followed by surgery and adjuvant gemcitabine for 6 months versus upfront surgery and adjuvant gemcitabine x 6 months. Target accrual is 310 patients with resectable disease, and primary outcome measure is relapse-free survival.

The Prep02/JSAP05 (UMIN000009634) randomized phase II/III study aims to accrue 360 patients with resectable pancreatic cancer. Randomization arms include 2 months of neoadjuvant gemcitabine + S1 followed by surgery and adjuvant S1 for 6 months versus surgery first and adjuvant S1 for 6 months. The phase II portion of the protocol with 40 patients per arm has resection rate as the primary endpoint, and the phase III component with 180 patients per arm has overall survival as the primary outcome measure.

NEONAX (AIO-PAK-0313, NCT02047513) is a randomized phase II study evaluating perioperative nab-paclitaxel plus gemcitabine delivered as neoadjuvant therapy × 2 months prior to surgery and additional 4 months after surgery versus the same regimen given only after surgery. Target accrual is 166 patients with resectable PDAC. Primary outcome measure is disease-free survival.

The NEPAFOX (NCT01272976) trial is a randomized, multicenter phase II/III design evaluating perioperative FOLFIRINOX. Patients in the investigational arm receive 6 cycles of neoadjuvant FOLFIRINOX and 6 cycles of postoperative adjuvant FOLFIRINOX compared to the control arm that receives standard adjuvant gemcitabine × 6 cycles. Estimated accrual is 126 patients with resectable disease, and primary outcome measure is overall survival.

The Southwest Oncology Group S1505 is a multicenter, randomized phase II perioperative trial NCT02562716) comparing neoadjuvant plus

Table 7.5 Selected ongoing trials in patients with resectable and borderline resectable PDAC

Study ID	Phase	Stage	*N*	Regimen	Primary endpoint
Adjuvant chemotherapy					
N01964430 APACT (completed)	III	Resected	866	Nab-paclitaxel + gemcitabine vs. gemcitabine	DFS
Neoadjuvant chemotherapy					
NCT01314027 NEOPAC	III	Resectable	310	Neoadjuvant GEMOX + adjuvant gemcitabine vs. adjuvant gemcitabine	RFS
UMIN000009634 Prep-02/JSAP05	II/III	Resectable	360	Neoadjuvant gemcitabine + S1 and adjuvant S1 vs. adjuvant S1	OS
MCT 02047513 NEONAX AIO-PAK-0313	II	Resectable	166	Neoadjuvant and adjuvant nab-paclitaxel + gemcitabine vs. adjuvant nab-paclitaxel + gemcitabine	DFS
NCT01272976 NEPAFOX	II/III	Resectable	126	Neoadjuvant FOLFIRINOX + adjuvant FOLFIRINOX vs. adjuvant gemcitabine	OS
NCT 02562716 SWOG 51505	II	Resectable	112	Neoadjuvant plus adjuvant FOLFIRINOX vs. neoadjuvant plus adjuvant nab-paclitaxel + gemcitabine	OS
NCT 02919787 NorPACT-1	III	Resectable	90	Neoadjuvant FOLFIRINOX × 4 + adjuvant gemcitabine + capecitabine x 4 vs. adjuvant gemcitabine/capecitabine x 6	OS
NCT 01150630 PACT-15	II/III	Resectable	98	Adjuvant gemcitabine vs. adjuvant PEXG vs. neoadjuvant + adjuvant PEXG	EVS, OS
NCT 02959879 PANACHE01/ PRODIGE 48	II	Resectable	160	ARM 1: neoadjuvant FOLFIRINOX × 4 + adjuvant × 4 months ARM 2: neoadjuvant FOLFOX × 4 + adjuvant chemotherapy × 4 months ARM 3: adjuvant chemotherapy only × 6 months	OS
Neoadjuvant chemoradiation					
NCT 01900327 NEOPA	III	Resectable	410	Neoadjuvant gemcitabine/XRT + adjuvant gemcitabine vs. adjuvant gemcitabine only	OS
NCT 02676349 PANDAS- PRODIGE44	II	Borderline Resectable	90	Neoadjuvant mFOLFIRINOX + capecitabine/XRT vs. neoadjuvant mFOLFIRINOX + adjuvant gemcitabine or modified LV5FU	RO
NCT 01458717 (Korea)	II/III	Borderline Resectable	116	Neoadjuvant gemcitabine/XRT + adjuvant gemcitabine vs. postop gemcitabine/XRT + adjuvant gemcitabine	OS
NCT 02839343 Alliance A 021501	II	Borderline Resectable	134	Neoadjuvant FOLFIRINOX + hypofractionated XRT and adjuvant FOLFOX vs. neoadjuvant FOLFIRINOX + adjuvant FOLFIRINOX	OS

adjuvant FOLFIRINOX versus neoadjuvant plus adjuvant nab-paclitaxel plus gemcitabine. Target accrual is 112 patients with resectable pancreatic cancer. Primary outcome measure is overall survival.

NorPACT-1 (NCT02919787) is a randomized phase III for resectable PDAC that compares neoadjuvant FOLFIRINOX × 4 cycles followed by surgery and then 4 cycles of adjuvant gemcitabine plus capecitabine versus surgery first followed by 6 cycles of adjuvant therapy with gemcitabine plus capecitabine. Expected enrollment is 90 patients. Primary outcome measure is overall survival.

PANACHE01/PRODIGE48 (NCT02959879) is a non-comparative three-arm randomized multicenter phase II trial evaluating four cycles of neoadjuvant FOLFIRINOX, four cycles of neoadjuvant FOLFOX, and upfront surgery with all patients receiving adjuvant chemotherapy for 4 months in the two neoadjuvant arms and 6 months in the surgery first arm. Enrollment will be 160 patients with resectable pancreatic cancer. Primary outcome measures are overall survival at 12 months and the number of patients who complete the chemotherapy treatment sequence.

The PACT-15 trial (NCT01150630) is a multicenter randomized phase II/III protocol evaluating perioperative PEXG (cisplatin, epirubicin, capecitabine, gemcitabine). Arm 1 patients receive standard adjuvant gemcitabine for 6 months. Patients in arm 2 receive adjuvant PEXG every 14 days for 6 months. Arm 3 includes neoadjuvant and adjuvant PEXG with up to 3 months prior to surgery and 3 months after surgery. Target accrual is 98 patients with resectable pancreatic cancer. Primary objective is to assess event-free survival at 1 year after neoadjuvant therapy (phase II) and overall survival (phase III).

Neoadjuvant Chemoradiation

NEOPA (NCT01900327) is a phase III trial that compares neoadjuvant chemoradiation 50.4 Gy using weekly low-dose (300 mg/m^2) radiosensitizing gemcitabine followed by surgery and adjuvant standard gemcitabine for six cycles to upfront surgery and adjuvant gemcitabine for six cycles. Enrollment target is 410 patients with resectable PDAC. Primary outcome measure is overall survival at 3 years.

PANDAS/PRODIGE44 (NCT02676349) is a randomized phase II trial evaluating neoadjuvant mFOLFIRINOX with or without preoperative concomitant chemoradiation 50.4 Gy with capecitabine. Following surgery, all patients will receive adjuvant chemotherapy with gemcitabine or modified LV5FU. Accrual goal is 90 patients with borderline resectable pancreatic cancer. Primary outcome measure is R0 resection.

A phase II/III trial with neoadjuvant chemoradiation in Korea (NCT02839343) uses low-dose (400 mg/m^2) gemcitabine plus XRT 54 Gy followed by surgery and adjuvant gemcitabine given for 4 months compared to surgery first followed by chemoradiation 54 Gy with low-dose gemcitabine and then adjuvant gemcitabine for 4 months in borderline resectable pancreatic cancer. Accrual target is 116 patients. Primary outcome measure is overall survival (2 years).

Alliance 021501 (NCT02839343) is a randomized phase II trial that compares perioperative FOLFIRINOX (8 cycles pre-and 4 cycles post-operatively) to 7 cycles of neoadjuvant FOLFIRINOX and hypo-fractionated preoperative radiation followed by 4 additional cycles of adjuvant FOLFIRINOX in 134 patients with borderline resectable PDAC. Primary outcome measure is overall survival (18 months).

In addition to the large-scale studies listed, there are smaller phase II trials that evaluate neoadjuvant/adjuvant FOLFIRINOX (NCT02047474, NCT01660711) in resectable PDAC, neoadjuvant FOLFIRINOX and chemoradiation (NCT 01821612, NCT01661088) for borderline resectable PDAC, and novel agents such as LDE-225 hedgehog inhibitor (NCT01431794), hydroxychloroquine (NCT01494155), pembrolizumab (NCT02305186), and vaccines such as GVAX (NCT00727441). Over the past several years, there has been an improvement in the treatment of metastatic pancreatic cancer, and there is increased interest to extrapolate those treatments to early stage disease and conduct research employing new strategies and novel therapies.

Conclusion

In summary, PDAC is a highly lethal malignancy with a propensity for both local and systemic metastases despite curative intent surgery. There is clear evidence to emphasize the role of systemic therapy and to some extent the role of radiotherapy as an adjunct to surgery in the curative intent treatment of localized PDAC. While it is important to ensure delivery of multimodality therapy to all patients with localized PDAC to maximize their chance of cure, it is equally important to develop a clear treatment plan with multidisciplinary input right from the time of initial diagnosis. Optimal treatment sequencing for each patient should be personalized, with the broader oncologic goal of eliminating both macroscopic and microscopic disease.

References

1. Siegel RL, Miller KD, Jemal A. Cancer statistics, 2017. CA Cancer J Clin. 2017;67(1):7–30.
2. Jemal A, et al. Global cancer statistics. CA Cancer J Clin. 2011;61(2):69–90.
3. Allen PJ, et al. Multi-institutional Validation Study of the American Joint Commission on Cancer (8th edition) changes for T and N staging in patients with pancreatic adenocarcinoma. Ann Surg. 2017;265(1):185–91.
4. Chun YS, Pawlik TM, Vauthey JN. 8th edition of the AJCC cancer staging manual: pancreas and hepatobiliary cancers. Ann Surg Oncol. 2018;25(4):845–7.
5. Al-Hawary MM, et al. Pancreatic ductal adenocarcinoma radiology reporting template: consensus statement of the society of abdominal radiology and the american pancreatic association. Gastroenterology. 2014;146(1):291–304.e1.
6. Ryan DP, Hong TS, Bardeesy N. Pancreatic adenocarcinoma. N Engl J Med. 2014;371(11):1039–49.
7. Neoptolemos JP, et al. Adjuvant chemoradiotherapy and chemotherapy in resectable pancreatic cancer: a randomised controlled trial. Lancet. 2001;358(9293):1576–85.
8. Neoptolemos JP, et al. A randomized trial of chemoradiotherapy and chemotherapy after resection of pancreatic cancer. N Engl J Med. 2004;350(12):1200–10.
9. Oettle H, et al. Adjuvant chemotherapy with gemcitabine vs observation in patients undergoing curative-intent resection of pancreatic cancer: a randomized controlled trial. JAMA. 2007;297(3):267–77.
10. Oettle H, et al. Adjuvant chemotherapy with gemcitabine and long-term outcomes among patients with resected pancreatic cancer: the CONKO-001 randomized trial. JAMA. 2013;310(14):1473–81.
11. Ueno H, et al. A randomised phase III trial comparing gemcitabine with surgery-only in patients with resected pancreatic cancer: Japanese Study Group of Adjuvant Therapy for Pancreatic Cancer. Br J Cancer. 2009;101(6):908–15.
12. Neoptolemos JP, et al. Adjuvant chemotherapy with fluorouracil plus folinic acid vs gemcitabine following pancreatic cancer resection: a randomized controlled trial. JAMA. 2010;304(10):1073–81.
13. Valle JW, et al. Optimal duration and timing of adjuvant chemotherapy after definitive surgery for ductal adenocarcinoma of the pancreas: ongoing lessons from the ESPAC-3 study. J Clin Oncol. 2014;32(6):504–12.
14. Neoptolemos JP, et al. Comparison of adjuvant gemcitabine and capecitabine with gemcitabine monotherapy in patients with resected pancreatic cancer (ESPAC-4): a multicentre, open-label, randomised, phase 3 trial. Lancet. 2017;389(10073):1011–24.
15. Conroy T, et al. FOLFIRINOX or gemcitabine as adjuvant therapy for pancreatic cancer. N Engl J Med. 2018;379(25):2395–406.
16. Kalser MH, Ellenberg SS. Pancreatic cancer. Adjuvant combined radiation and chemotherapy following curative resection. Arch Surg. 1985;120(8):899–903.
17. Klinkenbijl JH, et al. Adjuvant radiotherapy and 5-fluorouracil after curative resection of cancer of the pancreas and periampullary region: phase III trial of the EORTC gastrointestinal tract cancer cooperative group. Ann Surg. 1999;230(6):776–82; discussion 782–4.
18. Regine WF, et al. Fluorouracil vs gemcitabine chemotherapy before and after fluorouracil-based chemoradiation following resection of pancreatic adenocarcinoma: a randomized controlled trial. JAMA. 2008;299(9):1019–26.
19. Regine WF, et al. Fluorouracil-based chemoradiation with either gemcitabine or fluorouracil chemotherapy after resection of pancreatic adenocarcinoma: 5-year analysis of the U.S. Intergroup/RTOG 9704 phase III trial. Ann Surg Oncol. 2011;18(5):1319–26.
20. Gnerlich JL, et al. Microscopic margins and patterns of treatment failure in resected pancreatic adenocarcinoma. Arch Surg. 2012;147(8):753–60.
21. Iacobuzio-Donahue CA, et al. DPC4 gene status of the primary carcinoma correlates with patterns of failure in patients with pancreatic cancer. J Clin Oncol. 2009;27(11):1806–13.
22. Spitz FR, et al. Preoperative and postoperative chemoradiation strategies in patients treated with pancreaticoduodenectomy for adenocarcinoma of the pancreas. J Clin Oncol. 1997;15(3):928–37.
23. Mayo SC, et al. Management of patients with pancreatic adenocarcinoma: national trends in patient selection, operative management, and use of adjuvant therapy. J Am Coll Surg. 2012;214(1):33–45.
24. Evans DB, et al. Preoperative gemcitabine-based chemoradiation for patients with resectable adeno-

carcinoma of the pancreatic head. J Clin Oncol. 2008;26(21):3496–502.
25. Varadhachary GR, et al. Preoperative gemcitabine and cisplatin followed by gemcitabine-based chemoradiation for resectable adenocarcinoma of the pancreatic head. J Clin Oncol. 2008;26(21):3487–95.
26. Miura JT, et al. Use of neoadjuvant therapy in patients 75 years of age and older with pancreatic cancer. Surgery. 2015;158(6):1545–55.
27. Christians KK, et al. Neoadjuvant FOLFIRINOX for borderline resectable pancreas cancer: a new treatment paradigm? Oncologist. 2014;19(3):266–74.
28. Raut CP, et al. Neoadjuvant therapy for resectable pancreatic cancer. Surg Oncol Clin N Am. 2004;13(4):639–61, ix.
29. Takahashi H, et al. Preoperative chemoradiation reduces the risk of pancreatic fistula after distal pancreatectomy for pancreatic adenocarcinoma. Surgery. 2011;150(3):547–56.
30. Willett CG, et al. Resection margins in carcinoma of the head of the pancreas. Implications for radiation therapy. Ann Surg. 1993;217(2):144–8.
31. Cooper AB, et al. Does the use of neoadjuvant therapy for pancreatic adenocarcinoma increase postoperative morbidity and mortality rates? J Gastrointest Surg. 2015;19(1):80–6; discussion 86–7.
32. Christians KK, et al. Survival of patients with resectable pancreatic cancer who received neoadjuvant therapy. Surgery. 2016;159(3):893–900.
33. Winter JM, et al. Survival after resection of pancreatic adenocarcinoma: results from a single institution over three decades. Ann Surg Oncol. 2012;19(1):169–75.
34. Andriulli A, et al. Neoadjuvant/preoperative gemcitabine for patients with localized pancreatic cancer: a meta-analysis of prospective studies. Ann Surg Oncol. 2012;19(5):1644–62.
35. Assifi MM, et al. Neoadjuvant therapy in pancreatic adenocarcinoma: a meta-analysis of phase II trials. Surgery. 2011;150(3):466–73.
36. Gillen S, et al. Preoperative/neoadjuvant therapy in pancreatic cancer: a systematic review and meta-analysis of response and resection percentages. PLoS Med. 2010;7(4):e1000267.
37. Casadei R, et al. Neoadjuvant chemoradiotherapy and surgery versus surgery alone in resectable pancreatic cancer: a single-center prospective, randomized, controlled trial which failed to achieve accrual targets. J Gastrointest Surg. 2015;19(10):1802–12.
38. Golcher H, et al. Neoadjuvant chemoradiation therapy with gemcitabine/cisplatin and surgery versus immediate surgery in resectable pancreatic cancer: results of the first prospective randomized phase II trial. Strahlenther Onkol. 2015;191(1):7–16.
39. Mokdad AA, et al. Neoadjuvant therapy followed by resection versus upfront resection for resectable pancreatic cancer: a propensity score matched analysis. J Clin Oncol. 2017;35(5):515–22.
40. Evans DB, et al. Preoperative chemoradiation and pancreaticoduodenectomy for adenocarcinoma of the pancreas. Arch Surg. 1992;127(11):1335–9.
41. Staley CA, et al. Preoperative chemoradiation, pancreaticoduodenectomy, and intraoperative radiation therapy for adenocarcinoma of the pancreatic head. Am J Surg. 1996;171(1):118–24; discussion 124–5.
42. Pisters PW, et al. Rapid-fractionation preoperative chemoradiation, pancreaticoduodenectomy, and intraoperative radiation therapy for resectable pancreatic adenocarcinoma. J Clin Oncol. 1998;16(12):3843–50.
43. Hoffman JP, et al. Phase II trial of preoperative radiation therapy and chemotherapy for patients with localized, resectable adenocarcinoma of the pancreas: an Eastern Cooperative Oncology Group Study. J Clin Oncol. 1998;16(1):317–23.
44. White RR, et al. Neoadjuvant chemoradiation for localized adenocarcinoma of the pancreas. Ann Surg Oncol. 2001;8(10):758–65.
45. Pisters PW, et al. Preoperative paclitaxel and concurrent rapid-fractionation radiation for resectable pancreatic adenocarcinoma: toxicities, histologic response rates, and event-free outcome. J Clin Oncol. 2002;20(10):2537–44.
46. Moutardier V, et al. Assessment of pathologic response after preoperative chemoradiotherapy and surgery in pancreatic adenocarcinoma. Int J Radiat Oncol Biol Phys. 2004;60(2):437–43.
47. Talamonti MS, et al. A multi-institutional phase II trial of preoperative full-dose gemcitabine and concurrent radiation for patients with potentially resectable pancreatic carcinoma. Ann Surg Oncol. 2006;13(2):150–8.
48. Palmer DH, et al. A randomized phase 2 trial of neoadjuvant chemotherapy in resectable pancreatic cancer: gemcitabine alone versus gemcitabine combined with cisplatin. Ann Surg Oncol. 2007;14(7):2088–96.
49. Heinrich S, et al. Prospective phase II trial of neoadjuvant chemotherapy with gemcitabine and cisplatin for resectable adenocarcinoma of the pancreatic head. J Clin Oncol. 2008;26(15):2526–31.
50. Le Scodan R, et al. Preoperative chemoradiation in potentially resectable pancreatic adenocarcinoma: feasibility, treatment effect evaluation and prognostic factors, analysis of the SFRO-FFCD 9704 trial and literature review. Ann Oncol. 2009;20(8):1387–96.
51. O'Reilly EM, et al. A single-arm, nonrandomized phase II trial of neoadjuvant gemcitabine and oxaliplatin in patients with resectable pancreas adenocarcinoma. Ann Surg. 2014;260(1):142–8.
52. Kim SS, et al. Preoperative FOLFIRINOX for borderline resectable pancreatic cancer: is radiation necessary in the modern era of chemotherapy? J Surg Oncol. 2016;114(5):587–96.
53. Katz MH, et al. Preoperative modified FOLFIRINOX treatment followed by capecitabine-based chemoradiation for borderline resectable pancreatic cancer: alliance for clinical trials in oncology trial A021101. JAMA Surg. 2016;151(8):e161137.
54. Takahashi H, et al. Preoperative gemcitabine-based chemoradiation therapy for resectable and borderline resectable pancreatic cancer. Ann Surg. 2013;258(6):1040–50.

55. Kim EJ, et al. A multi-institutional phase 2 study of neoadjuvant gemcitabine and oxaliplatin with radiation therapy in patients with pancreatic cancer. Cancer. 2013;119(15):2692–700.
56. Kang CM, et al. Potential contribution of preoperative neoadjuvant concurrent chemoradiation therapy on margin-negative resection in borderline resectable pancreatic cancer. J Gastrointest Surg. 2012;16(3):509–17.
57. Barugola G, et al. Outcomes after resection of locally advanced or borderline resectable pancreatic cancer after neoadjuvant therapy. Am J Surg. 2012;203(2):132–9.
58. Stokes JB, et al. Preoperative capecitabine and concurrent radiation for borderline resectable pancreatic cancer. Ann Surg Oncol. 2011;18(3):619–27.
59. Chun YS, et al. Defining venous involvement in borderline resectable pancreatic cancer. Ann Surg Oncol. 2010;17(11):2832–8.
60. McClaine RJ, et al. Neoadjuvant therapy may lead to successful surgical resection and improved survival in patients with borderline resectable pancreatic cancer. HPB (Oxford). 2010;12(1):73–9.
61. Koprowski H, et al. Specific antigen in serum of patients with colon carcinoma. Science. 1981;212(4490):53–5.
62. Koprowski H, et al. Colorectal carcinoma antigens detected by hybridoma antibodies. Somatic Cell Genet. 1979;5(6):957–71.
63. Galli C, Basso D, Plebani M. CA 19-9: handle with care. Clin Chem Lab Med. 2013;51(7):1369–83.
64. Poruk KE, et al. Screening for pancreatic cancer: why, how, and who? Ann Surg. 2013;257(1): 17–26.
65. Poruk KE, et al. The clinical utility of CA 19-9 in pancreatic adenocarcinoma: diagnostic and prognostic updates. Curr Mol Med. 2013;13(3):340–51.
66. Zubarik R, et al. Screening for pancreatic cancer in a high-risk population with serum CA 19-9 and targeted EUS: a feasibility study. Gastrointest Endosc. 2011;74(1):87–95.
67. Orntoft TF, et al. Influence of Lewis alpha1-3/4-L-fucosyltransferase (FUT3) gene mutations on enzyme activity, erythrocyte phenotyping, and circulating tumor marker sialyl-Lewis a levels. J Biol Chem. 1996;271(50):32260–8.
68. Yu LC, et al. Correlation of a missense mutation in the human secretor alpha 1,2-fucosyltransferase gene with the Lewis(a+b+) phenotype: a potential molecular basis for the weak secretor allele (sew). Biochem J. 1995;312(Pt 2):329–32.
69. Kannagi R. Carbohydrate antigen sialyl Lewis a--its pathophysiological significance and induction mechanism in cancer progression. Chang Gung Med J. 2007;30(3):189–209.
70. Sanchez M, Gomes H, Marcus EN. Elevated CA 19-9 levels in a patient with Mirizzi syndrome: case report. South Med J. 2006;99(2):160–3.
71. Scoggins CR, et al. Supra-elevated CA 19-9 in a benign hepatic cyst adenoma. HPB (Oxford). 2004;6(1):43–4.
72. Berger AC, et al. Undetectable preoperative levels of serum CA 19-9 correlate with improved survival for patients with resectable pancreatic adenocarcinoma. Ann Surg Oncol. 2004;11(7):644–9.
73. Park HD, et al. The relationship between Lewis/Secretor genotypes and serum carbohydrate antigen 19-9 levels in a Korean population. Korean J Lab Med. 2010;30(1):51–7.
74. Bergquist JR, et al. Carbohydrate antigen 19-9 elevation in anatomically resectable, early stage pancreatic cancer is independently associated with decreased overall survival and an indication for neoadjuvant therapy: a National Cancer Database Study. J Am Coll Surg. 2016;223(1):52–65.
75. Mirkin KA, Hollenbeak CS, Wong J. Prognostic impact of carbohydrate antigen 19-9 level at diagnosis in resected stage I-III pancreatic adenocarcinoma: a U.S. population study. J Gastrointest Oncol. 2017;8(5):778–88.
76. Aldakkak M, et al. Pre-treatment carbohydrate antigen 19-9 does not predict the response to neoadjuvant therapy in patients with localized pancreatic cancer. HPB (Oxford). 2015;17(10):942–52.
77. Williams JL, et al. CA19-9 normalization during pre-operative treatment predicts longer survival for patients with locally progressed pancreatic cancer. J Gastrointest Surg. 2016;20(7):1331–42.

Neoadjuvant Chemoradiation for Localized Pancreatic Cancer

8

William A. Hall and Beth A. Erickson

Rationale for Neoadjuvant Therapy

Pancreatic cancer remains a devastating malignancy with high rates of mortality and low rates of overall survival. Patients managed with up-front surgical resection, without neoadjuvant therapy, have particularly poor outcomes. Common to an up-front surgical resection approach are high rates of R1 resections ranging from 14% to 60%, along with high rates of node positivity of approximately 60–80% [1–3]. The recently published European Study Group for Pancreatic Cancer (ESPAC-4) clinical trial, which included patients managed with up-front surgical resection, had a 60% rate of positive margins, and 80% of patients were found to be node positive [1]. This management approach was associated with a median overall survival of approximately 25–28 months, depending on the treatment arm [1]. Patients with positive margins had particularly poor outcomes [4]. An oncologic management approach with a 60% rate of positive margins is unprecedented in any other solid tumor and supports the use of neoadjuvant therapy. Notable is that the subsequent ESPAC-5 clinical trial design includes several permutations of neoadjuvant therapy. These include immediate surgery, gemcitabine/capecitabine chemotherapy followed by surgery, FOLFIRINOX chemotherapy followed by surgery, and chemoradiation (capecitabine-based) followed by surgery [5]. This design is presumably to help offset some of the adverse pathologic features associated with an up-front surgical resection approach.

Many patients treated with a surgery-first approach also have low rates of completing adjuvant therapy. These numbers are often difficult to estimate, given the frequent "absence of a denominator" effect in prospective adjuvant studies. In other words, it is difficult to know how many patients were treated with surgery and felt to be ineligible for study enrollment secondary to poor performance status. In publications that have included total numbers of surgical resections, the rates of patients completing adjuvant therapy are approximately 50–60%. In a study by Herman et al. from the Johns Hopkins, only 53% of patients underwent adjuvant therapy, this was despite exquisite care provided by a leading academic medical center [6]. It could only be postulated that, in a less experienced health care environment, the number of patients failing to undergo adjuvant therapy is larger. A second series by the Mayo Clinic demonstrated similar results with only 58% of patients receiving adjuvant therapy, following

W. A. Hall (✉) · B. A. Erickson
Department of Radiation Oncology, The Medical College of Wisconsin, Milwaukee, WI, USA
e-mail: whall@mcw.edu

S. Tsai et al. (eds.), *Management of Localized Pancreatic Cancer*,
https://doi.org/10.1007/978-3-319-98944-0_8

Table 8.1 Summary rationale for neoadjuvant versus adjuvant therapy for pancreatic cancer

Comparator variable	*Neoadjuvant*	*Adjuvant*	*Citations to support*
Rate of positive margins	2–10%	16–60%	[3, 8, 9]
Incidence of node positivity	17–35%	62–80%	[1, 8, 9]
Successful treatment completion	70–80%	50–60%	[6, 7, 9]
Local recurrence	5–9%	19–53%	[1, 3, 9]

up-front surgical resection [7]. While prospective adjuvant trials have attempted to make progress with novel systemic agents, the low number of patients able to undergo adjuvant therapy will make an adjuvant strategy difficult to advance overall survival in patients with pancreatic cancer (Table 8.1).

Neoadjuvant Therapy for Resectable Pancreatic Cancer

Even the earliest cases of pancreatic cancer, found when the cancer is surgically resectable, benefit from neoadjuvant therapy. One of the earliest reports of neoadjuvant therapy for resectable pancreatic cancer came from the University of Texas MD Anderson Cancer Center in 1992 [10]. In this series, a total of 28 patients underwent preoperative chemo-RT with concurrent 5-FU and 50.4 Gy of external beam radiation therapy. A total of 23 patients did not have any evidence of disease progression and subsequently underwent surgical resection. This series concluded that pancreaticoduodenectomy could be performed in patients with low overall toxicity and perhaps represented a promising area for future investigation [10]. Following this series, a rapid neoadjuvant therapy series examined the toxicity, radiographic, and pathologic outcomes for patients with resectable localized pancreatic cancer. In this series, by Pisters et al., patients underwent 30 Gy in 10 fractions of external beam radiation therapy with concurrent 5-FU chemotherapy [11]. Of note, patients in this series also received an intraoperative radiation therapy boost to a total dose of 10–15 Gy. Findings from this series were that this more rapid treatment course of external beam radiation therapy was associated with minimal toxicity and excellent local regional control. Variations in the type of chemotherapy were subsequently evaluated in the neoadjuvant setting. Pisters et al. examined the use of concurrent chemo-RT with paclitaxel-based concurrent therapy and a total of 30 Gy over 10 fractions given again with an intraoperative radiation therapy boost [12]. This series demonstrated that treatment with preoperative paclitaxel-based concurrent chemo-RT is feasible; however, the toxicity was higher than the preceding series with 5-FU-based chemotherapy [11, 12].

A subsequent prospective experience with neoadjuvant therapy in patients with resectable pancreatic cancer followed. Evans et al. enrolled a total of 86 patients with resectable pancreatic cancer in a prospective phase II study. Patients enrolled included those with uncinated process or pancreatic head tumors that had radiographically defined resectable disease and underwent concurrent gemcitabine-based chemo-RT. The radiation therapy in this trial was a total dose of 30 Gy given over 10 fractions. Several very important findings were confirmed in this trial. First, it was again noted that not all patients were able to undergo surgical resection. Indeed, a total of only 85% of the patients were able to successfully undergo surgical resection. However, for those patients who underwent surgical resection, the overall survival was an impressive 34 months. This series again highlighted an advantageous aspect of neoadjuvant therapy, which is the selection of patients who may benefit the most of from surgical resection.

The role for systemic chemotherapy in advance of neoadjuvant concurrent chemo-RT for patients with resectable pancreatic cancer was subsequently evaluated by Varadhachary et al. A total of 90 patients were enrolled in a phase II trial. First, patients underwent gemcitabine and cisplatin given every 2 weeks for a

Table 8.2 Summary of select neoadjuvant series for resectable pancreatic cancer

Series	N	Chemotherapy	Radiotherapy dose	Resected with PD	Not R0	Median OS if resected	Citation
Evans 1992	28	Fluorouracil, 300 mg/m^2 per day + XRT	50.4 Gy/28	17/28	18%	NR	[10]
Pisters 1998	35	Fluorouracil, 300 mg/m^2 per day + XRT	30 Gy/10 + IORT	20/35	10%	25	[11]
Hoffman 1998	53	Mitomycin 10 mg/m^2 day 2 and fluorouracil (5-FU) 1000 mg/m^2/d	50.4 Gy/28	24/53	25%	15.7	[48]
Pisters 2002	35	Paclitaxel (60 mg/m^2) + XRT	30 Gy/10 + IORT	20/35	32%	19	[12]
Evans 2008	86	Gemcitabine (400 mg/m^2) + XRT	30 Gy/10	73/86	11%	34	[9]
Varadhachary 2008	90	Gem + Cis → Gem Gemcitabine (400 mg/m^2) + XRT	30 Gy/10	52/90	4%	32	[13]
Kharofa 2014	69	Gem+Cis, FOLFIRINOX, FOLFOX, Gem+Cape Gem+Erlotinib	50.4 Gy/28 fractions, IMRT (Gem Con)	48/69	2%	26	[8]

IORT intraoperative radiation therapy, *PD* pancreaticoduodenectomy, *XRT* radiation therapy, *R0* margin-negative resection, *OS* overall survival, *Gem* gemcitabine, *Cis* cisplatin, *Con* concurrent

total of four doses; this was followed by concurrent chemo-RT with gemcitabine and a total dose of 30 Gy given over 10 fractions. The median survival of all patients in this series was 17.4 months, and in the 52 patients that underwent surgical resection, it was 31 months. Conclusions from this trial were that preoperative chemotherapy with gemcitabine and cisplatin followed by concurrent chemo-RT did not improve survival beyond that achieved with preoperative gemcitabine-based chemo-RT alone [13].

In a recent retrospective series, Kharofa et al. examined patients treated for both resectable and borderline resectable pancreatic cancer between 2009 and 2011. This series used modern era radiation therapy consisting of intensity modulated radiation therapy (IMRT) to a total dose of 50.4 Gy given with concurrent chemotherapy [8].These results again confirmed low rates of local failure and high rates of margin-negative resection using 50.4 Gy of neoadjuvant IMRT. Conclusions from this series were that neoadjuvant chemo-RT can facilitate margin-negative resections in patients with localized pancreatic cancer [8].A recent series by Christians et al. again showed that neoadjuvant treatment in patients with resectable pancreatic cancer was associated with an overall survival of 32 months [14]. A National Cancer Database (NCDB) by Mokdad et al. presented a propensity-matched cohort analysis comparing neoadjuvant therapy versus up-front surgical resection that concluded there is a potential overall survival benefit to the use of neoadjuvant therapy, as compared with a surgery-first approach, in patients with pancreatic cancer [15]. A summary of select series examining the role of neoadjuvant therapy in patients with resectable pancreatic cancer is presented in Table 8.2.

Neoadjuvant Therapy for Borderline Resectable Pancreatic cancer

The role of neoadjuvant therapy is more widely accepted and used in patients with borderline resectable pancreatic cancer. One of the largest challenges in the examination of patients with borderline resectable disease is the considerable heterogeneity of this categorization of pancreatic cancer [16, 17]. There exists a wide variety of both institution-specific and national guidelines that have varying definitions. Moreover, series examining borderline resectable pancreatic cancer often include groups of patients with locally advanced disease. Katz et al. presented a series of borderline resectable pancreatic cancer that examined a total of 125 patients who completed preoperative therapy and underwent repeat staging; a total of 66 (41%) underwent pancreatectomy. In the patients that completed all therapy, the median survival was a total of 40 months; this was in contrast to only 13 months for the patients that did not undergo pancreatectomy. Conclusions from this series were that a neoadjuvant approach allows for identification of a subset of patients that are most likely to benefit from surgery [18]. This set the stage for a large number of studies to follow over the coming decade that evaluated the role of neoadjuvant therapy in advance of surgical resection for patients with borderline resectable pancreatic cancer.

Several different variations in neoadjuvant chemotherapy have been used for patients with borderline resectable pancreatic cancer. Given the success of leucovorin, 5-FU, irinotecan, and oxaliplatin (FOLFIRINOX) in the metastatic setting [19], the use of neoadjuvant FOLFIRINOX has been tested in numerous clinical series. An earlier series using FOLFIRINOX in the neoadjuvant borderline resectable setting was presented by Christians and colleagues [20]. A total of 18 patients with borderline resectable pancreatic cancer diagnosed between 2010 to December 2012 were treated with neoadjuvant FOLFIRINOX chemotherapy, followed by concurrent gemcitabine or capecitabine chemoradiation. A total of 12 patients in this series were taken to surgical resection, and all 12 had negative margins, with a node positivity rate of only 17%. Conclusions from this series were that FOLFIRINOX followed by chemoradiation was safe and had favorable resection rates as compared with previous reports [20]. This was followed by several additional publications looking at the role of neoadjuvant FOLFIRINOX followed by concurrent chemo-RT [21–23]. Recently, a prospective clinical trial has been designed to evaluate this treatment strategy in the neoadjuvant setting [24].

Neoadjuvant Stereotactic Body Radiation Therapy (SBRT)

There has recently been considerable enthusiasm for the use of SBRT in a variety of malignancies [25]. When tumors are treated with SBRT, the total number of treatments is reduced typically to 5 or fewer. This means that patients can spend less time undergoing radiation therapy and more quickly resume systemic therapy. Indeed, SBRT provides a convenient manner in which high doses of radiation therapy can be delivered with considerable precision to a tumor. However, in pancreatic cancer, the use of SBRT in the neoadjuvant setting needs additional investigation. Pancreatic SBRT avoids treatment of several critical vascular and nodal regions that are at high risk of harboring micrometastatic disease from either nodal or perineural tumor spread. In one of the first series to examine the role of SBRT in the neoadjuvant setting, Chuong and colleagues retrospectively collected data for patients with both locally advanced and borderline resectable pancreatic cancer treated with preoperative SBRT [26]. From this series it was concluded that SBRT safely facilitates margin-negative resections while maintaining a high rate of local control. However, there are limitations and caution that should be applied to retrospectively collected data. This is particularly important when it comes to the accuracy of local recurrence given the possibility of heterogeneous or absent follow-up data. There is currently an ongoing prospective clinical trial lead by Paltaand colleagues at Duke University in the United States focused on a prospective evaluation of the role for SBRT [27]. Furthermore, a study being conducted by the Alliance (A021501) is evaluating the role of SBRT given for patients with borderline resectable pancreatic cancer [24]. Additional discussion of the ongoing

Alliance clinical trials is presented in the subsequent section on randomized clinical trials.

Neoadjuvant Radiotherapy and Concurrent Chemotherapy Intensification

There is relatively limited data examining the role of neoadjuvant radiotherapy dose intensification for patients with pancreatic cancer. Similarly there are few series that have examined the role for neoadjuvant, concurrent, chemotherapeutic intensification. Shaib et al. conducted a phase I study in a total of 13 patients that treated pancreatic cancer patients with neoadjuvant FOLFIRINOX followed by four different radiation therapy dose levels delivered in three fractions to the planning target volume with a simultaneous boost to the posterior resection margin. Conclusions from this series were that 45 Gy delivered over 3 fractions to the posterior resection margin was safe and well-tolerated and the dose-limiting toxicity was not reached. More recent radiotherapy dose intensification strategies have been published. Wang and colleagues retrospectively reviewed cases of borderline resectable and some locally advanced patients that underwent a radiotherapy vascular boost; a total of 23 patients underwent a vascular boost, with a range of 54–64 Gy, and 78% received no boost. Conclusions from this series were that dose escalation appeared to result in an improvement in surgical resection rate, although this improvement was not statistically significant [28]. Huang and colleagues also retrospectively examined the role for an IMRT vascular boost strategy using a SIB boost to areas very to be at high risk as defined on PET. Conclusions from this series were that this treatment strategy is feasible and seems to improve the likelihood of an R0 resection without compromising the organs at risk [29]. Kim and colleagues evaluated the use of preoperative full-dose gemcitabine, oxaliplatin, and radiation therapy in a total of 23 patients with resectable disease and 39 patients with borderline resectable disease [30]. A total of 43 patients underwent surgical resection (total of 63%), and complete R0 resection was seen in 36 of those 43 patients. Conclusions from this chemotherapeutic intensification series were that preoperative full-dose gemcitabine and oxaliplatin and radiation therapy was feasible [30]. Given the increasing popularity of proton therapy, Hong and colleagues recently published a phase II trial in which 50 patients were enrolled and were treated with 5 daily doses of 5GyE times 5 fractions and 35 patients were treated in the phase II portion of the study. The local failure rate was reported as 16.2%, and distant disease recurrence was the predominant mode of failure at 72.9%.Treatment with this strategy was felt to have favorable local control, and the rate of grade 3 toxicity was reported as only 4.1% [31].

Randomized Clinical Trials of Evaluating the Role of Neoadjuvant Therapy

Given the presence of multiple retrospective and prospective single-arm series that have supported the role for neoadjuvant therapy in resectable pancreatic adenocarcinoma, there has been a substantial interest in conducting a randomized trial comparing these approaches. Such sequencing studies have defined the standard of care in other disease sites, such as rectal adenocarcinoma with the German colorectal trial [32]. One of the first attempts to conduct such a trial was performed by Doi et al. in Japan. In this multi-institutional prospective clinical trial, a total of 42 patients were randomly assigned to receive either surgery up front (20 patients) or radiochemotherapy (22 patients) followed by surgery. This total number of randomized patients was considerably smaller than the initial intended accrual goal of 150 patients. The trial reported being stopped early secondary to a clear overall survival benefit seen in the surgically resected patients [33]. However, given the small size of the trial, the particularly poor survival of patients in the radiotherapy arm (8.9 months), it is difficult to draw reliable conclusions from this series [33]. Golcher and colleagues designed a randomized phase II trial that was intended to accrue a total of 254 patients; however, the trial was stopped after 73 patients secondary to slow accrual [34]. Given the limited accrual of this clinical trial, it is also difficult to arrive at any firm conclusions; however, the trial did determine that neoadjuvant chemoradiation is safe with regard to toxicity, perioperative morbidity, and mortality [34]. The Dutch are currently conducting a phase III clinical trial designed to test the hypothesis that median overall survival can be improved with the use of neoadjuvant radiochemotherapy [35]. Titled the PREOPANC clinical trial, patients are randomized to either neoadjuvant therapy with 15 fractions of 2.4 Gy (total of 36 Gy) given with concurrent gemcitabine or up-front surgical resection. Each arm in the trial is followed by either six cycles of adjuvant chemotherapy or four cycles of adjuvant chemotherapy in patients who underwent neoadjuvant therapy [35]. In addition, as discussed above, the Alliance cooperative group is conducting a randomized phase II clinical trial evaluating the role of neoadjuvant SBRT (33–40 Gy in 5 fractions) in the treatment of patients with borderline resectable pancreatic cancer. The goal of this trial is to accrue a total of 134 patients with borderline resectable pancreatic cancer to evaluate 18-month overall survival of patients enrolled onto each of the two treatment arms as compared with a historical control rate [24]. Finally, the Neoadjuvant Treatment in Resectable Pancreatic Cancer (NEOPA) is ongoing. This randomized, two-armed, open label, multicenter, phase III trial is estimating a 3-year overall survival increase by 12% compared to patient undergoing up-front surgery for resectable pancreatic cancer, NCT01900327 [36].

Practical Considerations of Neoadjuvant Radiation Therapy Delivery

Radiation therapy must be delivered with considerable care, given that organs in the upper abdomen are extremely sensitive to treatment with radiation therapy. Significant progress has been made in defining the treatment targets and shaping the dose distribution to cover the areas that need radiation and avoiding the normal adjacent structures. Advanced imaging used for radiation planning, including CT, MRI, and PET scans, allows improved target definition along with dose escalation to key parts of the target volume. This can also result in further reduction of the irradiated volumes in the sensitive upper abdomen [37]. While many historic series used three-dimensional conformal radiotherapy (3DCRT), this treatment paradigm has recently shifted to treatment with IMRT. IMRT is an advanced version of 3DCRT that uses a computer-controlled radiation beam delivery through varying beam intensities within each beam portal. This results in a substantial improvement in the conformity of the dose distribution to the shape of the tumor. Furthermore, IMRT can result in avoidance of adjacent normal organs [38]. IMRT treatment planning is performed using inverse treatment planning. In this process, planning target volume dose is specified as well as the allowable doses/volumes to the adjacent normal organs. This allows for tighter margins and permits the ability to sculpt and bend dose around normal organs. Image-guided radiation therapy centers around the acquisition of daily images to direct conformal radiation therapy treatment plans [38]. This may also allow for adaptation and change in daily radiotherapy treatment plans to account for variations in patient shape or changes in tumor size.

One of the challenges of using IMRT is accurately defining both the tumor and the prophylactic target volume. This is particularly challenging and critical in pancreatic cancer. There often exists heterogeneity among even expert radiation oncologists regarding the location and extent of gross pancreatic tumor [39]. The success of IMRT is dependent on accurate target delineation and treatment delivery. There are several helpful atlases that can be used to assist in the identification of treatment volumes when patients are treated with IMRT. A consensus postoperative atlas was created to help ensure consistency in contouring (RTOG Consensus Panel Contouring Atlas for the Delineation of the Clinical Target Volume in the Postoperative Treatment of Pancreatic Cancer (https://www.rtog.org)).

Dholakia et al. have published an excellent version of this atlas [40]. Recent pancreatic contouring guideline publications have integrated MRI to assist in the process of gross tumor identification [39, 41]. While these atlases are very useful for gross tumor volume and local normal structures, precisely understanding the volumes to be treated in the preoperative setting remains challenging.

At the Medical College of Wisconsin, in the neoadjuvant setting, several important contouring approaches are taken (e.g., Figs. 8.1, 8.2, 8.3, 8.4, 8.5, and 8.6). Depending on the location of the gross tumor volume, the clinical target volume is designed to include the entire pancreatic head, body, or tail. These regions of the pancreas are targeted, rather than just the visible gross tumor volume. The creation of this primary clinical target volume is used primarily as a result of the difficulty in visualizing the location and extent of pancreatic gross tumor. Coverage of a region of the pancreas helps to ensure that both microscopic and perineural diseases are treated. With regard to vascular clinical target volume, the celiac axis and superior mesenteric artery and vein are generally contoured with a variable margin that is influenced by the clinical suspicion for perivascular involvement. The expansion of these vascular structures is primarily to account for nodal involvement or perineal spread [8] (Figs. 8.1, 8.2, 8.3, 8.4, 8.5, and 8.6). Lesions that are near the portal vein, portal venous confluence, IVC, aorta, or the branches of the celiac artery (common hepatic artery) are also selectively targeted, if close to or involved by the primary lesion. If any suspicious nodes are present, those are also targeted and those nodal regions can be considered for inclusion in the target volumes.

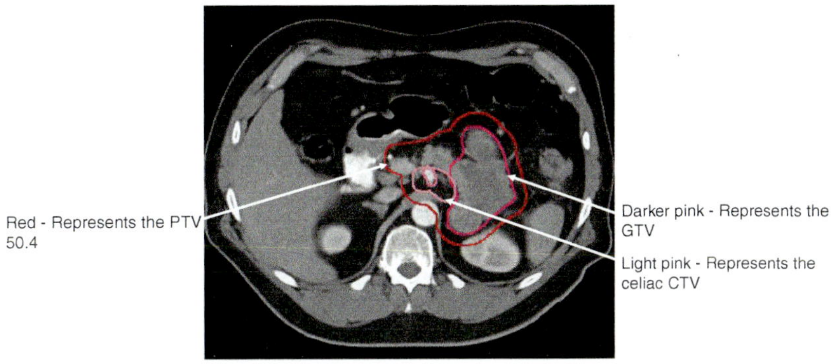

Fig. 8.1 Pancreatic tail lesion treated with neoadjuvant therapy. Summary: Primary tumor in the pancreatic tail which abuts the left kidney and also is inseparable from the left adrenal gland. There is encasement of the splenic artery to its origin from the celiac artery

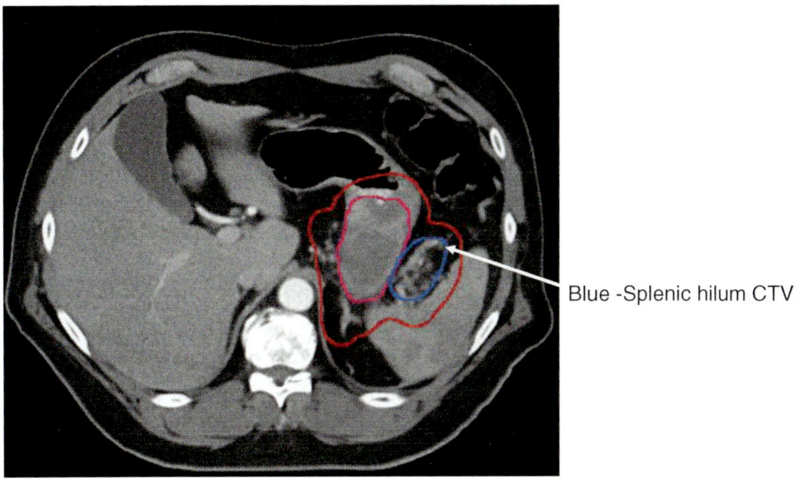

Fig. 8.2 Example treatment volumes for a typical patient being treated with neoadjuvant concurrent chemoradiation therapy for pancreatic cancer

Fig. 8.3 Example treatment volumes for a typical patient being treated with neoadjuvant concurrent chemoradiation therapy for pancreatic cancer

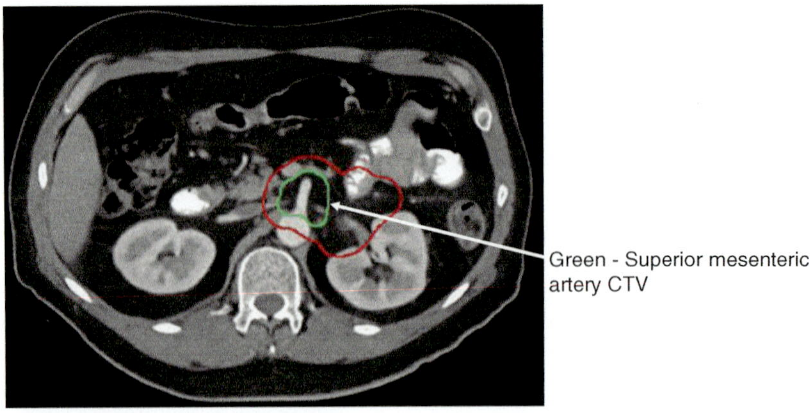

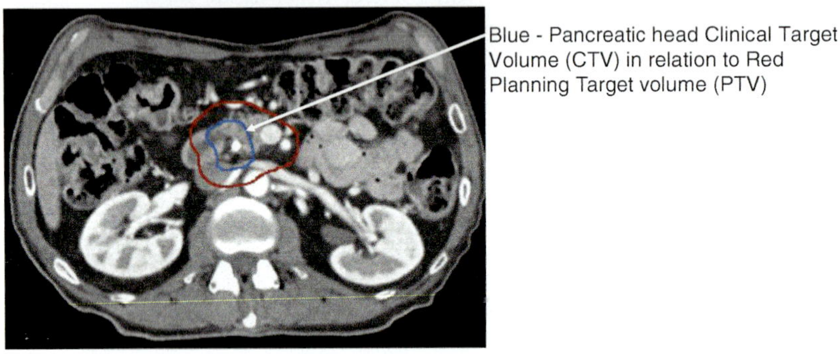

Fig. 8.4 Resectable pancreatic head cancer being treated with neoadjuvant therapy. Summary: Imaging showed a head of pancreas mass without arterial abutment or encasement, there was noted to be mild SMV abutment, no lymph nodes appreciated, and plan to treat with neoadjuvant concurrent chemo-RT

Fig. 8.5 Example treatment volumes for a typical patient being treated with neoadjuvant concurrent chemoradiation therapy for pancreatic cancer

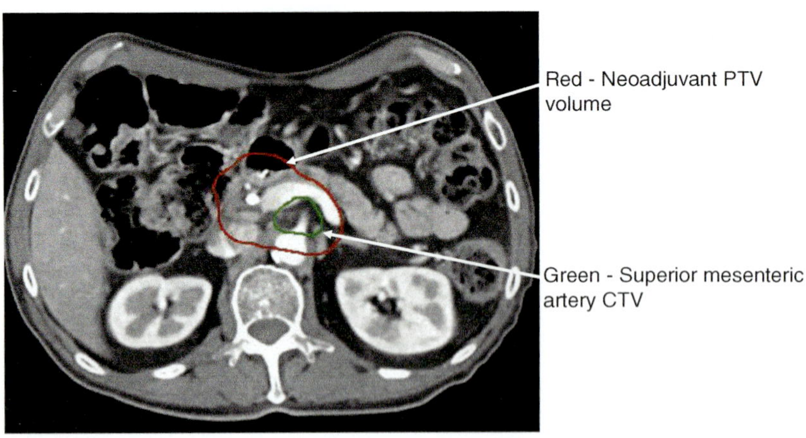

A summary of CTV expansions and treatment volumes used at the Medical College of Wisconsin is summarized in Table 8.3.

As previously mentioned, there is an evolving role for MRI in the management of patients with pancreatic cancer. CT often underestimates target volume, whereas MR may offer better soft tissue determination and more accurate target definition [42]. There have been several recent publications that have focused on the use of MRI in the

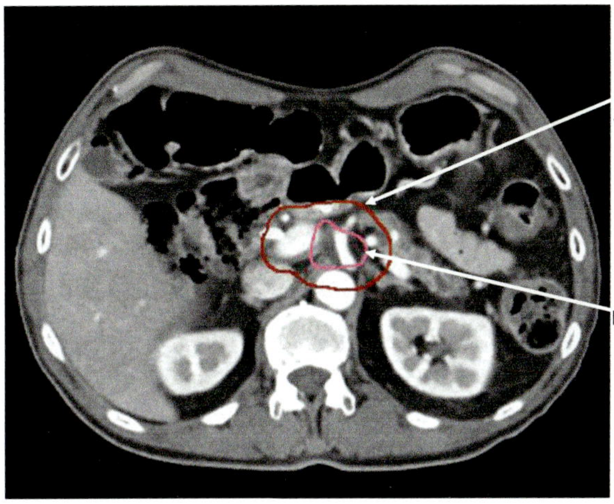

Fig. 8.6 Example treatment volumes for a typical patient being treated with neoadjuvant concurrent chemoradiation therapy for pancreatic cancer

Table 8.3 Medical College of Wisconsin, Pancreatic clinical target volumes

	Descriptions
Primary tumor CTV	The primary tumor and region of the pancreas that contains the primary tumor should be identified and contoured in its entirety. This should include all available clinical information, including endoscopic reports, CT scans, MRIs, PET, along with tumor board discussion
Primary nodal CTV	All visible nodes should be contoured and identified' nodal regions felt to contain highly suspicious nodes should be included
Celiac CTV	The proximal 1.0 cm of the celiac artery from the origin at the aorta is contoured and expanded a total of 1.5–3.0 cm to the right, 1.0–2.0 cm to the left, 1.0–1.5 cm anterior, 1.0 cm posterior, 1.0 cm superior, and 1.0–2.0 cm inferior to create CTV celiac, variations in expansion based on clinical suspicion for perineural involvement, equivocal nodal involvement, or primary tumor extension
SMA CTV	The proximal 2.0–3.0 cm of the SMA is contoured from the origin at the aorta and expanded a total of 1.0–3.0 cm to the right, 1.0–2.0 cm to the left, 1.0–1.5 cm anterior, 1.0 cm posterior, 1.0 cm superior, and 1.0–2.0 cm inferior to create CTV SMA
SMV CTV	The 1.0 cm of the SMV in closest proximity to the tumor will be contoured and expanded by a total of 0.5–1.0 cm to create CTV SMV; this can be excluded if there is a low degree of clinical suspicion for involvement
CTV 50.4	The above structures are Booleaned together to create CTV 50.4
Variations	For pancreatic tail lesions, the splenic hilum is often prophylactically included and radiated

process of gross tumor volume identification [39, 41, 42]. While MRI may not be routinely indicated, it can provide clarity if tumors are difficult to visualize on CT.

Various methods of neoadjuvant radiation therapy dose escalation are enabled by advanced radiotherapy techniques including IMRT. Dose painting, or simultaneous integrated boost (SIB) techniques, is possible with IMRT [43]. Dose escalation is often difficult as the normal tissues adjacent to the pancreas are very dose sensitive. IMRT, with daily image guidance, can allow for delivery of higher doses than 3D conformal plans with better dose sparing of the adjacent stomach, duodenum, bowel, and kidneys. Radiation therapy can be escalated around pivotal portions of the tumor, such as the retroperitoneal margin, while pulling dose away from the adjacent normal organs [44].

An advantage of IMRT is to produce a greater conformity and precision of the dose distribution as compared with 3D-CRT. This enables dose manipulation to create a sharp dose falloff near the boundaries of tumor and critical normal organs. This may also allow for a higher dose to be delivered to the tumor and a lower dose to the organs at risk of radiation injury or both. IMRT has also been shown to lead to less acute and late toxicity in multiple series [45–47]. Additionally, this enables excellent target volume coverage and, if needed, dose escalation to critical portions of the tumor near adjacent blood vessels.

Conclusions and Future Directions

While controversial, there is considerable evidence as to the role of neoadjuvant therapy in patients with pancreatic cancer. More data is needed to understand the optimal type of neoadjuvant therapy that should be given for these patients. Notable is the considerable heterogeneity of radiation therapy management schedules that exist in the neoadjuvant setting with doses including 5 Gy × 5, 2.4 Gy × 15, 3.0 Gy × 10, and 1.8 Gy × 28 fractions. Further notable is the absence of any randomized data to compare these dose and fractionation schedules. In addition, there are a range of boost schedules that exist for these patients. To our knowledge, there has never been a randomized trial evaluating differences in these fractionation schedules when given in the neoadjuvant setting. This is despite important differences in radiobiological effectiveness of these doses. Additional research is needed to understand differences in the outcomes between these various dose and fractionation schedules.

References

1. Neoptolemos JP, Palmer DH, Ghaneh P, Psarelli EE, Valle JW, Halloran CM, et al. Comparison of adjuvant gemcitabine and capecitabine with gemcitabine monotherapy in patients with resected pancreatic cancer (ESPAC-4): a multicentre, open-label, randomised, phase 3 trial. Lancet. 2017;389(10073):1011–24.
2. Oettle H, Neuhaus P, Hochhaus A, Hartmann JT, Gellert K, Ridwelski K, et al. Adjuvant chemotherapy with gemcitabine and long-term outcomes among patients with resected pancreatic cancer: the CONKO-001 randomized trial. JAMA. 2013;310(14):1473–81.
3. Uesaka K, Boku N, Fukutomi A, Okamura Y, Konishi M, Matsumoto I, et al. Adjuvant chemotherapy of S-1 versus gemcitabine for resected pancreatic cancer: a phase 3, open-label, randomised, non-inferiority trial (JASPAC 01). Lancet. 2016;388(10041):248–57.
4. Ghaneh P, Kleeff J, Halloran CM, Raraty M, Jackson R, Melling J, et al. The impact of positive resection margins on survival and recurrence following resection and adjuvant chemotherapy for pancreatic ductal adenocarcinoma. Ann Surg. 2019;269(3):520–9.
5. Available from: http://www.isrctn.com/ISRCTN89500674.
6. Herman JM, Swartz MJ, Hsu CC, Winter J, Pawlik TM, Sugar E, et al. Analysis of fluorouracil-based adjuvant chemotherapy and radiation after pancreaticoduodenectomy for ductal adenocarcinoma of the pancreas: results of a large, prospectively collected database at the Johns Hopkins Hospital. J Clin Oncol. 2008;26(21):3503–10.
7. Corsini MM, Miller RC, Haddock MG, Donohue JH, Farnell MB, Nagorney DM, et al. Adjuvant radiotherapy and chemotherapy for pancreatic carcinoma: the Mayo Clinic experience (1975–2005). J Clin Oncol. 2008;26(21):3511–6.
8. Kharofa J, Tsai S, Kelly T, Wood C, George B, Ritch P, et al. Neoadjuvant chemoradiation with IMRT in resectable and borderline resectable pancreatic cancer. Radiother Oncol. 2014;113(1):41–6.
9. Evans DB, Varadhachary GR, Crane CH, Sun CC, Lee JE, Pisters PW, et al. Preoperative gemcitabine-based chemoradiation for patients with resectable adenocarcinoma of the pancreatic head. J Clin Oncol. 2008;26(21):3496–502.
10. Evans DB, Rich TA, Byrd DR, Cleary KR, Connelly JH, Levin B, et al. Preoperative chemoradiation and pancreaticoduodenectomy for adenocarcinoma of the pancreas. Arch Surg. 1992;127(11):1335–9.
11. Pisters PW, Abbruzzese JL, Janjan NA, Cleary KR, Charnsangavej C, Goswitz MS, et al. Rapid-fractionation preoperative chemoradiation, pancreaticoduodenectomy, and intraoperative radiation therapy for resectable pancreatic adenocarcinoma. J Clin Oncol. 1998;16(12):3843–50.
12. Pisters PW, Wolff RA, Janjan NA, Cleary KR, Charnsangavej C, Crane CN, et al. Preoperative paclitaxel and concurrent rapid-fractionation radiation for resectable pancreatic adenocarcinoma: toxicities, histologic response rates, and event-free outcome. J Clin Oncol. 2002;20(10):2537–44.
13. Varadhachary GR, Wolff RA, Crane CH, Sun CC, Lee JE, Pisters PW, et al. Preoperative gemcitabine and cisplatin followed by gemcitabine-based chemoradiation for resectable adenocarcinoma of the pancreatic head. J Clin Oncol. 2008;26(21):3487–95.
14. Christians KK, Heimler JW, George B, Ritch PS, Erickson BA, Johnston F, et al. Survival of patients with resectable pancreatic cancer who received neoadjuvant therapy. Surgery. 2016;159(3):893–900.
15. Mokdad AA, Minter RM, Zhu H, Augustine MM, Porembka MR, Wang SC, et al. Neoadjuvant therapy followed by resection versus upfront resection for resectable pancreatic cancer: a propensity score matched analysis. J Clin Oncol. 2017;35(5):515–22.

16. Papavasiliou P, Chun YS, Hoffman JP. How to define and manage borderline resectable pancreatic cancer. Surg Clin North Am. 2013;93(3):663–74.
17. Varadhachary GR, Tamm EP, Crane C, Evans DB, Wolff RA. Borderline resectable pancreatic cancer. Curr Treat Options Gastroenterol. 2005;8(5):377–84.
18. Katz MH, Pisters PW, Evans DB, Sun CC, Lee JE, Fleming JB, et al. Borderline resectable pancreatic cancer: the importance of this emerging stage of disease. J Am Coll Surg. 2008;206(5):833–46; discussion 46–8.
19. Conroy T, Desseigne F, Ychou M, Bouche O, Guimbaud R, Becouarn Y, et al. FOLFIRINOX versus gemcitabine for metastatic pancreatic cancer. N Engl J Med. 2011;364(19):1817–25.
20. Christians KK, Tsai S, Mahmoud A, Ritch P, Thomas JP, Wiebe L, et al. Neoadjuvant FOLFIRINOX for borderline resectable pancreas cancer: a new treatment paradigm? Oncologist. 2014;19(3):266–74.
21. Paniccia A, Edil BH, Schulick RD, Byers JT, Meguid C, Gajdos C, et al. Neoadjuvant FOLFIRINOX application in borderline resectable pancreatic adenocarcinoma: a retrospective cohort study. Medicine (Baltimore). 2014;93(27):e198.
22. Blazer M, Wu C, Goldberg RM, Phillips G, Schmidt C, Muscarella P, et al. Neoadjuvant modified (m) FOLFIRINOX for locally advanced unresectable (LAPC) and borderline resectable (BRPC) adenocarcinoma of the pancreas. Ann Surg Oncol. 2015;22(4):1153–9.
23. Petrelli F, Coinu A, Borgonovo K, Cabiddu M, Ghilardi M, Lonati V, et al. FOLFIRINOX-based neoadjuvant therapy in borderline resectable or unresectable pancreatic cancer: a meta-analytical review of published studies. Pancreas. 2015;44(4):515–21.
24. Katz MHG, Ou FS, Herman JM, Ahmad SA, Wolpin B, Marsh R, et al. Alliance for clinical trials in oncology (ALLIANCE) trial A021501: preoperative extended chemotherapy vs. chemotherapy plus hypofractionated radiation therapy for borderline resectable adenocarcinoma of the head of the pancreas. BMC Cancer. 2017;17(1):505.
25. Lo SS, Fakiris AJ, Chang EL, Mayr NA, Wang JZ, Papiez L, et al. Stereotactic body radiation therapy: a novel treatment modality. Nat Rev Clin Oncol. 2010;7(1):44–54.
26. Chuong MD, Springett GM, Freilich JM, Park CK, Weber JM, Mellon EA, et al. Stereotactic body radiation therapy for locally advanced and borderline resectable pancreatic cancer is effective and well tolerated. Int J Radiat Oncol Biol Phys. 2013;86(3):516–22.
27. Palta M. Gemcitabine/Nab-Paclitaxel with HIGRT in resectablepancreatic cancer 2017. Available from: https://clinicaltrials.gov/ct2/show/NCT02318095?term=palta&cond=Pancreatic+Cancer&rank=1.
28. Wang LS, Shaikh T, Handorf EA, Hoffman JP, Cohen SJ, Meyer JE. Dose escalation with a vessel boost in pancreatic adenocarcinoma treated with neoadjuvantchemoradiation. Pract Radiat Oncol. 2015;5(5):e457–63.
29. Huang X, Knoble JL, Zeng M, Aguila FN, Patel T, Chambers LW, et al. Neoadjuvant gemcitabine chemotherapy followed by concurrent IMRT simultaneous boost achieves high R0 resection in borderline resectable pancreatic cancer patients. PLoS One. 2016;11(12):e0166606.
30. Kim EJ, Ben-Josef E, Herman JM, Bekaii-Saab T, Dawson LA, Griffith KA, et al. A multi-institutional phase 2 study of neoadjuvant gemcitabine and oxaliplatin with radiation therapy in patients with pancreatic cancer. Cancer. 2013;119(15):2692–700.
31. Hong TS, Ryan DP, Borger DR, Blaszkowsky LS, Yeap BY, Ancukiewicz M, et al. A phase 1/2 and biomarker study of preoperative short course chemoradiation with proton beam therapy and capecitabine followed by early surgery for resectable pancreatic ductal adenocarcinoma. Int J Radiat Oncol Biol Phys. 2014;89(4):830–8.
32. Sauer R, Becker H, Hohenberger W, Rodel C, Wittekind C, Fietkau R, et al. Preoperative versus postoperative chemoradiotherapy for rectal cancer. N Engl J Med. 2004;351(17):1731–40.
33. Doi R, Imamura M, Hosotani R, Imaizumi T, Hatori T, Takasaki K, et al. Surgery versus radiochemotherapy for resectable locally invasive pancreatic cancer: final results of a randomized multi-institutional trial. Surg Today. 2008;38(11):1021–8.
34. Golcher H, Brunner TB, Witzigmann H, Marti L, Bechstein WO, Bruns C, et al. Neoadjuvant chemoradiation therapy with gemcitabine/cisplatin and surgery versus immediate surgery in resectable pancreatic cancer: results of the first prospective randomized phase II trial. Strahlentherapie und Onkologie : Organ der DeutschenRontgengesellschaft [et al]. 2015;191(1):7–16.
35. Versteijne E, van Eijck CH, Punt CJ, Suker M, Zwinderman AH, Dohmen MA, et al. Preoperative radiochemotherapy versus immediate surgery for resectable and borderline resectable pancreatic cancer (PREOPANC trial): study protocol for a multicentre randomized controlled trial. Trials. 2016;17(1):127.
36. Tachezy M, Gebauer F, Petersen C, Arnold D, Trepel M, Wegscheider K, et al. Sequential neoadjuvantchemoradiotherapy (CRT) followed by curative surgery vs. primary surgery alone for resectable, non-metastasized pancreatic adenocarcinoma: NEOPA- a randomized multicenter phase III study (NCT01900327, DRKS00003893, ISRCTN82191749). BMC Cancer. 2014;14:411.
37. Reese AS, Lu W, Regine WF. Utilization of intensity-modulated radiation therapy and image-guided radiation therapy in pancreatic cancer: is it beneficial? Semin Radiat Oncol. 2014;24(2):132–9.
38. Jaffray DA. Image-guided radiotherapy: from current concept to future perspectives. Nat Rev Clin Oncol. 2012;9(12):688–99.
39. Hall WA, Heerkens HD, Paulson ES, Meijer GJ, Kotte AN, Knechtges P, et al. Pancreatic gross tumor volume contouring on computed tomography (CT) compared with magnetic resonance imaging (MRI): results of

an international contouring conference. Pract Radiat Oncol. 2018;8(2):107–15.
40. Dholakia AS, Kumar R, Raman SP, Moore JA, Ellsworth S, McNutt T, et al. Mapping patterns of local recurrence after pancreaticoduodenectomy for pancreatic adenocarcinoma: a new approach to adjuvant radiation field design. Int J Radiat Oncol Biol Phys. 2013;87(5):1007–15.
41. Heerkens HD, Hall WA, Li XA, Knechtges P, Dalah E, Paulson ES, et al. Recommendations for MRI-based contouring of gross tumor volume and organs at risk for radiation therapy of pancreatic cancer. Pract Radiat Oncol. 2017;7(2):126–36.
42. Hall WA, Mikell JL, Mittal P, Colbert L, Prabhu RS, Kooby DA, et al. Tumor size on abdominal MRI versus pathologic specimen in resected pancreatic adenocarcinoma: implications for radiation treatment planning. Int J Radiat Oncol Biol Phys. 2013;86(1):102–7.
43. Shaib WL, Hawk N, Cassidy RJ, Chen Z, Zhang C, Brutcher E, et al. A phase 1 study of stereotactic body radiation therapy dose escalation for borderline resectable pancreatic cancer after modified FOLFIRINOX (NCT01446458). Int J Radiat Oncol Biol Phys. 2016;96(2):296–303.
44. Krishnan S, Chadha AS, Suh Y, Chen HC, Rao A, Das P, et al. Focal radiation therapy dose escalation improves overall survival in locally advanced pancreatic cancer patients receiving induction chemotherapy and consolidative chemoradiation. Int J Radiat Oncol Biol Phys. 2016;94(4):755–65.
45. Abelson JA, Murphy JD, Minn AY, Chung M, Fisher GA, Ford JM, et al. Intensity-modulated radiotherapy for pancreatic adenocarcinoma. Int J Radiat Oncol Biol Phys. 2012;82(4):e595–601.
46. Bittner MI, Grosu AL, Brunner TB. Comparison of toxicity after IMRT and 3D-conformal radiotherapy for patients with pancreatic cancer - a systematic review. RadiotherOncol: Journal of the European Society for Therapeutic Radiology and Oncology. 2015;114(1):117–21.
47. Lee KJ, Yoon HI, Chung MJ, Park JY, Bang S, Park SW, et al. A comparison of gastrointestinal toxicities between intensity-modulated radiotherapy and three-dimensional conformal radiotherapy for pancreatic cancer. GutLiver. 2016;10(2):303–9.
48. Hoffman JP, Lipsitz S, Pisansky T, Weese JL, Solin L, Benson AB 3rd. Phase II trial of preoperative radiation therapy and chemotherapy for patients with localized, resectable adenocarcinoma of the pancreas: an Eastern Cooperative Oncology Group Study. J Clin Oncol. 1998;16(1):317–23.

New Classification of Locally Advanced Pancreatic Cancer

9

Kathleen K. Christians

Background The eighth edition of the American Joint Committee on Cancer (AJCC) staging system for pancreatic cancer was released in late 2016 and is the system that clinicians and patients are most familiar [1]. In this staging system, the primary tumor (T) is classified as T1 through T4 based on size of the tumor and involvement of the celiac axis (CA), superior mesenteric artery (SMA), and/or common hepatic artery (CHA) (Table 9.1).Tumors are then assigned a stage (I–IV) based on a combination of tumor stage, the number of nodes involved by tumor, and the presence or absence of metastatic disease (Table 9.2). While the TNM stage is a very accurate assessment of the pathologic (resected) stage, it does not aid surgeons in determining whether the patient's tumor can be surgically removed. The only current meaningful chance for patients with pancreatic cancer to have prolonged survival is to achieve an R0 (or R1) margin-negative surgical resection. It is well documented that survival is poor (similar to inoperable patients) for those who undergo incomplete (R2) resection; therefore, staging patients by resection status is a critical component to their management [2–5]. Rather than utilizing TNM stage, the patient's tumors

Table 9.1 AJCC eighth edition TNM definitions

T1	Tumor ≤2 cm in greatest dimension
T1a	Tumor ≤0.5 cm in greatest dimension
T1b	Tumor >0.5 cm and <1 cm in greatest dimension
T1c	Tumor 1–2 cm in greatest dimension
T2	Tumor >2 cm and ≤4 cm in greatest dimension
T3	Tumor >4 cm in greatest dimension
T4	Tumor involves the CA, SMA, and/or CHA regardless of size
N0	No regional nodal metastases
N1	1–3 regional nodal metastases
N2	≥4 regional nodal metastases
M0	No distant metastases
M1	Distant metastases

CA celiac axis, *SMA* superior mesenteric artery, *CHA* common hepatic artery

Table 9.2 AJCC Stage based on TNM status

T	N	M	Stage
T1	N0	M0	IA
T1	N1	M0	IIB
T1	N2	M0	III
T2	N0	M0	IB
T2	N1	M0	IIB
T2	N2	M0	III
T3	N0	M0	IIA
T3	N1	M0	IIB
T3	N2	Mo	III
T4	Any N	M0	III
Any T	Any N	M1	IV

K. K. Christians (✉)
Division of Surgical Oncology, Department of Surgery, The Medical College of Wisconsin, Milwaukee, WI, USA
e-mail: kchristi@mcw.edu

S. Tsai et al. (eds.), *Management of Localized Pancreatic Cancer*,
https://doi.org/10.1007/978-3-319-98944-0_9

are classified as clinically resectable, borderline resectable, locally advanced, or metastatic. This is not based on a judgment call made at the time of laparotomy but rather objective radiographic criteria acquired by multidetector computed tomography or magnetic resonance images, largely driven by the presence or absence of vascular involvement [6, 7]. Abutment is defined as tumor involvement that touches/involves the vessel ≤180°, and encasement is considered any tumor-vessel involvement that is >180°. The clinical staging criteria for localized pancreatic cancer utilized by the Medical College of Wisconsin pancreatic cancer team is seen in Table 9.3.

While the controversy raged on for many years regarding the concept of delivering neoadjuvant, as opposed to adjuvant therapy to patients with pancreatic cancer, most clinicians now support the use of neoadjuvant therapy for (at least) patients with borderline resectable pancreatic cancer [8, 9]. These patients, by definition, have an operable tumor that involves a larger, more technically complex, and often high-risk operation as compared to patients with resectable disease. Knowing that survival is improved with multimodality therapy, it only makes sense that the most toxic therapy (surgery) would fall last in the treatment sequencing line. In contrast to resectable and borderline resectable pancreatic cancers, locally advanced pancreatic cancers are a relatively small subset of patients who have no evidence of metastatic disease but whose tumor encases critical visceral arterial or venous structures. In most centers, locally advanced pancreatic cancer patients have been largely considered inoperable, and the median overall survival has been limited to 1–2 years with chemotherapy +/− radiation alone. As cancer treatments have improved, an increasing subset of patients with locally advanced disease have received extensive chemotherapy and have potentially even been radiated, without evidence of local or distant disease progression. Our group at the Medical College of Wisconsin has therefore sought to not only challenge the definition of what is "inoperable" but also provide patients a probability for resection from the date of initial diagnosis. Locally advanced type A patients are those patients who have tumor-vessel involvement which may allow for a potential surgical resection after an extended course of neoadjuvant chemotherapy and chemoradiation, whereas those patients categorized as having locally advanced type B tumors have extensive tumor-vessel involvement and are unlikely to ever be taken to the operating room for resection. These categories were created based on our experience that a plane between the adventitia of the artery and the surrounding neural tissue can often be developed and thereby the tumor separated from the vessel. In order for this to be true, the tumor must not encompass the vessel by 360°, or one would cut through tumor to do so. Importantly, all patients were treated with at least 4–6 months of chemotherapy followed by chemoradiation prior to ever being taken to the operating room for resection. We would never consider taking a locally advanced pancreatic cancer patient to the operating room for up-front surgery. In addition, these patients had to

Table 9.3 Medical College of Wisconsin pancreas cancer clinical staging system

Vessel involvement	Resectable	Borderline resectable	Locally Advanced Type A	Locally Advanced Type B
SMA	None	≤180° involved	>180°but ≤270°	>270°
CA	None	≤180° involved	>180°but no extension to the aorta and CA resection (+/− reconstruction) possible	>180° and abuts/encases the aorta
HA	None	Short segment, not extending to CA or HA bifurcation	>180° with extension to the CA and reconstruction possible	>180° with extension beyond the bifurcation of the proper HA into the right and left HA
SMV/PV	<50% if present	>50%; if occluded, suitable PV above and SMV below to reconstruct	Occlusion but can be reconstructed	Occlusion without option for reconstruction
Other		Biopsy-proven N1 disease or indeterminate distant disease (lung/liver)		

SMA superior mesenteric artery, *CA* celiac artery, *HA* hepatic artery, *SMV* superior mesenteric vein, *PV* portal vein demonstrate a performance status <2 (preferably 0-1), a falling (preferably normalized) carbohydrate antigen 19-9 (CA 19-9), and a lack of any comorbidities, which may preclude a major operation with concomitant vascular resection/reconstruction. The discreet anatomic definitions of locally advanced type A and locally advanced type B pancreatic cancer are seen in Table 9.3, and imaging examples of these findings are provided in Figs. 9.1a–d and 9.2a–d.

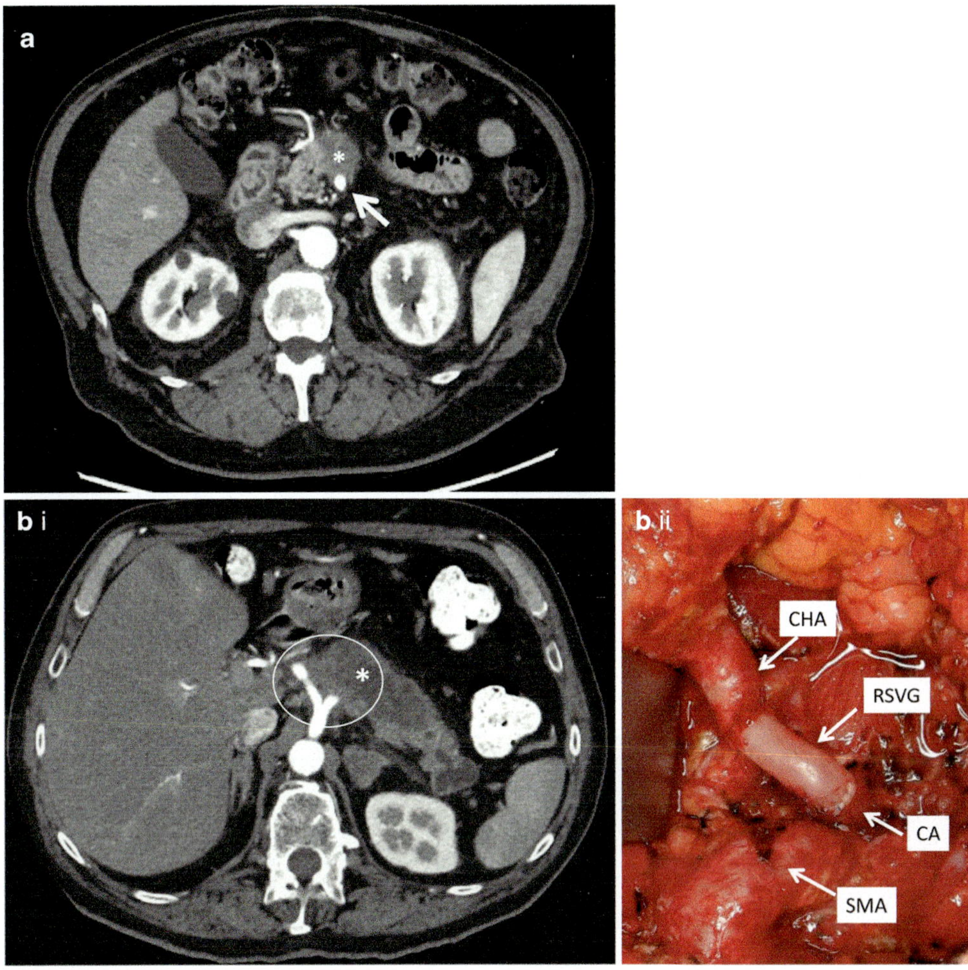

Fig. 9.1 Locally advanced Type A pancreatic cancer. (**a**) Axial computed tomography image of a locally advanced pancreatic neck tumor that involves the SMA >180° but <270° and is therefore considered Type A and potentially resectable (arrow points to SMA; asterisk marks tumor). (**b**) (i) Axial computed tomography image of a pancreatic body tumor that involves the bifurcation of the celiac axis into the common hepatic artery and splenic artery. The celiac trunk is uninvolved making this tumor potentially resectable (asterisk marks tumor; circle encompasses celiac axis). (ii) We prefer to revascularize ("supercharge") the common hepatic artery by placing a reverse saphenous vein graft between the celiac trunk and distal common hepatic artery just before the takeoff of the gastroduodenal artery as shown in this intraoperative photograph. This maneuver restores forward arterial flow through the common hepatic artery therefore not relying on reverse flow through the superior mesenteric artery and pancreaticoduodenal arcade to supply the stomach and liver as occurs with a standard Appleby (CHA, common hepatic artery; RSVG, reversed saphenous vein graft; CA, celiac axis; SMA, superior mesenteric artery). (**c**) (i) Axial CT image of a large pancreatic body tumor that involves the common and proper hepatic arteries (oval shape encircles). (ii) The bifurcation into the right and left hepatic arteries seen on this axial CT image is free of disease making this tumor potentially resectable (arrow points to uninvolved bifurcation). (**d**) (i) This axial CT image of a locally advanced pancreatic neck tumor illustrates focal near occlusion of the superior mesenteric vein (asterisk marks tumor; arrow points to nearly occluded SMV). (ii) The superior mesenteric vein reconstitutes and provides an appropriate distal target for reconstruction (arrow points to the SMV)

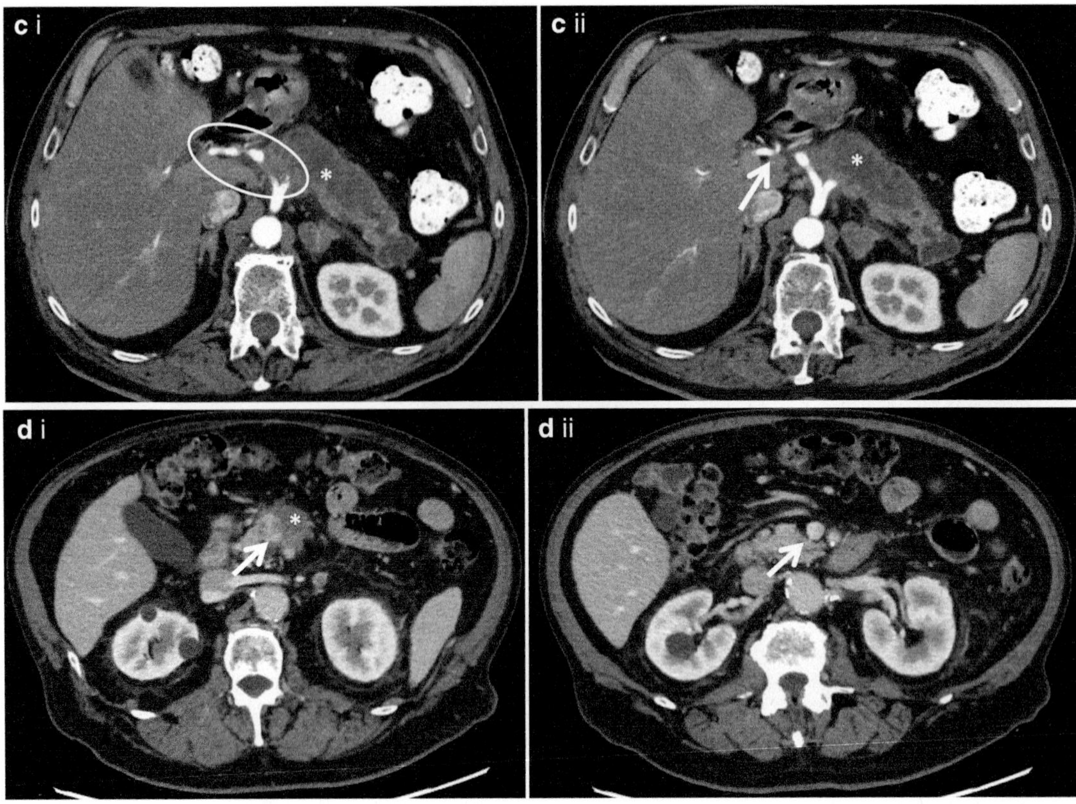

Fig. 9.1 (continued)

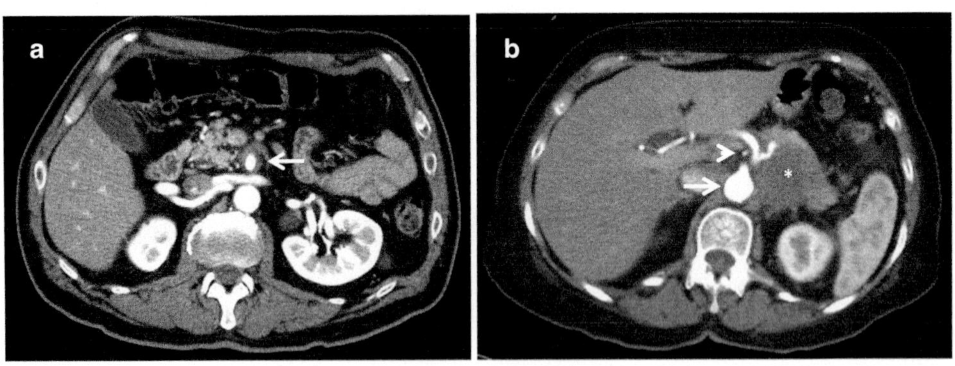

Fig. 9.2 Locally advanced Type B pancreatic cancer. (**a**) Axial computed tomography image revealing 360° tumor encasement of the superior mesenteric artery (SMA).The tumor involves the SMA >270° and is therefore, by definition, considered Locally advanced Type B (arrow points to SMA). (**b**) Axial computed tomography image illustrating tumor involvement of the celiac axis; the patient is considered Type B due to tumor extension to the aorta (asterisk marks tumor; arrow head points to celiac axis; arrow points to the aorta). (**c**) (i) Axial computed tomography image illustrating tumor encasement of the common hepatic artery (oval). (ii) Axial computed tomography extension of the tumor beyond the bifurcation into the right and left branches. Tumor that extends to this bifurcation is considered inoperable and therefore Locally advanced Type B (oval illustrates tumor engulfing the proper hepatic artery; arrow points to bifurcation into right and left hepatic artery branches). (**d**) Locally advanced pancreatic neck tumor causing cavernous transformation of the portal vein. There is no superior target for vascular resection/reconstruction, and therefore the tumor is considered Locally advanced Type B (asterisk marks tumor; arrow points to collaterals formed from portal vein occlusion)

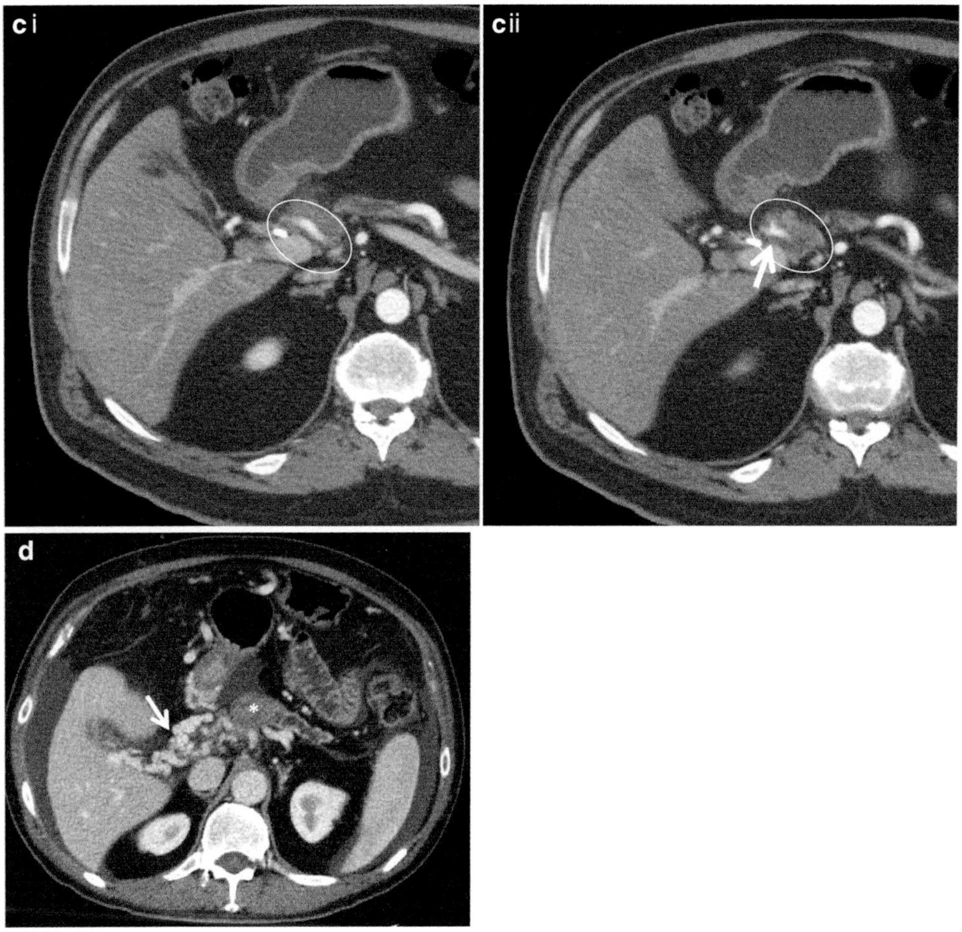

Fig. 9.2 (continued)

Rationale for Type A and Type B by Vascular Involvement

SMA In general, any involvement of the SMA >270° is considered locally advanced type B as there is no option (in the absence of resection/reconstruction) to remove the tumor without cutting through it, an oncologically unacceptable maneuver. Please note that the authors do not advocate for SMA resection and reconstruction for pancreatic cancer at this time due to the high risk of mortality if the vessel occludes and the extreme morbidity of denervation of the midgut which results in rapid transit and debilitating diarrhea in many.

Celiac Axis A 360° involvement of the celiac axis with preservation of the origin of the celiac artery off the aorta is considered locally advanced type A. Once the tumor involves the aorta, the chance of cutting through tumor is nearly 100% and thus considered Type B. If the tumor can be separated from the celiac axis and its branches (with the removal of all of the associated tumor-infiltrated perineurium), this is preferred over resection and reconstruction. If the tumor is inseparable from these vessels, the tumor is resected en bloc with the celiac axis if either the left gastric artery can be preserved (preferred) or the gastroduodenal artery can be preserved in order to provide retrograde flow via the pancreaticoduodenal arcades to the gastroepiploic (stomach). In the absence of either a preserved left gastric artery or gastroduodenal artery, the risk of gastric necrosis with resection of the celiac axis is high. The authors will not perform a total gastrectomy along with a total pancreatectomy due to the associated morbidity; therefore, either the left gastric artery or the gastroduodenal artery must be uninvolved with tumor or the operation will not be undertaken.

Common Hepatic Artery The tumor can sometimes be separated from this vessel by dissecting the plane between the adventitia and neural tissue that surrounds it (Fig. 9.3). Preoperative radiation has been observed to facilitate this dissection. Importantly, the neural tissue must then be resected en bloc with the main pancreatic tumor, or it would become the source of local disease recurrence. If the tumor cannot be separated from the vessel, then the vessel is resected and reconstructed with a reversed saphenous vein graft (preferred vascular conduit for the common hepatic artery due to size). Once the proper hepatic artery branches into the right and left branches, the anastomosis becomes one that requires microvascular work, and the risk of occlusion is increased. We therefore mandate that the distal proper hepatic artery must be free of tumor before branching into the right and left hepatic arteries to be considered locally advanced type A. Tumor infiltration beyond the bifurcation into the right and left hepatic arteries is therefore considered locally advanced type B.

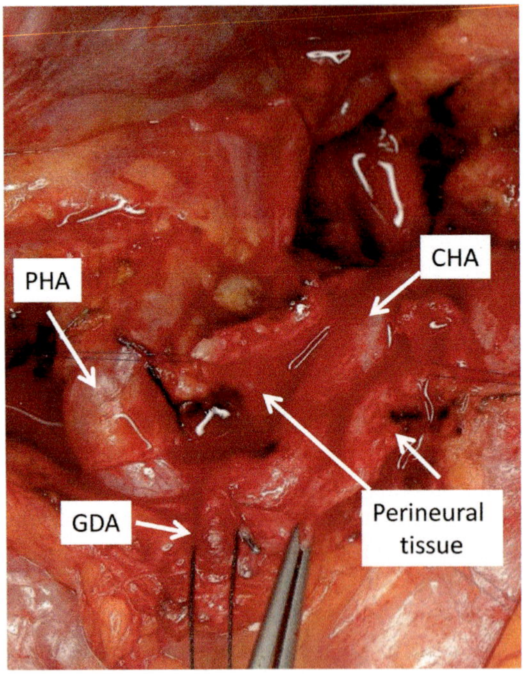

Fig. 9.3 Intraoperative photograph illustrating dissection of the tumor-infiltrated perineurium from the underlying common hepatic artery. This tissue is then resected en bloc with the main pancreatic tumor to achieve an R0 resection (PHA, proper hepatic artery; CHA, common hepatic artery; GDA, gastroduodenal artery)

Superior Mesenteric Vein/Portal Vein The SMV/PV classification is similar to that of borderline resectable patients. The patients are considered Type A if there is acceptable PV above and caliber/length of the SMV below the occlusion for resection/reconstruction. If either the PV above or the SMV below is not of adequate caliber or length to reconstruct, then the patient is considered locally advanced type B. This is a modification from our initial work on this subject [10].

It goes without saying that most locally advanced pancreatic cancer patients rarely present with a single artery involved but rather a combination of artery(ies) and PV-SMV involvement which greatly increases the complexity and risk of the operation. The authors have written extensively about the nuances of these operations and utilize various shunts to facilitate safe exposure and resection/reconstruction of the involved vasculature [11–14].

Utilizing this new classification for locally advanced pancreatic cancer in the context of an extended course of neoadjuvant chemotherapy and chemoradiation, we have been able to achieve an overall resectability rate of 42%, 85% when considering only those who were taken to surgery and given general anesthesia[11]. Sixty-two percent of the locally advanced type A patients underwent surgical resection resulting in a median survival of 55.6 months, whereas 24% of the locally advanced type B patients were resected achieving a median survival of 37.5 months. The overall median survival of Type A and B patients was 38.9 months for those who were able to complete all neoadjuvant therapy and surgery [11]. These numbers rival earlier stages of this disease, outperform the survival seen utilizing chemotherapy and/or radiation alone, and support the concept that not all locally advanced pancreatic cancer is, or should be, considered inoperable.

Conclusion

Treatment for pancreatic cancer continues to evolve. New therapies are emerging in the arena of molecular profiling and targeted therapies and will soon incorporate knowledge from the realm of genetics and epigenetics. It is quite likely that pancreatic surgeons will see more and more patients with tumors involving complex vascular anatomy that a able to live longer with improved multimodality therapies. Our data illustrates that not all locally advanced pancreatic cancer is inoperable, but discrete anatomic findings on axial imaging will allow clinicians to predict which locally advanced patients will be able to complete all multimodality therapy including surgery and give patients the chance for survival beyond that afforded by chemotherapy and radiation alone.

References

1. Kakar S, Pawlik TM, Allen PJ, Vauthey JN. Exocrine Pancreas. In: Amin MB, et al., editors. AJCC cancer staging manual, vol. 28. 8th ed. Cham: Springer; 2017. p. 337–47.
2. Millikan KW, Deziel DJ, Silverstein JC, et al. Prognostic factors associated with resectable cancer of the head of the pancreas. Am Surg. 1999;65:618–23; discussion 623–4.
3. Sohn TA, Yeo CJ, Cameron JL, et al. Resected cancer of the pancreas—616 patients: results, outcomes, and prognostic indicators. J Gastrointest Surg. 2000;4:567–79.
4. Neoptolemos JP, Stocken DD, Dunn JA, et al. Influence of resection margins on survival for patients with pancreatic cancer treated by adjuvant chemoradiation and/or chemotherapy chemotherapy in the ESPAC-1 randomized controlled trial. Ann Surg. 2001;234:758–68.
5. Kuhlmann KF, de Castro SM, Wesseling JG, et al. Surgical treatment of pancreatic cancer; actual survival and prognostic factors in 343 patients. Eur J Cancer. 2004;40:549–58.
6. Varadhachary GR, Tamm EP, Abbruzzese JL, et al. Borderline resectable pancreatic cancer: definitions, management, and role of preoperative therapy. Ann Surg Oncol. 2006;13(8):1035–46.
7. Callery MP, Chang KJ, Fishman EK, et al. Pretreatment assessment of resectable an borderline resectable pancreatic cancer: expert consensus statement. Ann Surg Oncol. 2009;16:1727–33.
8. NCCN clinical practice guidelines in oncology. Pancreatic cancer. Version 1; 2017. February 24, 2017. https://www.nccn.org/professionals/physician_fls/f_guidelines.asp#pancreatic.pdf.
9. Fathi A, Christians KK, George B, et al. Neoadjuvant therapy for localized pancreatic cancer: guiding principles. J Gastrointest Oncol. 2015;6:418–29.
10. Tsai S, Christians KK, Ritch P, et al. Multimodality therapy in patients with borderline resectable or locally advanced pancreatic cancer: importance of locoregional therapies for a systemic disease. J Oncol Pract. 2016;12(10):915–23.
11. Chatzizacharias N, Tsai S, Griffin M, et al. Locally advanced pancreas cancer: staging and goals of therapy. Surgery. 2018;163:1053–62; 160 Epub ahead of print.
12. Younan G, Tsai S, Evans DB, Christians KK. Techniques of vascular resection and reconstruction in pancreatic cancer. Surg Clin North Am. 2016;96(6):1351–70.
13. Pilgrim CH, Tsai S, Tolat P, Patel P, Rilling W, Evans DB, Christians KK. Optimal management of the splenic vein at the time of venous resection for pancreatic cancer: importance of the inferior mesenteric vein. J Gastrointest Surg. 2014;18(5):917–21.
14. Pilgrim CH, Tsai S, Evans DB, Christians KK. Mesocaval shunting: a novel technique to facilitate venous resection and reconstruction and enhance exposure of the superior mesenteric and celiac arteries during pancreaticoduodenectomy. J Am Coll Surg. 2013;217(3):e17–20.

10 Treatment Sequencing for Locally Advanced Pancreatic Cancer

Kathleen K. Christians and Beth A. Erickson

Historically, patients with locally advanced pancreatic cancer (LAPC) lived 9–13 months and had a 5-year survival of <5%. They were considered inoperable largely due, by definition, to the major vasculature involved (superior mesenteric artery [SMA], celiac axis, common hepatic artery [CHA], portal vein/superior mesenteric vein [PV/SMV]). Involvement of these vessels not only significantly escalated the operative risk and potential surgical complications but also required knowledge of the anatomic nuances of this region and surgical skill and techniques neither taught in most surgical residencies nor in advanced fellowships. Researchers have also shown that seeding of distant organs occurs before, and in parallel to, tumor formation at the primary site [1]. In a disease with micrometastatic disease (at least) at diagnosis, a surgery alone or even a surgery-first approach is therefore not logical.

Chemotherapy addresses the issue of metastatic disease at presentation. Gemcitabine was Food and Drug Administration (FDA)-approved in 1997 as first-line therapy for pancreatic cancer based on a phase III study showing clinical benefit (23.8% vs. 4.8%) relative to 5-fluorouracil (5FU), with a median survival of 5.6 versus 4.4 months and a 1-year survival of 18% vs. 2% [2]. While an improvement from palliation alone, single-agent gemcitabine resulted in only a meager benefit to the patient. This led researchers to try multiple gemcitabine-based therapies with most showing prolonged survival in mainly good performance status (PS) patients [3–5]. Eventually, it was discovered that the combination of gemcitabine with nab paclitaxel improved intratumoral delivery of both drugs facilitated by albumin. This resulted in improvement in median overall survival (OS) of 8.5 vs. 6.7 months, progression-free survival (PFS) of 5.5 vs. 3.7 months, and 1-year survival of 35% vs. 22% [6, 7]. Within a similar time frame, FOLFIRINOX (5FU, leucovorin, irinotecan, oxaliplatin) emerged as a combination therapy for pancreatic cancer resulting in an OS of 11.1 vs. 6.8 months, PFS of 6.4 vs. 3.3 months, and a 1-year survival of 48.4% vs. 20.6% [8] (Table 10.1). However, while an improvement from the single-agent gemcitabine era, systemic chemotherapy as a standalone treatment for pancreatic cancer still provided pancreatic cancer patients with an anticipated <1-year survival.

Radiation therapy had similar early mixed reviews in the treatment of pancreatic cancer. Older studies not only failed to show a benefit but also underscored the potential toxicities. These

K. K. Christians (✉)
Division of Surgical Oncology, Department of Surgery, The Medical College of Wisconsin, Milwaukee, WI, USA
e-mail: kchristi@mcw.edu

B. A. Erickson
Department of Radiation Oncology, The Medical College of Wisconsin, Milwaukee, WI, USA

S. Tsai et al. (eds.), *Management of Localized Pancreatic Cancer*,
https://doi.org/10.1007/978-3-319-98944-0_10

Table 10.1 FDA-approved drug combinations for pancreatic cancer

Drugs	*N*	OS in months	*P* value
Gem vs. 5FU	126	5.65 vs. 4.4	0.0025
Gem erlotinib vs. gem	569	6.2 vs. 5.9	0.038
Gem abraxane vs. gem	861	8.5 vs. 6.7	<0.001
FOLFIRINOX vs. gem	342	11.1 vs. 6.8	<0.001

Gem gemcitabine, *FOLFIRINOX* 5FU, leucovorin, irinotecan, oxaliplatin

early studies were fraught with a lack of standardization, utilizing suboptimal doses, treatment delivery methods, and treatment duration, and swayed many clinicians away from the use of radiation for pancreatic cancer. However, more recent trials such as the Eastern Cooperative Oncology Group (ECOG) 4201 and the Selective Chemoradiation in Advanced Localized Pancreatic (SCALOP) cancer trials both revealed a survival advantage [9, 10]. ECOG 4201 compared gemcitabine to gemcitabine plus chemoradiation and showed an 11.1 month vs. 9.2 month ($P = 0.017$) improved median OS in those receiving chemoradiation. Similarly, the SCALOP trial was a randomized phase II trial where LAPC patients received induction gemcitabine plus capecitabine. In those who responded, another cycle of chemotherapy was administered, and patients were then treated with either gemcitabine- or capecitabine-based chemoradiation (50.4 Gy in 28 fractions). Median OS was 14.6 months for those who were treated with chemoradiation and 8.1 months for those who were unable to receive the intended chemoradiation and treated with chemotherapy alone. The SCALOP trial reinforced two important concepts in pancreatic cancer treatment (1) the use of chemotherapy first to select responders for local therapy and (2) the survival benefit for those who were able to receive chemoradiation. Key also to the success of the SCALOP trial was a central review of a pretrial test case in which the contours of the planned radiation tumor target as well as the radiation plan were reviewed for adherence to protocol guidelines. Furthermore, Krishnan et al. [11] highlighted the benefit of dose-escalated chemoradiation wherein 47 of 200 patients were treated with capecitabine radiation with dose escalation to a biologic effective dose of >70 Gy utilizing a simultaneous integrated boost technique, motion management with an inspiration breath-hold technique, and daily image-guided (computed tomography) radiation therapy (IGRT). The authors demonstrated a 17.8 month vs. 15.0 month OS advantage for the dose-escalated patients as well as an improved regional recurrence free survival (10.2 vs. 6.2 months [$P = 0.05$]). Chung SY et al. also demonstrated that patients who received higher doses of radiation therapy (EQD2 > 61 Gy) even after propensity matching had improved OS, improved PFS, and improved local failure rate with similar toxicities to standard chemoradiation doses [12].

In addition to dose escalation, an emerging treatment in the realm of radiation therapy is stereotactic body radiotherapy (SBRT). A recent study in *Cancer* reviewed the survival impact of SBRT on unresected, nonmetastatic pancreatic cancer. A National Cancer Data Base (NCDB) review revealed that prior to matching, median survival for chemotherapy alone was 9.9 months, three-dimensional standard dose fractionated external beam radiation therapy (EBRT) was 10.9 months, intensity modulated radiation therapy (IMRT) was 12 months, and SBRT was 13.9 months. In separate matched analysis, SBRT was superior to chemotherapy alone (log rank $P < 0.0001$) and ERBT (log rank $P = 0.180$). After matching, survival did not differ between IMRT and SBRT (log rank $P = 0.0492$)[13]. Proponents of SBRT cite the advantages of being able to deliver the therapy in 3–5 days, without the requirement of concurrent chemotherapy and with tumor control that is equivalent to, or perhaps better, than standard chemoradiotherapy [14]. Further dose escalation using SBRT or IMRT with a simultaneous integrated boost may improve outcomes, especially with the addition of evolving MR-guided radiation techniques. The unknowns with this emerging therapy include (1) the safety of vascular resection and reconstruction following SBRT and dose intense IMRT and (2) local-regional control, as radiation fields are currently not standardized and often, in an effort to reduce morbidity, not designed to include nodes and perineural tissue that are frequently positive in borderline resectable and locally advanced cases.

While it is true that systemic chemotherapy continues to evolve/improve and chemoradiation via IMRT and SBRT techniques with/without dose escalation results in improved OS for patients with LAPC, it is clear that chemotherapy alone and chemoradiation alone have not resulted in long-term (>2 year) survivors. Patients with LAPC whose tumors progress on first-line chemotherapy have three options: (1) switch chemotherapeutic agents, (2) participate in a clinical trial, or (3) best supportive care. However, those who show treatment response after 4–6 months of chemotherapy, defined as less pain, improved performance status, drop/normalization of cancer antigen 19-9(CA 19-9), and stable or shrinking primary tumor, are the subset of patients with favorable biology where folding in a local therapy may play an important role in OS. Autopsy series show that nearly one third of patients die of locally destructive disease progression rather than metastatic disease [15]. There is also evidence that local control, or at least delay in local progression, is paramount to both preventing disease progression and improving OS [16].

Our pancreatic cancer group has taken the discussion of the best treatment algorithm for LAPC one step further. We recently described two categories of LAPC – type A and type B (Table 10.2). These categories were created based on discreet anatomic definitions with varying probabilities of completing all multimodality treatment (neoadjuvant chemotherapy plus chemoradiation, followed by surgical resection). LAPC type A was defined as SMA involvement that was >180° but ≤270°; celiac axis involvement that was >180° of the vessel, but not touching the aorta and with a viable option for resection with/without reconstruction; and>180° involvement of the CHA with extension to the

Table 10.2 Staging of locally advanced pancreatic cancer

Vascular structures, any of which, can determine the stage of PC	Locally advanced PC	
	Type A	Type B
SMA	>180°, but ≤270° encasement	>270° encasement
Celiac	>180° but doesn't extend to the aorta, resectable w/wo reconstruction	>180° and abuts/encases the aorta
Hepatic artery	>180° and extends to celiac but reconstructable	>180° encasement and extends beyond bifurcation of proper into right and left HA
SMV/PV	Occlusion but reconstructable	Occluded, can't reconstruct

PC pancreatic cancer, *SMA* superior mesenteric artery, *SMV/PV* superior mesenteric vein/portal vein, *HA* hepatic artery

celiac axis, but still amenable to resection/reconstruction and PV/SMV occlusion with an option for reconstruction (Fig. 10.1). LAPC type B was defined as SMA involvement >270°; celiac involvement >180°, but involving the aorta; CHA involvement from celiac axis to the level of the bifurcation into the right and left hepatic artery (presuming standard anatomy); and occlusion of the PV/SMV without option for reconstruction (Fig. 10.2). While resection of the PV/SMV has become relatively commonplace among high volume pancreatic surgeons, resection of visceral arteries carries an even higher magnitude of risk and is not commonly done. However, planned major visceral arterial resection can be performed safely with good outcomes when done in appropriately selected patients by experienced pancreatic surgeons. Resection is also the backbone of definitive and potentially curative therapy for LAPC. Arterial involvement can be surgically treated in tw@ @o ways (1) skeletonize the vessel and separate it from the tumor, or (2) resect the tumor en bloc with the involved vessel and reconstruct the vessel. In regard to skeletonization, it is important to

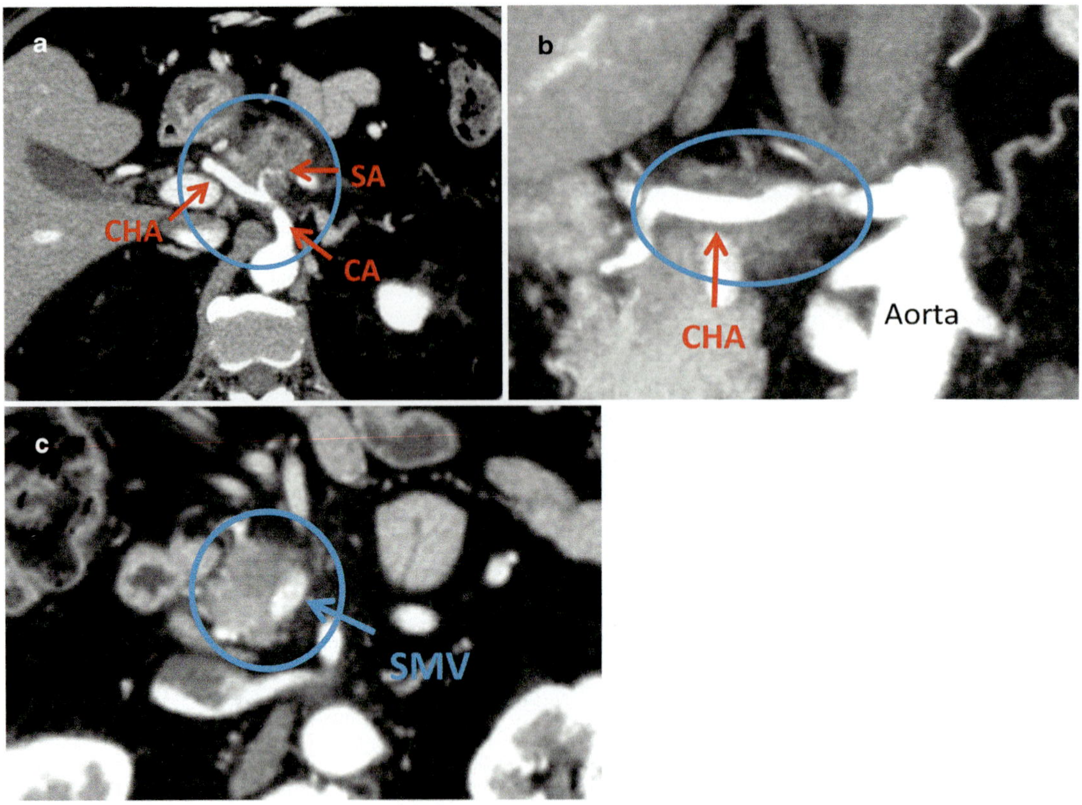

Fig. 10.1 Locally advanced type A pancreatic cancer: (**a**) axial computed tomography (CT) image of tumor involving the celiac axis (CA), common hepatic artery (CHA), and splenic artery (SA), (**b**) curved planar reformat CT image of tumor involving the length of the CHA, and (**c**) axial CT image of tumor abutting/distorting the superior mesenteric vein (SMV). The tumor is considered type A as it involves the celiac axis but remains resectable

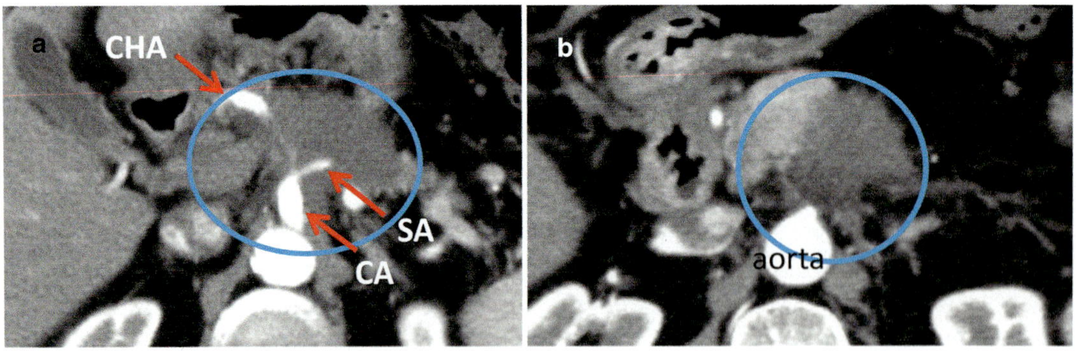

Fig. 10.2 Locally advanced type B pancreatic cancer: (**a**) axial CT image of a tumor that engulfs the celiac axis (CA), as well as the origin of the common hepatic artery (CHA) and splenic artery (SA), (**b**) axial CT image of tumor engulfing the celiac axis to the level of the aorta, (**c**) curved planar CT reformats illustrating extent of involvement of SMA (>180°), and (**d**) coronal CT images of tumor occlusion of the portal vein with associated cavernous transformation (red arrows).This patient's tumor is considered type B due to aortic involvement and the lack of a cephalad target for reconstruction of the portal vein. (SMA superior mesenteric artery, SMV superior mesenteric vein)

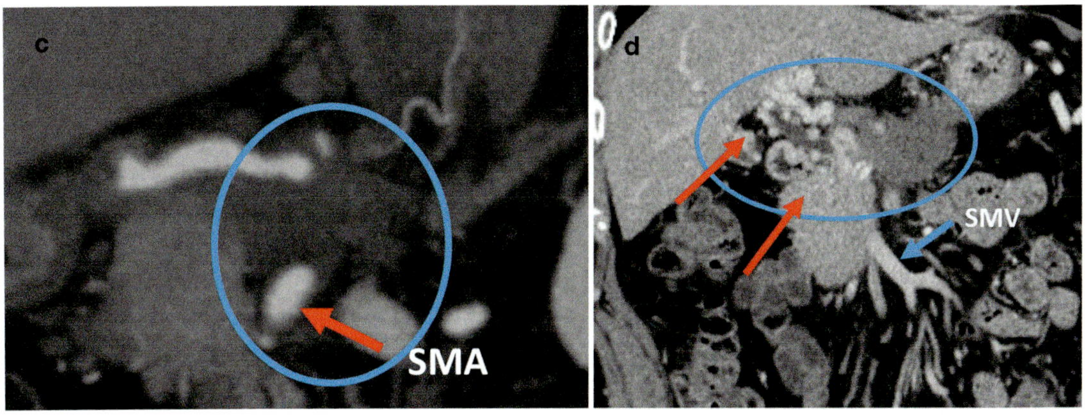

Fig. 10.2 (continued)

note that visceral arteries are enveloped by a perineural sheath. Tumors that involve this nerve sheath often spread longitudinally through this neural layer. Failure to recognize this fact can result in R1 or even R2 resections and persistence or early recurrence of disease. Conversely, finding the natural plane that exists between the arterial adventitia and the nerve sheath may allow removal of the tumor without arterial resection in some patients (Fig. 10.3). This dissection is enhanced by neoadjuvant chemoradiation, not only making the plane between the two more apparent but also sterilizing the periphery of these tumors allowing R0 margins even in the presence of arterial abutment [17, 18]. One caveat to the ability to skeletonize visceral arteries for complete tumor extirpation is the morbidity of doing so to the SMA. If this maneuver is done to the SMA, the patient is at risk for rapid gastrointestinal transit due to deinnervation of the midgut as the autonomic nerves regulating small bowel motility are divided/removed. Patients can develop incapacitating diarrhea and severe nutritional deficiencies requiring the use of total parenteral nutrition and multiple anti-motility agents. We therefore try to not 360° skeletonize the SMA, and we do not advocate SMA resection/reconstruction (in addition to the risk of intestinal ischemia if the graft occluded) for pancreatic cancer. If a tumor encases the entire circumference of an artery, dissection will require cutting through the tumor to reach this peri-adventitial plane which is oncologically

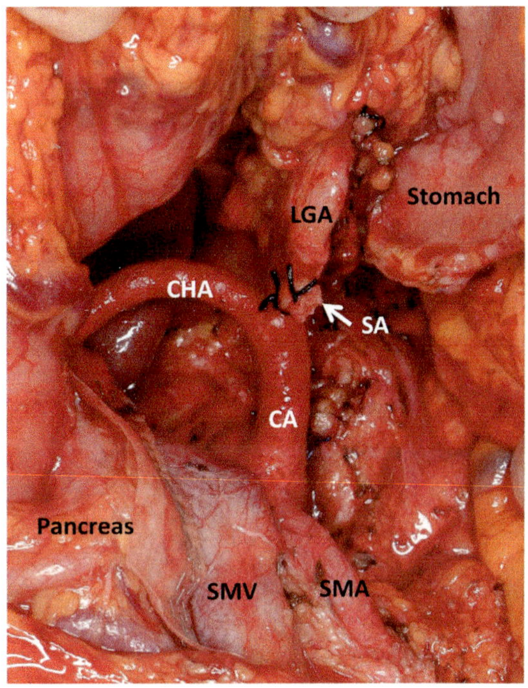

Fig. 10.3 Intraoperative photograph of a skeletonized celiac axis with preserved left gastric artery (LGA), common hepatic artery (CHA), and celiac axis (CA). In this patient, a distal subtotal pancreatectomy, en bloc splenectomy, and complete microdissection of all nerve tissue and surrounding nodes were completed. The splenic artery (SA) has been ligated just past its origin at the celiac axis. (SMA superior mesenteric artery, SMV superior mesenteric vein)

unacceptable at least at the present time. This forms the basis for the designation of LAPC Type A and B tumors; LAPC type A tumors can be removed without cutting through the tumor, and the LAPC type B tumors would require tremendous treatment response for this to ever be the case.

In patients where the tumor has invaded or is inseparable from the vessel, such as many pancreatic body tumors with celiac axis involvement, resection of the celiac trunk is required. This means that retrograde blood flow through the gastroduodenal artery (GDA) and the pancreatic arcade must then provide hepatic arterial blood flow through the proper hepatic artery (PHA) and gastric perfusion through the right gastric and right gastroepiploic arteries. We therefore prefer a "supercharged" Appleby procedure consisting of distal pancreatectomy, splenectomy, en bloc celiac axis resection, plus reversed saphenous vein interposition grafting between the celiac and distal CHA before it divides into the GDA and PHA (Fig. 10.4). Interposition grafting augments hepatic and gastric blood flow and, we believe, enhances gastric emptying. Supercharging theoretically prevents delayed gastric emptying resulting from "relative" gastric ischemia when the left gastric artery needs to be resected with the celiac artery. A replaced right hepatic artery during an Appleby procedure precludes the need for supercharging the hepatic arterial flow but obviously does not affect gastric perfusion. If the left gastric artery is resected, gastric atony may occur in the absence of a larger head of pressure in the right gastric and right gastroepiploic arteries. Variations in mesenteric arteries occur quite frequently, and thus pancreatic surgeons dealing with LAPC must be well-versed in the nuances of these variations in addition to the technical challenges of the "average" locally advanced case [19, 20].

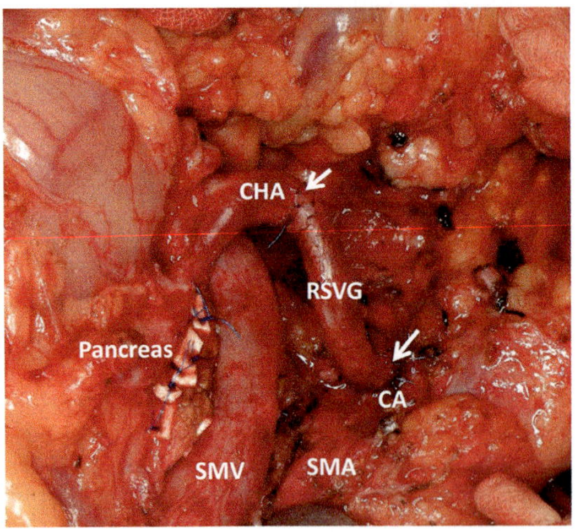

Fig. 10.4 Intraoperative photograph of a "supercharged Appleby" illustrating a celiac axis (CA) resection with reconstruction of the common hepatic artery (CHA) via reversed saphenous vein interposition graft (RSVG). The tumor was removed with a distal subtotal pancreatectomy, celiac axis resection, and splenectomy. The celiac ganglion and all nerve and lymphatic tissue were removed en bloc with the specimen. (SMA superior mesenteric artery, SMV superior mesenteric vein)

Chemotherapeutic drugs are improving, radiation delivery and dosages are more refined, and surgeons have developed techniques to safely remove these tumors from complex anatomic regions. Utilizing the advantages of each treatment modality (chemotherapy's systemic effects, radiation's sterilization of the tumor periphery and nodal basins and surgery's removal of the tumor) follows a logical paradigm utilized in many other cancer disease sites (i.e., breast, rectum, others) to maximize the chances of the patient's OS.

Our pancreatic cancer treatment algorithm at the Medical College of Wisconsin in Milwaukee consists of 4–6 months of chemotherapy, followed by chemoradiation via a standard fractionation preoperative IMRT technique targeting the pancreatic head or body/tail and the primary tumor, enlarged nodes, major vascular trunks, and any visible perineural spread, followed by surgical resection. Patients are restaged including physical examination, tumor markers (Ca19-9, carcinoembryonic antigen [CEA]), and axial imaging at 2-month intervals, and proceed to the next phase of care after multidisciplinary review, provided they show clinical improvement in terms of pain and performance status (PS), a stable or falling (preferred) Ca 19-9, and stable or diminishing tumor size. Provided these things are true, the patients are taken to the operating room for diagnostic laparoscopy to rule out metastatic disease followed by the same anesthetic resection if no metastatic disease is found (Fig. 10.5). Following this treatment plan, we found that patients with type A LAPC had a 62% chance of completing all treatments and had an expected

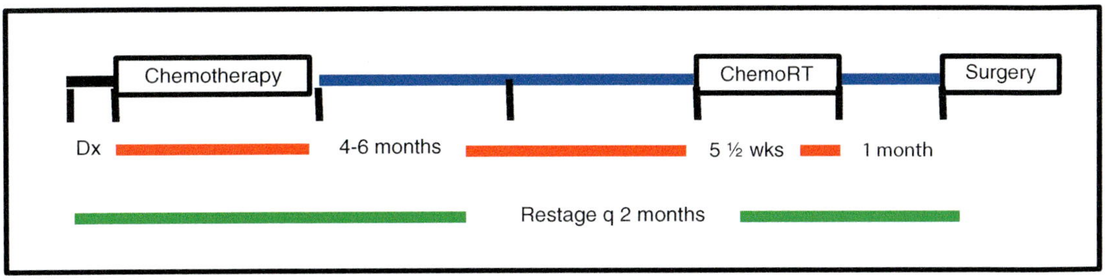

Fig. 10.5 Treatment algorithm for LAPC employing multimodality therapy starting with chemotherapy for 4–6 months, followed by chemoradiation, and finally surgical resection. Restaging, which includes physical examination, axial imaging (CT or MRI), and tumor markers, is completed every 2 months and between modalities of care. (Dx diagnosis, q every, wks weeks, chemo RT chemoradiation)

median OS of 55.6 months. Patients with type B LAPC had a 24% chance of completing all treatment and had an OS of 37.5 months in those with treatment response who were successfully resected. Taking both LAPC type A and B together, median OS was 38.9 months for this trimodal approach to this advanced stage of disease, which is nearly two to three times that of best chemotherapy, or chemoradiation alone [21]. Separating these two stages also gives patients and providers a probability for completion of all therapy and sets realistic treatment goals for the patient from the outset.

Summary

The management of LAPC is complex and still evolving. Special expertise is required in each phase of care. Careful delivery and management of potentially toxic chemotherapy agents with the necessary supportive care is essential as the first phase of treatment. If successful, a smooth hand-off following restaging imaging to radiation oncologists skilled in preoperative or dose-escalated radiation is essential. Image-based treatment planning with accurate delineation of the tumor and its extensions is pivotal to future margin-negative surgery. Advanced treatment planning and daily image-guided radiation ensures that the complex plan is actualized. Supportive care is necessary to sustain the patient for future surgical intervention if restaging is affirmative. Finally, evaluation for resection requires a surgical oncologist with a complete understanding of the complexities of the existing anatomy and the necessary surgical skills to completely remove the tumor and its perineural extensions, restoring the necessary blood supply to the remaining upper abdominal organs. Skilled care intraoperatively and postoperatively is essential for full recovery, as is carefully planned follow-up and surveillance. This comprehensive team approach is essential to the exceptional reported outcomes herein and can only be successfully achieved in centers committed to this series of interwoven and highly complex treatments.

References

1. Rhim AD, Mirek ET, Aiello NM, et al. EMT and dissemination precede pancreatic tumor formation. Cell. 2012;148:348–61.
2. Burris HA, Moore MJ, Andersen J, Green MR, Rothenberg ML, Modiano MR, Cripps MC, Portenoy RK, Storniolo AM, Tarassoff P, et al. Improvements in survival and clinical benefit with gemcitabine as first-line therapy for patients with advanced pancreas cancer: a randomized trial. J Clin Oncol. 1997;15:2403–13.
3. Heinemann V, Quietzsch D, Gieseler F, Gonnermann M, Schonekas H, Rost A, Neuhaus H, Haag C, Clemens M, Heinrich B, et al. Randomized phase III trial of gemcitabine plus cisplatin compared with gemcitabine alone in advanced pancreatic cancer. J Clin Oncol. 2006;24:3946–52.
4. Boeck S, Hoehler T, Seipelt G, Mahlberg R, Wein A, Hochhaus A, Boeck HP, Schmid B, Kettner E, Stauch M, et al. Capecitabine plus oxaliplatin (CapOx) versus capecitabine plus gemcitabine (CapGem)versus

gemcitabine plus oxaliplatin (mGemOx): final results of a multicenter randomized phase II trial in advanced pancreatic cancer. Ann Oncol. 2008;19:340–7.
5. Fine RL, Fogelman DR, Schreibman SM, Desai M, Sherman W, Strauss J, Guba S, Andrade R, Chabot J. The gemcitabine, docetaxel, and capecitabine (GTX) regimen for metastatic pancreatic cancer: a retrospective analysis. Cancer Chemother Pharmacol. 2008;61:167–75.
6. Von Hoff DD, Ervin T, Arena FP, Chiorean EG, Infante J, Moore M, Seay T, Tjulandin SA, Ma WW, Saleh MN, et al. Increased survival in pancreatic cancer with nab-paclitaxel plus gemcitabine. N Engl J Med. 2013;369:1691–703.
7. Goldstein D, El-Maraghi RH, Hammel P, Heinemann V, Kunzmann V, Sastre J, Scheithauer W, Siena S, Tabernero J, Teixeira L, et al. nab-Paclitaxel plus gemcitabine for metastatic pancreatic cancer: long-term survival from a phase III trial. J Natl Cancer Inst. 2015;107:dju413.
8. Conroy T, Desseigne F, Ychou M, Bouche O, Guimbaud R, Becouarn Y, Adenis A, Raoul JL, Gourgou-Bourgade S, de la Fouchardiere C, et al. FOLFIRINOX versus gemcitabine for metastatic pancreatic cancer. N Engl J Med. 2011;364:1817–25.
9. Loehrer P, Powell ME, Cardenes HR, et al. A randomized phase III study of gemcitabine in combination with radiation therapy versus gemcitabine alone in patients with localized unresectable pancreatic cancer: E4201. J Clin Oncol. 2008;26(Suppl):abstract 4506.
10. Mukherjee S, Hurt CN, Bridgewater J, et al. Gemcitabine-based or capecitabine-based chemoradiotherapy for locally advanced pancreatic cancer (SCALOP): a multicentre, randomised, phase 2 trial. Lancet Oncol. 2013;14:317–26.
11. Krishna S, Chadha AS, Suh Y, et al. Focal radiation therapy dose escalation improves overall survival in locally advanced pancreatic cancer patients receiving induction chemotherapy and consolidation chemoradiation. Int J Radiat Oncol Biol Phys. 2016;94(4):755–65.
12. Chung SY, Chang JS, Lee BM, et al. Dose escalation in locally advanced pancreatic cancer patients receiving chemoradiotherapy. Radiother Oncol. 2017;123:438–45.
13. De Geus SWL, Eskander MF, Kasumova GG, et al. Stereotactic body radiotherapy for unresected pancreatic cancer: a nationwide review. Cancer. 2017;123(21):4158–67.
14. Rosati LM, Herman JM. Role of stereotactic body radiotherapy in treatment of elderly and poor performance patients with pancreatic cancer. J Oncol Pract. 2017;13(3):157–66.
15. Iacobuzio-Donahue CA, Fu B, Yachida S, et al. DPC4 gene status of the primary carcinoma correlates with patterns of failure in patients with pancreatic cancer. J Clin Oncol. 2009;27:1806–13.
16. Gutt R, Liauw SL, Weichselbaum RR. The role of radiotherapy in locally advanced pancreatic carcinoma. Nat Rev Gastroenterol Hepatol. 2010;7:437–47.
17. Evans DB, George B, Tsai S. Non-metastatic pancreatic cancer: resectable, borderline resectable, and locally advanced-definitions of increasing importance for the optimal delivery of multimodality therapy. Ann Surg Oncol. 2015;22(11):3409–13.
18. Kang CM, Chung YE, Park JY, et al. Potential contribution of preoperative neoadjuvant concurrent chemoradiation therapy on margin-negative resection in borderline resectable pancreatic cancer. J Gastrointest Surg. 2012;16(3):509–17.
19. Pilgrim C, Tsai S, Ritch P, George B, Evans DB, Christians KK. Arterial resection at the time of pancreatectomy for cancer. Surgery. 2014;155(5):919–26.
20. Younan G, Tsa S, Evans DB, Christians KK. Techniques of vascular resection and reconstruction. Surg Clin N Am. 2016;96:1351–70.
21. Chatzizacharias N, Tsai S, Griffin M, Tolat P, Ritch P, George B, Barnes C, Aldakkak M, Khan AH, Hall W, Erickson B, Evans DB, Christians KK. Locally advanced pancreatic cancer: staging and goals of therapy. Surgery. 2018;pii: S0039-6060(17):30633–5. https://doi.org/10.1016/j.surg.2017.09.012.

Role of Radiation for Locally Advanced Pancreatic Cancer

11

Beth A. Erickson and William A. Hall

Introduction

Pancreatic cancer is the fourth leading cause of cancer death for both men and women in the United States [1]. Despite aggressive multimodality therapy, the 5-year survival rate remains less than 8% [1]. The majority of patients (80–85%) present with locally advanced and metastatic disease [2]. Of these locally advanced patients, approximately 30–40% present without metastatic disease with a median survival of 1-year (9–13 months) and a 5-year survival of <5% [2]. The definition of locally advanced pancreatic cancer (LAPC) is somewhat variable and dependent upon surgeon, institutional practice patterns, and response to neoadjuvant therapy. Historically, tumors have been classified as unresectable due to encasement or occlusion of the superior mesenteric vein (SMV), SMV/portal vein confluence, or direct involvement of the superior mesenteric artery (SMA), celiac axis, inferior vena cava, or aorta. These dictums, however, are evolving based on more effective neoadjuvant therapies and more advanced vascular reconstruction surgical techniques [3]. These patients are now approached initially with systemic chemotherapy, given their propensity to metastasize, and radiation is used selectively based on response to chemotherapy, performance status, and lack of distant dissemination [4, 5]. Even with systemic therapy, local progression in the absence of metastatic disease remains a significant problem. In LAP 07, local disease progression occurred in 32% of patients treated with chemotherapy and radiation (chemo–RT) and 46% of patients with chemotherapy alone. This improvement in local control was not associated with any increase in grade 3 or 4 toxicity [6]. In addition, isolated local/regional disease progression remains a primary cause of death in approximately one third of pancreatic cancer patients studied at the time of autopsy [7]. These patients die with symptoms of pain, fatigue, loss of appetite, and weight loss. Additionally, failure to control the primary tumor not only increases morbidity but may also increase mortality. In a multivariate analysis of Murphy et al., local failure was an independent predictor of overall survival (OS), even when distant metastatic disease was a covariate. This supports the premise that local control or a delay in local progression is key in preventing tumor progression and improving OS [8, 9].

It has been shown that standard radiation (50.4–60 Gy) delivered with concurrent chemotherapy continuous infusion 5-fluorouracil (CI 5-FU), given as a palliative intervention,

B. A. Erickson (✉) · W. A. Hall
Department of Radiation Oncology, The Medical College of Wisconsin, Milwaukee, WI, USA
e-mail: berickson@mcw.edu

S. Tsai et al. (eds.), *Management of Localized Pancreatic Cancer*,
https://doi.org/10.1007/978-3-319-98944-0_11

can improve the length and quality of survival in patients with LAPC over observation alone [10]. Conventional single-agent chemotherapy and concurrent low-dose radiation as a treatment for LAPC are no longer considered the standard of care [5, 11]. The emergence of more effective systemic therapy, given prior to radiation, may help to decrease the risk of failure outside of the pancreas and make radiation more pivotal in contributing to cure [4, 11]. Early studies using radiation were compromised by suboptimal doses, treatment planning and delivery methods, and treatment duration. This swayed many clinicians away from the use of radiation for pancreatic cancer given the seeming lack of a survival benefit compared with the toxicity. Though still debated, the advent of contemporary advanced radiation therapy technology allows for escalation of radiation dose to much higher levels than achievable historically with improved local control and acceptable toxicity [12]. Select patients with unresectable pancreatic cancer may be curable with high-dose chemoradiation if they do not develop metastatic disease. Survival may be improved by intensification of local therapy. The best evidence for the impact of durable local tumor control on survival comes from the surgical literature: resection leads to a substantial median survival benefit and cure in 20% of patients. Similar outcomes can be achieved in select patients with the use of carefully planned dose-escalated radiation. Chemotherapy alone is not a durable solution with a number of US clinical trials using gemcitabine-based chemotherapy, without radiation, reporting median survival durations of 9.1–9.9 months. In other international trials combining chemotherapy first followed by chemoradiation, these median survivals increase to 12 and 14.3 months [13, 14]. Further escalation of radiation dose and improvements in systemic therapy are needed to reach more durable survival figures. Considerable challenges remain, however, in selecting the optimal patients and accomplishing dose escalation in the upper abdomen which involve both treatment planning and treatment delivery.

Sequencing of Treatment Modalities

Induction chemotherapy is favored prior to chemoradiation to address the high risk of micrometastatic disease and provide early systemic intervention. By excluding patients with rapid distant progression, induction chemotherapy selects patients with LAPC who will benefit the most from consolidative irradiation and spares those who will not, the rigors of locoregional irradiation [5, 11]. There has not been an increase in toxicity from the combination of up-front chemotherapy followed by chemoradiation. Induction chemotherapy for LAPC, prior to radiation, has traditionally consisted of gemcitabine (Gem)-based regimens [5]. The LAP 07 trial evaluated Gem alone versus Gem followed by radiation in patients with LAPC [6, 15]. In this trial, 442 patients were first randomized to Gem alone or Gem plus erlotinib for 4 months. Patients without progression (60%) were then randomized to 2 additional months of chemotherapy or chemoradiation (54 Gy/30 fractions). There was no improvement in survival with the addition of radiation following Gem (15.2 mo. vs. 16.5 mo., $p = 0.83$). Criticisms of this trial include the low-radiation doses used in comparison to single institutional data, the off-protocol use of chemoradiation, and the low rate of radiation protocol adherence (32%) [16]. On secondary analysis, however, chemoradiation was associated with decreased local progression (32 vs. 46%, $p = 0.3$) [6]. In contrast to LAP 07, a phase III trial by the Eastern Cooperative Oncology Group (ECOG) 4201 showed a survival advantage to the combination of radiotherapy and Gem over Gem alone [17]. The study was closed early because of slow accrual; however, in the 74 patients enrolled, median survival improved from 9.2 to 11.1 months with the addition of modest doses of radiation (50.4 Gy) following Gem ($P = 0.017$). The Selective

Chemoradiation in Advanced Localized Pancreatic Cancer (SCALOP) trial also revealed a survival advantage for the addition of chemoradiation following chemotherapy [18]. This was a randomized phase II trial where LAPC patients received 12 weeks of induction Gem plus capecitabine (Cape). In those who responded, another cycle of chemotherapy was administered, and patients were then treated with either Gem- or Cape-based chemoradiation (50.4 Gy/28 fractions). Not all the 114 patients who were registered received the concurrent chemoradiation phase of the study. Median OS was 14.6 months for those who were treated with chemoradiation and 8.1 months for those who were treated with chemotherapy alone. In the 74 patients who were able to get chemoradiation, the median OS was 15.2 months in the Cape arm and 13.4 months in the Gem arm, with more toxicity in the Gem arm. Though not a primary endpoint, the SCALOP trial revealed a survival benefit for those who received chemoradiation and also reinforced the use of chemotherapy first to select responders for local therapy. Key also to the success of the SCALOP trial was a central review of a pre-trial test case in which the contours of the planned radiation tumor target as well as the radiation plan were reviewed for adherence to protocol guidelines. A later update to the SCALOP trial continued to show improved outcomes with the Cape arm. Additionally, a CA19.9 < 46 after induction chemotherapy predicted improved OS and progression-free survival (PFS) in those receiving radiation and may help to select those patients most likely to benefit from the addition of radiation [19]. A phase III clinical trial for patients with metastatic disease has demonstrated that the multidrug regimen FOLFIRINOX (fluorouracil, oxaliplatin, leucovorin, and irinotecan) was statistically significantly superior to Gem with respect to response rate (31.6% vs. 9.4%), PFS (6.4 months vs. 3.3 months), and OS (11.1 months vs. 6.8 months) for patients with metastatic disease [20]. This drug combination is now used in the neoadjuvant setting for patients with resectable and borderline resectable pancreas cancer [21–23] and prior to radiation in patients with locally advanced disease (50.4 Gy) with excellent outcomes [22, 24, 25].

Radiation Treatment Planning

Simulation

Radiation treatment planning begins with simulation. Patients are typically simulated near the end of their course of systemic chemotherapy. It is important for them to maintain a stable body mass (weight) in the interval from simulation through the end of radiation to have consistent absorption of the planned radiation throughout its course. Weight gain can lead to underdosage of the radiation targets, and weight loss can lead to overdosage to the normal organs within the radiation fields. This can be especially problematic for the kidneys, spinal cord, and bowel. Patients should be NPO for at least 2–4 hours prior to simulation and treatment. If they have delayed gastric emptying, even longer periods of fasting may be required as may the addition of motility agents to promote gastric emptying. A small volume of oral contrast (~ 8 ounces) should be ingested prior to simulation to define the stomach and duodenum. The second portion of the duodenum can be difficult to see even with ingestion of oral contrast. At some institutions, water is used instead of oral contrast to distend the duodenum. Patients will also ingest this each day before treatment to push the outer wall of the duodenum further from the pancreas. Intravenous contrast is essential for CT-based planning as it helps to define the vessels that are often intimately related to the pancreatic tumor and also helps to define the tumor within the pancreatic tissues. It also helps to localize any suspicious lymph nodes. If IV contrast administration is not feasible at the time of simulation, the diagnostic CT scans can be fused with the radiation planning CT scans to facilitate contouring of the tumor and its extensions. Simulation can also be done using MR rather than CT images and improves visualization of tumor and its extensions [26]. This will be discussed in the Imaging and Radiation Targets section. For dose escalation patients, the essentials include respiratory motion management, NPO status prior to simulation and treatment, MRI simulation in the treatment position, accurate target and OAR delineation, and daily image guidance with good soft-tissue resolution. This may lead to improved outcomes for this challenging disease presentation [26, 27].

Motion Management

Radiation of the upper abdomen is challenging due to the inherent motion within the abdominal cavity. This motion comes from the diaphragms, which move with respiration, as well as bowel motility, stomach/duodenal peristalsis, and other random motion. Motion control is important as it allows for margin reduction and dose escalation. Methods to control for motion can include immobilization and abdominal compression devices as well as respiratory gating or breath-hold techniques or tracking of key structures [28]. The first step in controlling motion is immobilization at the time of simulation and at each treatment. This can include body molds (Alpha cradles, full body vac fix, etc.) and compression belts which limit abdominal wall movement [27]. Additionally, controlling PO status prior to simulation and daily radiation treatments can also lead to more reproducible onboard imaging. An enlarged stomach can move the pancreas as well as the nearby vessels [29]. Another key step is measurement of respiratory motion which is considerable in the upper abdomen. The most significant motion is in the superior-inferior direction, followed by the AP direction, with very little lateral motion [30]. With free breathing, this has been reported ranging from 2 mm to over 20 mm and can be inter-fractional as well as intra-fractional [31, 32]. Four-dimensional computed tomography (4DCT) and 4D MRI are used to measure this motion and to plan gated and other motion-managed treatments. Gated treatment provides reconstruction of 3D scans at various phases in the respiratory cycle. Sorting of these images following simulation will provide the optimal phases for contouring and treatment. Both free-breathing and breath-hold images can be obtained at the time of simulation with both MR and CT. If superior-inferior motion is >8 mm, gated treatment delivery is required [33]. Typically, gated treatments are given using the 50% (end expiration) phase of the breathing cycle. The pancreas can move as much as 2–3 cm from inspiration to expiration. The motions of the pancreatic head, body, and tail are all different. The celiac and superior mesenteric arteries move less than the pancreas [29]. Taniguchi et al. found that duodenal dose was higher if patients were treated on the inspiratory rather than the expiratory phase of respiration. They concluded that expiratory gating may be preferable to inspiratory breath-hold or free-breathing strategies for minimizing risk to the duodenum [34]. Cine MRI has also been used to measure this motion with similar finding to 4DCT. The end-exhale position (50%) was the most stable position in the breathing cycle, and tumors spent the most time in this position [28]. Future use of MR-guided radiation will give a more complete understanding of intra- and inter-fraction motion, with MR imaging throughout each entire radiation fraction. Currently, a daily CT image is obtained prior to each radiation treatment. This real-time verification, known as image-guided radiation therapy (IGRT), is essential for executing radiation with tight margins and high doses.

Imaging of Pancreatic Cancer

It is very important to correctly identify the pancreatic tumor and its extensions when planning dose-escalated radiation. This is especially true given the tight margins that necessarily accompany a dose escalation strategy. Traditionally, this has been done using contrast-enhanced CT imaging. Pancreatic tumors usually are hypo-attenuating with ill-defined borders. CT has limitations in identifying pancreatic tumors within the pancreatic parenchyma, and often times the borders of the tumor may blend imperceptively with the pancreatic parenchyma. Even after contrast delivery, the Hounsfield unit difference between cancer and normal pancreatic tissue is only 44 and 42, respectively. There may be more of a difference in the Hounsfield units in the center of the tumor where there may be a visible hypodensity, but these differences diminish at the periphery of the tumor with blending with the normal pancreas [35]. Five to 14% of pancreatic cancers are isoattenuating [36]. Most of these are located in the head of the pancreas and can usually be detected with endoscopic ultrasound (EUS) [37]. Godfrey et al. reported the use of triphasic contrast-enhanced CT simulation with bolus tracking for contouring of the pancreatic gross tumor volume (GTV). They reported that the later arterial and portal venous phases made the GTV more conspicuous [38]. On comparison of the maximal CT tumor dimensions with the fresh gross specimen following surgery, Arvold et al. found that 84% of patients in their series had a tumor that was larger on gross specimen analysis than on CT. Duodenal invasion was evident in 5% on CT but was found in 70% at the time of specimen analysis. Duodenal invasion is usually viewed as a contraindication to dose escalation. An expansion formula for margin added beyond the visible tumor on CT for contouring was suggested. Recognition of this disparity between CT and the gross specimen is especially important when tight margins of 2–3 mm from GTV to planning target volume (PTV) are used for dose escalation strategies [37]. Qui et al. confirmed the underestimation of tumor size on conventional CT but a much more accurate representation of maximal tumor dimension using 3D CT [39]. A similar underestimation of tumor size was reported by Hall et al. when comparing tumor size on MR to that found when the pathologic specimen was evaluated [40].

Pancreatic tumors are known to be hypoxic, which may be due to hypoperfusion. This has been proven with intra-tumoral oxygen tension measurements [41]. The dense fibrous desmoplastic stroma and relatively sparse vascularity of most pancreatic cancers, which lead to hypoxia, may explain the resistance to both chemotherapy and radiation. When radiation is given in the setting of hypoxia, the dose must be increased by a factor of 2.5–3.0 to achieve the same degree of cell killing in comparison to fully oxygenated conditions. This hypoperfusion may make chemotherapy unable to reach its target [42]. Park et al. reported on the use of perfusion CT to predict tumor response to concurrent chemotherapy and radiation. Patients with high pretreatment K^{trans} values, indicating higher intra-tumoral flow, tended to respond better to chemoradiation than those with lower values [43].

This is also the reason that even following high-dose radiation, there may be little change in size of these connective tissue-rich neoplasms [44]. If there is going to be shrinkage, it may take up to 12 weeks after radiation for this to be seen [9]. It is also the explanation for the characteristic imaging findings on contrast-enhanced MR and CT. Normal pancreatic tissue typically demonstrates maximum enhancement in the early/arterial phase of contrast enhancement. The relative hypoperfusion/non-enhancement of the pancreatic tumor in comparison to the normal pancreas makes it most conspicuous during the early phase of contrast enhancement [36].

The superior contrast resolution/tissue differentiation of MRI may make this easier not only to detect pancreatic cancer but also to more accurately distinguish the tumor volume (GTV) from the normal pancreas [45, 46]. Not only is post-contrast MR imaging superior to CT for defining the intraglandular extent of pancreatic tumors, but there are other MR imaging sequences that are very helpful for distinguishing normal glandular tissue from tumor. The aqueous protein within the pancreatic acini has high signal on T1-weighted imaging and can be used to differentiate tumor, which is dark, from normal parenchyma, which is bright [47]. In addition, fluid sensitive T2-weighted sequences allow for very high-resolution imaging of the pancreatic duct and the ductal disruption associated with pancreatic adenocarcinoma. The duodenum is also bright on T2 and easy to differentiate from the pancreas.

Functional imaging is also available with MRI. Initial experience with diffusion-weighted imaging (DWI) of the pancreas has been very encouraging. Early investigations have yielded very high sensitivity and specificity for the detection of pancreatic cancer [48]. DWI is a very useful sequence for evaluating pancreatic cancer because it is very sensitive for detecting tissue that has relatively restricted diffusion in comparison with the adjacent normal tissue [46]. Pancreatic cancer has increased cellularity and a higher nucleus to cytoplasm ratio than normal pancreatic tissue. Therefore, the Brownian motion of water is significantly reduced compared to the adjacent normal pancreatic parenchyma. This results in higher signal in areas of the pancreas displaying restricted diffusion and making it quite sensitive for the detection of pancreatic cancer [48]. Impeded or restricted diffusion results in a low apparent diffusion coefficient (ADC) on ADC maps and high signal intensity on DW MR images. Free or unimpeded diffusion results in a high ADC on ADC maps and low signal intensity on DW MR images. Pancreatic cancer is usually associated with low ADCs because of the presence of fibrosis and increased cell density. Necrosis, which may be a component of large tumors or which can occur after treatment, is associated with increased ADCs [49]. In addition, DWI appears to be quite promising for monitoring early treatment response/cell death prior to a change in tumor size [43]. Decreases in DWI signal can be correlated with treatment response/cell death prior to a reduction in tumor size and may be a more accurate way to assess response than simply a change in size as available with CT [50]. Some of the seeming lack of response to treatment when using CT size criteria may, in fact, be a result of the shortcomings of CT in assessing response rather than the shortcomings of the treatment. Cuneo et al. compared pretreatment ADC parameters with CT and pathologic response. They found a significant correlation between pretreatment mean tumor ADC values and the amount of tumor cell destruction after chemoradiation. Tumors with a low ADC mean value at baseline responded poorly to standard chemoradiation [50]. These findings were confirmed by Dalah with changes in pre- and posttreatment ADC correlated with pathological treatment response following chemoradiation [51].

Dynamic contrast enhancement (DCE) MR perfusion imaging may also provide some prognostic information regarding survival [52] and treatment response [53]. In a recently published study, higher perfusion values for the rate of transfer of gadolinium-based contrast to and from the extracellular space (K^{trans}) in pancreatic tumors were correlated with better response to anti-angiogenic chemotherapy. Considering that tumor response to radiation therapy is dependent upon tissue oxygenation for the generation of the cytotoxic-free radicals, measuring tumor perfusion may also yield important prognostic information prior to initiating radiation therapy.

PET imaging has also been explored in the staging of pancreatic tumors and is now an approved disease site for this test. PET imaging utilizes fluorodeoxyglucose (FDG) which is a glucose analog tagged with the fluorine-18 (^{18}F) isotope. FDG is preferentially taken up by cells with high metabolic activity such as pancreatic cancer. Changes in PET activity may correlate and be a means to assess tumor response after radiation [54]. FDG PET may also be prognostic. In the series of Chang et al., patients with an SUV < 3.5 and/or SUV decline >60% had significantly better OS and PFS than those having none [55]. In the series of Schellenberg et al., SUV max was an independent predictor for OS and PFS [56].

Radiation Target Identification

Radiation to the upper abdomen must be delivered with careful planning and great accuracy to adeptly irradiate the defined pancreatic tumor volumes while partially avoiding the many normal organs which live in close proximity to the pancreas. Significant progress has been made in defining the treatment targets and shaping the dose distribution to securely cover the areas that need radiation and partially avoid the normal adjacent structures. Advanced multi-planar imaging used for radiation planning, including CT, MRI, and PET scans, enables excellent target definition, selective dose escalation to key parts of the target volume, and reduction of the irradiated volumes in the radiosensitive upper abdomen. This leads to better patient tolerance and reduced complications [29]. Definition of the gross tumor volume (GTV) and subsequent determination of the best clinical target volume (CTV) and planning target volume (PTV) margin are pivotal. These margins are used to compensate for the uncertainties in accurate GTV definition on multi-planar images and for significant and challenging organ motion in the upper abdomen. Accurate tumor contouring as a part of treatment planning is vital as contouring errors can result in systematic underdosage of the target and/or preventable toxicity to the organs at risk (OAR). Differences in interpretation of multi-planar images can also lead to variations in contours, even among experienced radiation oncologists [57]. Yamazaki et al. reported significant inter-observer variation in a multi-institutional trial where eleven radiation oncologists contoured the GTV using CT on two cases of LAPC. The ratio of the largest to smallest contours was 9:3 for the two cases, demonstrating significant inter-observer variability [58].

A standardized pancreatic cancer protocol abdominal MRI with and without intravenous contrast should be used to stage, assist in treatment planning, and monitor treatment response for patients undergoing MR-based radiation. Standardized approaches to MR simulation are available for both 1.5 T and 3.0 T scanners [26, 27]. The three MR sequences utilized for contouring the radiation targets are T2 (duodenal wall delineation), fat-suppressed T1 (normal gland delineation), and late arterial phase post-contrast, fat-suppressed T1 (tumor boundary and lymph node delineation; e.g., tumor appears dark, and lymph nodes appear bright) because these sequences offer the best contrast resolution between tumor and normal pancreatic parenchyma (Fig. 11.1a–c). Normal pancreatic tissue is bright/high signal on T1-weighted imaging. A pancreatic tumor appears as a hypo-intense or dark area when surrounded by normal pancreatic tissue on T1-weighted imaging. A detailed approach to MR-based delineation is provided for both 1.5 and 3.0 T images [27]. Delineation of the GTV on both CT and MR was performed by

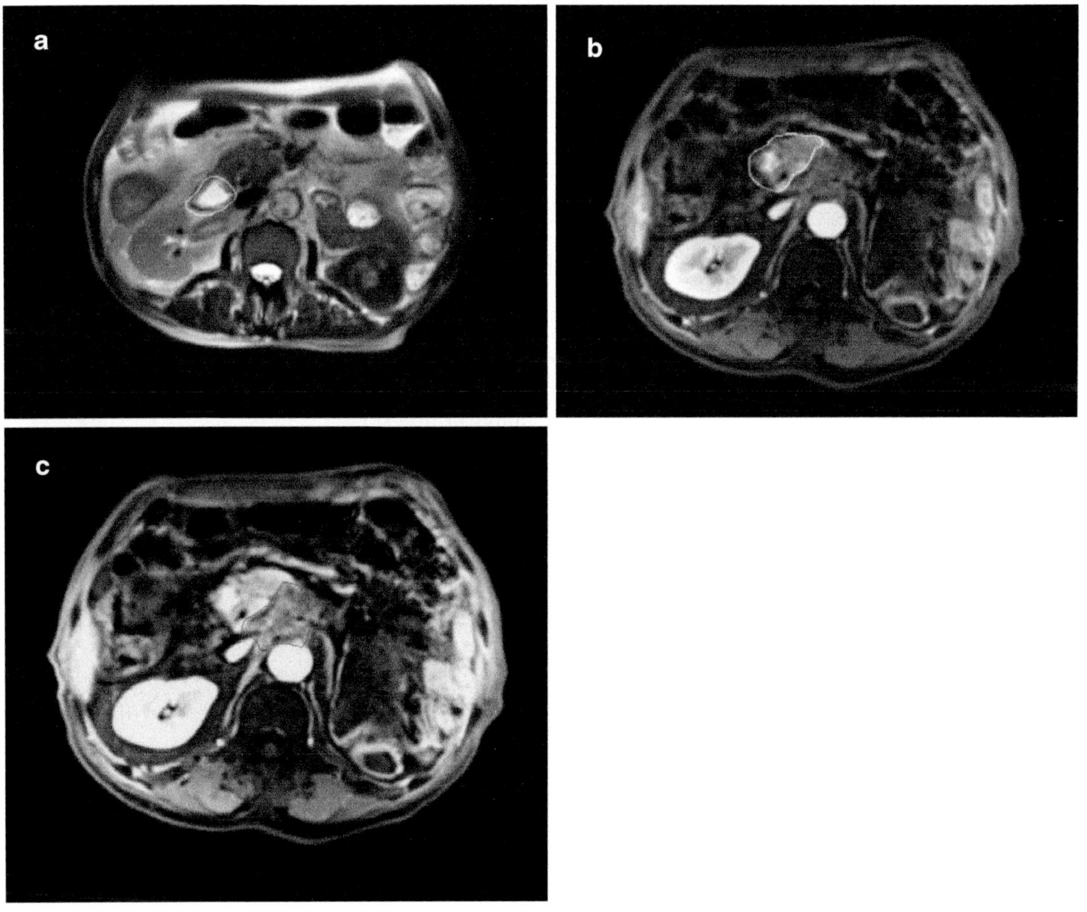

Fig. 11.1 The three MR sequences utilized for contouring the radiation targets are (**a**) T2 (duodenal wall delineation, yellow), (**b**) fat-suppressed T1 (normal gland delineation, white), and (**c**) late arterial phase post-contrast, fat-suppressed T1 (tumor boundary and lymph node delineation, e.g., tumor appears dark, and lymph nodes appear bright, red) because these sequences offer the best contrast resolution between tumor and normal pancreatic parenchyma

a group of 12 international radiation oncologists experienced in GI radiation oncology. A stepwise process was identified that led to significant agreement in the delineations between the participants. Despite areas of agreement, displayed on count maps, there were definite areas of disagreement among the participants. The MR-defined GTVs were smaller volume than the CT-defined GTVs which could be helpful in the setting of dose escalation [57]. Dalah et al. also found inconsistencies in defining the GTV on CT, PET, DCE-MRI, and ADC-DWI [59]. Some of this can be due to image registration but it is not recommended to use any of the functional imaging studies for GTV definition due to inaccuracies in defining the boundaries of these lesions on these imaging series [27].

Radiation Plan Design

A trend toward treating only the visible tumor (involved field radiation) rather than elective volumes (large field radiation) has evolved for the treatment of LAPC although there is still considerable variation in the volumes treated [11]. In a review of large field irradiation, which included the primary tumor and surrounding pancreas as well as the regional nodes, vs. treating the GTV only with a limited margin (5–10 mm) without the regional nodes, only 5% relapsed in the untreated nodes, and local recurrences were reported in 17–49% which was similar to studies using only large field irradiation. These high rates of local failure were in series with doses ≤54 Gy [30]. One of the most comprehensive guides for LAPC planning is a joint effort from the RTOG and GERCOR [30]. In this summary, the recommendation was to include the primary gross tumor volume (GTV) and any enlarged lymph nodes over 1 cm. Both IV and oral contrast were recommended at simulation to best define the tumor and its extensions as well as the adjacent GI tract. The planning target volume (PTV) was recommended to be 1.5–2.0 cm around the GTV in the AP and lateral directions and 2.0–3.0 cm in the craniocaudal directions to account for motion. These margins could be reduced if motion was either measured or controlled through the use of 4DCT or respiratory gating. Prophylactic irradiation of uninvolved nodes was optional and recommended only to include the peripancreatic, SMA, and celiac regions with the porta hepatis included only for head lesions and the splenic hilum only for tail lesions. Conventional fractionation was recommended [30]. The UK SCALOP study was also very prescriptive in defining the radiation volumes. Patients underwent CT simulation with IV contrast and drank 200–300 ml of water. The GTV consisted of the CT-defined tumor and any node with short axis diameter > 1 cm. The PTV included the GTV with a margin of 2.0 cm in the craniocaudal directions and 1.5 cm in all other directions. Prophylactic irradiation of the nodes was not done. A radiotherapy atlas which defined the appropriate way to contour both a pancreatic head and body tumor, according to the protocol guidelines, was available for participating radiation oncologists to review prior to contouring participating patients. Both the contours and the radiation plan were then sent for central review and the need for revisions communicated back to the radiation oncologist. The development and insistence of adherence to protocol guidelines was a novel aspect of this important study [18]. In the series of Ben-Josef et al. using intensity-modulated radiation therapy (IMRT) and a simultaneous integrated boost (SIB) with full-dose Gem, there was no elective lymph node irradiation, and the CT-defined GTV was expanded by 1.0 cm to form the PTV. Active breathing control was used to reduce breathing motion. Without including the elective nodes, only 5% of patients had peripancreatic node failures, and none experienced a regional lymph node failure outside of the 80% isodose line [9, 12]. The volume of the PTV also correlated with toxicity with severe GI toxicity >260 cc when given with full-dose Gem [9]. Badiyan et al. used similar expansions (GTV + 5–10 mm) and had PTVs ranging from 101 to 531 cm^3 [22]. Contrastingly, Ito et al. used more traditional large fields covering the primary tumor and the regional lymphatics. PTVs in this series ranged from 357 cc to 1215 cc with a median value of 555 cc. The total volume of the PTV was significantly correlated to acute intestinal toxicity with the highest incidence of grade 3+ in patients with a PTV volume > 500 cc [60]. The MD Anderson technique, "hypofractionation using a stereotactic body radiation therapy (SBRT) technique," is described by Crane [13, 14]. This includes a SIB technique with three different PTVs that include a microscopic dose, a SIB to the entire GTV, and a higher SIB dose to the hypoxic center of the GTV in select tumors optimally positioned away from the GI tract (Fig. 11.2). The SIB to the entire GTV (67.5 Gy in 15 fractions or 70 Gy in 28 fractions) is treated with a 0- to 5-mm PTV. A reduction of that volume by 10 mm is used to create the PTV to the hypoxic center. The hypoxic center of the tumor receives the higher dose of 75 Gy in 15 fractions or 98 Gy in 28 fractions. Most of the time, the tumor is too small, or the bowel is too close for this central high dose to be given. The decision to use 0 to 5 mm for the PTV of the high-dose SIB is based on the proximity of the bowel. The microscopic PTV is treated with a 15-mm margin on the GTV, celiac axis, and superior mesenteric artery. The microscopic dose at the periphery is 37.5 Gy in 15 fractions or 50.4 Gy in 28 fractions. They begin the planning process with larger expansions of the high-dose PTV and reduce these margins rather than the total doses to achieve plans that are within bowel tolerance. The decision between 15 and 28 fractions is made to maximize the GTV coverage to the prescription dose. When the tumor is ≤1cm from bowel, 28 fractions are always used to spare the bowel and achieve the highest minimum dose to the tumor. When the tumor is >1cm from the bowel, they use 15 fractions. Bowel dose constraints, with the inspiratory breath-hold gating and CT image guidance, are based on the work of Kelly et al. [61]. They use a maximum point dose of 60 Gy in 28 fractions and 45 Gy in 15 fractions for the stomach and descending duodenum. For the transverse duodenum and jejunum, they use a 10% lower constraint, 55 Gy and 40 Gy, because those structures are out of reach of an endoscopic argon plasma laser procedure, making the consequences of bleeding greater. Using these constraints, they have not had a significant bleeding event in 4 years [13, 14]. They have also not seen any arterial or biliary complications at these doses, but they do exclude the arteries from the ultrahigh dose volumes [14]. In most SBRT series, the GTV is contoured with a tight margin added (3–5 mm) to create the

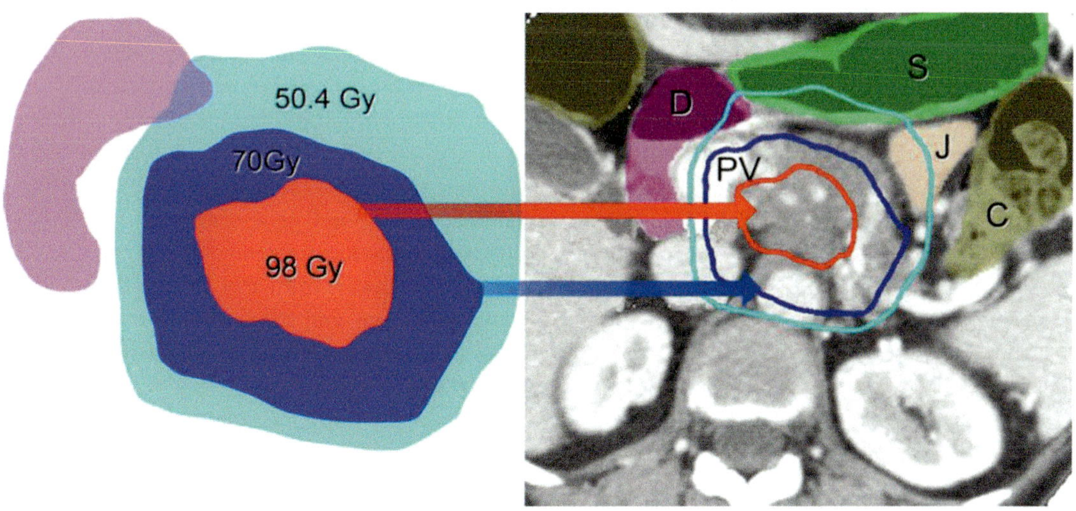

Fig. 11.2 Simultaneous integrated boost (SIB) and simultaneous integrated protection (SIP) in the treatment planning of LAPC. This figure illustrates the proximity of gastrointestinal organs to a pancreatic tumor. This patient was treated with a dose of 70 Gy in 28 fractions to the GTV and 98 Gy to the hypoxic center, using feedback-assisted inspiration breath-hold gating and daily diagnostic-quality CT imaging to verify stomach position. GTV gross tumor volume, S stomach, J jejunum, D duodenum, C colon, PV collaterals from an occluded portal vein. (With permission from Crane *Journal of Radiation Research* 57(S1):pi55, 2016)

PTV. There is a great need for motion management with these tight margins, or the GTV will be underdosed. If a 4DCT is not available to evaluate tumor motion during treatment planning, Goldstein et al. recommend asymmetric expansions of 1.0, 0.7, and 0.6 cm along the SI, AP, and medial-lateral directions rather than 3–5 mm. They also found that the biliary stents were not reliable surrogates for the position of the GTV during treatment with the stent and tumor motion poorly correlated [44, 50].

IMRT

Radiation to the upper abdomen must be delivered with careful planning and great accuracy to adeptly irradiate the defined pancreatic tumor volumes while partially avoiding the many normal organs which live in close proximity to the pancreas. Significant progress has been made in defining the treatment targets and shaping the dose distribution to securely cover the areas that need radiation and partially avoid the normal adjacent structures. As described, advanced multi-planar imaging used for radiation planning, including CT, MRI, and PET scans, enables excellent target definition, selective dose escalation to key parts of the target volume, and reduction of the irradiated volumes in the sensitive upper abdomen. The success of IMRT is very dependent on accurate target delineation and treatment delivery [29]. The use of 3D image-based conformal radiotherapy (3DCRT) has been closely followed by development of intensity-modulated radiation therapy (IMRT). IMRT is an advanced version of 3DCRT that entails the use of sophisticated computer-controlled radiation beam delivery by varying beam intensities within each beam portal to improve the conformity of the dose distribution to the shape of the tumor with associated avoidance of adjacent normal organs. IMRT treatment planning is performed using inverse treatment planning where the PTV dose is specified as well as the allowable doses/volumes to the adjacent normal organs. The computer program then calculates a customized intensity pattern to best meet the specified dose-volume constraints for the PTV and normal organs [36]. IMRT allows for a reduction in morbidity as well as for dose escalation and is the standard technique used for definitive irradiation for LAPC [36].

Dose escalation is challenging as the normal tissues adjacent to the pancreas are very dose sensitive. IMRT along with daily image guidance can allow for delivery of higher doses than 3D conformal plans with better dose sparing of the adjacent stomach, duodenum, bowel, and kidneys. Dose can be escalated to pivotal portions of the tumor while pulling dose away from the adjacent normal organs such as the stomach and duodenum [62]. Bittner et al. provided a systematic review of IMRT vs. 3D conformal radiation and found that nausea, vomiting, diarrhea, and late GI toxicity were significantly reduced with IMRT [63]. Prasad et al. retrospectively evaluated 205 patients with LAPC treated with IMRT (71 pts) vs. 3D-CRT(71 pts). 3D-CRT had significantly higher grade 2+ GI toxicity (34%) vs. IMRT(16%) [64].

IGRT

In addition to accurate target definition, image-guided radiation therapy (IGRT) is the process of positioning the patient on the treatment table and using onboard imaging to localize the tumor and adjacent organs at risk before each delivered radiation treatment. This allows for tighter margins and also assesses and corrects for pancreatic motion due to breathing and variable GI filling and motility. IGRT is essential to IMRT [29]. During RT, the location and shape of the pancreas vary significantly from day to day due to daily setup variations and physiological changes [65]. This is also true for the closely positioned loops of bowel. Singh et al. reported that due to the large inter-fraction anatomical changes, the day-to-day V80% (volume covered by 80% isodose line) for the duodenum and non-duodenal small bowel varied in the ranges of 30–100% and 1–20%, respectively [65]. IGRT based on soft-tissue registration can address setup error and these inter-fractional shifts [29]. Furthermore, online adaptive RT (ART), where the radiation plan is adapted to the daily target and organ positions, has the potential to fully account for these inter-fraction variations, including organ deformation [32]. With the respiratory motion eliminated/reduced by a respiration management technique such as gating, the PTV margin can be reduced from 1–2 cm to 0.3–0.5 cm by the use of IGRT and/or online ART. Because the PTV often overlaps with the duodenum and small bowel, such a drastic reduction in PTV margin would potentially reduce toxicities or allow RT doses to be escalated to eradicate the bulk of the tumor and improve treatment outcomes.

Radiation Dose and Dose Fractionation: Targets and Organs at Risk

The challenge of controlling pancreatic cancer with radiation is the coexistence of tumor radioresistance with the radiosensitivity of the surrounding duodenum and stomach [35]. High doses of radiation are needed but must be expertly controlled. Both standard fractionation and stereotactic body radiation therapy (SBRT) have been used for dose escalation. With standard fractionation, the dose to the target can be elevated in comparison to the other adjacent structures at risk such as the SMA, celiac axis, or adjacent pancreas with a technique referred to as a simultaneous integrated boost (SIB). This allows for dose painting based on the volume of tumor present, with the higher dose per fraction going to gross disease, and the lower dose per fraction to microscopic disease. This also affords a biologically higher dose to be given over a shorter period of time to the gross tumor. SBRT has been advocated as a better approach than fractionated radiation allowing precise delivery of high doses to limited volumes over 1–5 fractions. SBRT has the advantage of a more rapid treatment course and is typically given without concurrent chemotherapy. This offers a welcome break for patients who have received months of prior chemotherapy. The doses delivered are felt to have a different method of cell kill than conventionally fractionated radiation with an ablative impact that is effective against radioresistant cells. With these large fraction sizes, however, it is very important to spare the adjacent stomach, duodenum, jejunum, and colon. This has led to treatment of the defined tumor (GTV) with a very tight margin of 3–5 mm. The accuracy of defining tumors based on CT imaging has been previously questioned. There are also patients in whom lower-dose palliative irradiation can be given with both SBRT and other lower-dose, hypofractionated approaches. This may be appropriate for frail patients or those with metastatic disease but symptomatic primaries. To date, the most common dose fractionation for SBRT has been 660 cGy X 5. A multi-institutional trial using this dose fractionation has proven it safe, but local control and survival were not moved beyond that seen with standard fractionation [66]. Treatment with standard fractionation (50.4 Gy: BED 10–59.47 Gy) and low-dose hypofractionated SBRT (25–33 Gy/5 fractions: BED10–53.65 Gy) have led to little or no chance of long-term tumor control or median survival benefit [14]. A synthesis of SBRT and SIB ("hypofractionation using an SBRT technique") has been proposed by Crane as previously described. This high- and low-dose inhomogeneity allows areas in the tumor abutting the GI tract to receive a lower dose and those further away to receive an ablative dose. It is unclear if it is the fraction size or the total dose that improves outcome. A BED 10 of 100 Gy is proposed as the ideal for optimal tumor control, which is at least twice as high as standard doses [13, 14].

Despite combinations of chemotherapy and radiation, local control in addition to distant failure continues to be a challenge for patients with locally advanced unresectable pancreatic cancer. Given the propensity for local failure, there has been interest in improving outcomes in LAPC through dose escalation. An analysis of recently published data was performed to assess the usefulness of dose escalation [67]. Multiple series with various dose fractionation schemes were analyzed for a dose response. Inclusion in the analysis required histologic/cytologic confirmation of unresectable pancreatic cancer without distant metastases. Only results published after 1997 were included. Studies not reporting tumor response or those combining conventional radiation schedules with a large boost dose were excluded. Radiation treatment was usually combined with different chemotherapy treatments, yet due to the lack of sufficient studies for separate analysis, no distinc-

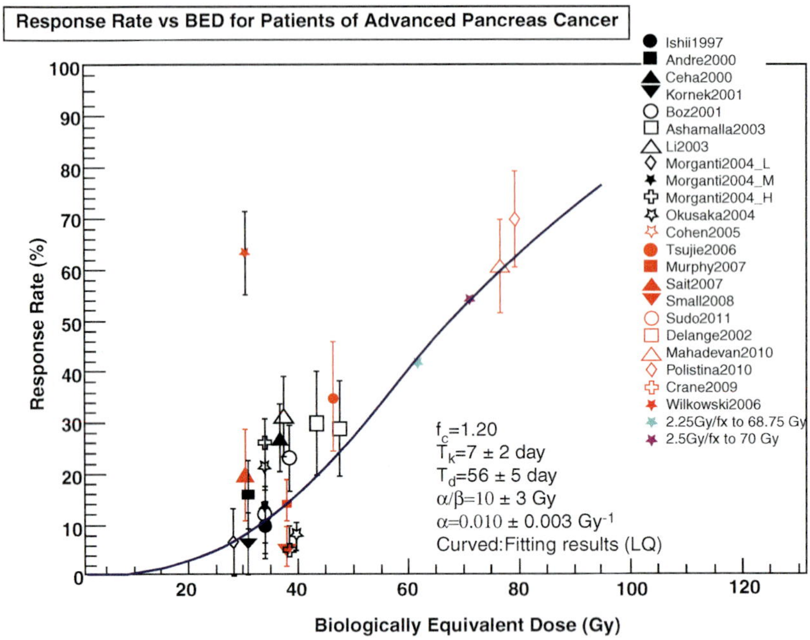

Fig. 11.3 (**a**) Tumor local control versus biologically effective dose for radiation therapy of advanced unresectable pancreatic cancer. (**b**) Tumor response rate vs. biologically effective dose for radiation therapy of advanced unresectable pancreatic cancer. The data are fitted with a modified linear quadratic (LQ) model. The points (pink star, green star, and blue star) show the expected response for potential dose escalation schemes. (For color version, see online at www.practicalradonc.org) (With permission from Moraru et al. *Practical Radiation Oncology* 4:16, 2014)

tion was made between the various agents. In order to properly compare the data, a biologically equivalent dose (BED) was calculated for each trial based on the fractionation scheme and treatment duration, using estimates for the radiobiological parameters. Even though there was no survival advantage with increasing the radiation dose, the results reveal that there is a benefit of increased tumor response with higher dose radiation, as illustrated in Fig. 11.3. A BED >70 Gy correlated with improved response.

Clinical Series Using Dose Escalation

Conventionally fractioned doses of radiation of 50–54 Gy must be considered palliative in LAPC [30]. Dose escalation in the upper abdomen has been approached with great care. The Groupe Cooperateur Multidisciplinaire en Oncologie (GERCOR) retrospectively evaluated 181 patients with LAPC who were prospectively enrolled on multiple phase II and III clinical trials and had received chemotherapy for at least 3 months. In patients without disease progression (128 patients), the treating physician determined whether to continue chemotherapy or proceed with chemoradiation to 55 Gy with concurrent infusion 5-FU. The groups were balanced for initial characteristics and induction chemotherapy. In the group receiving CRT vs. chemotherapy alone, the progression and median overall survival times were 10.8 vs. 7.4 months and 15.0 vs. 11.7 months. The radiation in this trial was advanced 3D conformal with contouring of the targets (GTV and associated pancreas and regional nodes) and organs at risk. Dose-volume histograms were generated. Both initial large (45 Gy/25 fx) and subsequent boost fields (10 Gy/8 fx) were created [4]. This became the backbone trial for the LAP 07 trial previously described, which did not show a survival advantage for the subsequent addition of radiation (54 Gy) following chemotherapy [6, 15]. Contrastingly, in a phase III radiation first vs. chemotherapy alone study, Chauffert et al. reported on 119 patients with LAPC randomized to intensive induction chemoradiation (60 Gy/30 fractions with concurrent 5-FU and cisplatin) vs. induction Gem without radiation. Maintenance Gem was then given in both arms. There was no survival advantage in the radiation arm vs. chemotherapy alone arm with median overall survivals of 8.6 and 13 months and a worse toxicity profile in the radiation arm. Large radiation fields were used in this study which included the primary and elective nodes, and toxicity was problematic with concurrent cisplatin and 5-FU coupled with these large volumes. This combination had never been tested in a phase I or II trial first [68]. In another 3D series, Ceha et al. treated 44 patients with unresectable disease with doses of 70–72 Gy in a phase II study using small volume treatment (PTV = GTV + 1 cm) and no concurrent chemotherapy. GI toxicity included three grade 3, two grade 4, and three grade 5 (fatal GI bleeding) complications. In six of these eight patients, there was also progressive local disease [69].

IMRT was used in a phase I/II trial at the University of Michigan, to escalate the dose from 50 to 60 Gy in 25 fractions delivered concurrently with full-dose Gem (1000 mg/m2 weekly on weeks 1, 2, 4, and 5 of radiotherapy) [12]. The trial accrued 50 patients and demonstrated that high-dose radiotherapy (55Gy in 25 fractions) can be delivered safely with concurrent full-dose Gem, with the use of IMRT. The rate of severe toxicity (24%) observed at this dose compares favorably with toxicities reported with other contemporary regimens. The median and 2-year survival in this trial (14.8 months and 30%, respectively) was significantly better than historical controls (11.2 months and 13%, respectively) [9]. High-dose radiotherapy also improved the 2-year local control from 38% (historical controls) to 59%. Additionally, 12 of 50 patients (24%) receiving high-dose radiotherapy were able to undergo resection with good outcomes; 10 patients (83%) had R0 resections, and 5 patients (42%) had a major pathological response. The median survival in these patients was 32 months. The trial also confirmed that elective lymph node irradiation is not required in this setting as only the CT-defined GTV was treated with a 1.0 cm margin with active breathing control [12]. Investigators at Washington University also reported a favorable progression-free and overall survival (13.9 and 23.1 months, respectively) for 25 patients with locally advanced disease and seven with borderline resectable disease following intensified IMRT radiation with 55 Gy in 25 fractions with full-dose gemcitabine. All of these patients received induction FOLFIRINOX or gemcitabine-based chemotherapy [22]. Chung et al. also demonstrated that patients who received modestly higher doses of radiation therapy (EQD2 of 61Gy), even after propensity matching, had improved OS, improved PFS, and improved local failure rate with similar toxicities to standard chemoradiation doses. They used 3D conformal techniques for the patients receiving 50.4 Gy/28 fractions (EQD2 49.56 Gy) and IMRT techniques for the higher-dose patients: 57–58.42 Gy/20–23 fractions (EQD2 61 Gy) [70]. At MD Anderson, Krishnan et al. highlighted the benefit of dose-escalated chemoradiation following induction chemotherapy. Of the 200 patients with LAPC treated between 2006 and 2014, 47 had tumors >1cm from luminal organs and were chosen for dose-escalated IMRT and concurrent Cape to a biologically effective dose (BED) > 70 Gy. The choice of dose fractionation was determined by evaluating tumor coverage vs. the proximity of the stomach, duodenum, and jejunum. A more fractionated and lower-dose regimen was used when tumors were closer to GI mucosa with a range of fractions from 5–39 with total doses of 50 Gy–70.4 Gy [62]. The authors demonstrated a 17.8-month versus 15.0-month OS advantage ($p = 0.03$) for patients who received a BED >70 Gy as well as an improved regional recurrence-free survival (10.2 versus 6.2 months [$P = 0.05$]) as compared to those with a BED <70 Gy. With exclusion of patients with tumors adjacent to bowel, they were able to achieve median gross tumor volume (GTV) coverage of 96% of the prescription dose. Of note, with tumors abutting the bowel, these high doses could also be delivered, but the GTV coverage would necessarily be lower to meet the organs-at-risk constraints. To date, the extent of GTV coverage with the prescription dose does not appear to affect outcome with GTV coverage as low as 70% in some patients, but more data is forthcoming relative to this cohort. For the 47 patients treated with tumors >1cm from the GI tract, there was no difference in median recurrence-free survival, time to local recurrence, distant recurrence-free survival, or the time to distant recurrence. There was no increase in toxicity in the high-dose group. Higher dose (BED) was the only predictor of improved OS on multivariate analysis. There was a threefold increase in overall survival at 3 years (31% vs. 9%) [13, 14]. Rudra et al. reported the first series of patients treated with high-dose adaptive MRI-guided radiation therapy from three institutions. Thirty-six patients were treated according to institutional guidelines. On multivariate analysis, BED >70 was predictive of improved OS even after controlling for CA 19–9 at diagnosis and use of induction chemotherapy ($p = 0.045$). In the BED <70, OS was 8.8 months, while OS had not been reached for the BED ≥70 [71]. These trials demonstrate that intensification of local therapy with the use of high-dose radiation and highly conformal techniques can be delivered safely and results in encouraging local control rates and OS.

A National Cancer Data Base (NCDB) review of unresected, nonmetastatic pancreatic cancer patient treated in the United States revealed that prior to matching, median survival for chemotherapy alone was 9.9 months, external beam radiation therapy (EBRT) was 10.9 months, intensity-modulated radiation therapy (IMRT) was 12 months, and SBRT was 13.9 months. In separate matched analysis, SBRT was superior to chemotherapy alone (log rank $P < 0.0001$) and ERBT (log rank $P = 0.180$). After matching, survival did not differ between IMRT and SBRT (log rank $P = 0.0492$) [72]. Petrelli et al. did a systematic review and pooled analysis of 19 SBRT trials which included 1009 patients. The pooled 1-year OS was 51.6% in 13 trials. The median OS ranged from 5.7 months to 47 months (median 17 months). The LRC rate at 1 year was 72.3%, and severe adverse events did not exceed 10%. LRC appeared to correlate with the total SBRT dose and the number of fractions [73]. A recent review of SBRT dose fractionation schemes and outcomes is provided by Rosati et al. [74].

Considerations for Doses to Normal Structures

Duodenal toxicity is of concern when treating unresectable pancreatic cancer and has often restricted radiation dose escalation strategies due to this intimately related organ. Similar challenges exist for the stomach and other portions of the small bowel. Singh et al. characterized duodenal and non-duodenal small bowel organ motion between fractions of pancreatic radiation therapy by obtaining multiple weekly CT scans during the radiation course. They concluded that the duodenum may be more vulnerable than other small bowel segments due to its attachments and relative immobility. The duodenum is fixed to the pancreas by the pancreatic duct and to the gallbladder by the common bile duct. The ligament of Treitz also positions the pancreas close to the duodenum [65]. The mobile non-duodenal small bowel may be less threatened by high doses to large volumes than the relatively fixed duodenum. Additionally, the presence of stomach acid may also make the duodenum more vulnerable to ulceration after radiation [61]. There is concern over ulceration, bleeding, and even perforation with high radiation doses. When there is duodenal invasion by tumor, the risk of perforation is even higher and is considered a contraindication to SBRT. There has been very little data on duodenal dose constraints. Huguet et al. suggest caution when doses approach 55 Gy [30].

The Quantitative Analysis of Normal Tissue Effects in the Clinic (QUANTEC) review by Kavanagh et al. presents useful consensus guidelines for small bowel dose-volume effects for conventionally fractionated doses of the 45–50 Gy and suggests that the volume of the small bowel irradiated to 15 Gy, V_{15}, should be less than 120 cc. For SBRT, the absolute volume of small bowel receiving >12.5 Gy in a single fraction should be less than 30 cc with avoidance of circumferential coverage above that dose. For a three- to five-fraction regimen, the maximum point dose should be <30 Gy. For stomach, doses of conventional fractionation of 45 Gy to the entire stomach are associated with late toxicity in 5–7%. For SBRT, the volume of stomach receiving >22.5 Gy should be <4% or 5cc with a maximum point dose of <30 Gy [75].

In an effort to look for dose/volume correlates of toxicity for both SBRT and conventional fractionation radiation, Prior et al. performed modified linear quadratic (*MLQ*) based on iso-effective dose calculations using duodenum/small bowel dose-response data from reports whose fractionation schedules ranged from 1.5 to 25 Gy/fx [76]. Published duodenum/small bowel dose-response data using a dose per fraction of 1.5–25 Gy were converted to MLQ equivalent dose in 2 Gy fractions ($MLQED_2$) using parameters obtained by modified Lyman model fitting. Furthermore, a method of converting dose-response data at one level of NTCP to another NTCP level was also presented. It was concluded that these converted dose-response data from conventionally fractionated radiotherapy (CFRT) and stereotactic body radiation therapy (SBRT) reports were reasonably consistent with one another in the range of 55–65 Gy.

There have been a number of retrospective series that have evaluated duodenal toxicity when treating upper abdominal malignancies. Three of these are based on para-aortic irradiation from the gynecologic literature. Verma et al. at MD Anderson studied 105 patients who had para-aortic IMRT with doses of 45–50.4 Gy to large fields and sequential boost doses up to 60–66 Gy at 1.8–2.2 Gy/fx. The 3-year actuarial rate of any duodenal toxicity (≥G2) was 11.7% with nine patients with complications. The 3-year actuarial rates of duodenal toxicity with V55 above and below 15 cm^3 were 48.6% and 7.4% ($p = <0.1$). In recursive partitioning analysis, a V55 less than 13.94% segregated all patients with duodenal toxicity. A V55 < 15cm^3 was recommended [77]. Xu et al. at Pittsburg reported no duodenal complications in their 76 patients who received para-aortic irradiation for gynecologic cancers. These patients received 45–50 Gy to the entire para-aortic region, and then SIB boosts to positive nodes to 55 Gy at 2.2 Gy/fx. No patients in their series had a V55 Gy > 15 cm^3, and two patients had a V55 > 5cm^3, and 7, a V55 > 1cm^3 without complications. They suggested careful editing of the high-dose PTV from the duodenum and limiting this overlap to 4–5 mm [78]. Poorvu et al. at Brigham and Women's Hospital also reported their experience with para-aortic irradiation and duodenal toxicity in 46 patients. These patients received 41.4–65 Gy at 1.8–2.0 Gy/fx using a sequential boost technique. There were no duodenal complications in their 6.5% incidence of both acute and late GI toxicities [79].

There is also important data from the pancreas radiation literature:

SBRT A dosimetric model of NCI Common Terminology Criteria for Adverse Events (CTC) v3.0 duodenal toxicity had been developed by Murphy et al. using SBRT dose-volume data from 73 pancreatic cancer patients treated with Cyberknife [80]. This study reported an association between 12-month actuarial estimates of grade ≥ 2 CTCAE duodenal toxicity (including ulceration, stricture, gastrointestinal (GI) hemorrhage, and perforation), dose-volume parameters V10–V25, and the maximum dose to 1 cc of duodenum, $D_{1\,cc}$. This series used a single fraction dose of 25 Gy which is no longer in use. Bae et al. used a 45 Gy/three-fraction SBRT regimen for a number of abdominal tumors and sites and found that Dmax was predictive of toxicity with a recommendation to limit Dmax <35 Gy. A pre-existing history of ulcers or cirrhosis can lower the threshold for toxicity [81].

Conventional Fractionation Nakamura et al. identified several dosimetric parameters that correlated with acute upper gastrointestinal toxicity and upper gastrointestinal bleeding in 40 patients with LAPC treated with 54 Gy/30 fractions with low-dose Gem. For acute GI toxicity, a V50 > 16cm^3 of the stomach was the best predictor, and the actual incidence was 9% vs. 61% above or below this threshold. For upper GI bleeding, a V50 of ≥33 cm^3 of a composite stomach/duodenum was the best predictor [82].

Huang et al. reported dosimetric predictors of GI toxicity in a group of 46 LAPD patients receiving 36 Gy in 2.4 Gy per fraction and full-dose concurrent Gem. The authors report a 12-month GI toxicity rate of 8% provided the $V_{25} \leq 45\%$. On multivariate analysis, the V25 Gy and V35 Gy > 20% were the best predictors for GI toxicity [83].

Kelly et al. reported on duodenal toxicity after fractionated chemoradiation for LAPC. All patients received neoadjuvant as well as concurrent chemotherapy. Of the 106 patients treated, 78 were treated with standard dose/fractionation of 50.4 Gy/28 fractions, and 28 received dose-escalated radiation (IMRT) of 57.5–75.4 Gy/28–39 fractions. Twenty patients had treatment-related duodenal toxicities. On multivariate analysis, only V55 ≥ 1 cm^3 was statistically significant [66].

Cattaneo et al. treated 61 patients with an altered fractionation regime half treated with 44.25 Gy/15 fx with an SIB to a tumor subvolume infiltrating the vessels to 48–58 Gy. The other half received just the 44.25/15 fx. Only the tumor and any suspicious regional nodes were treated. All of the patients received chemotherapy first and then concurrent chemotherapy. They found that the stomach V20 was an independent predictor of acute GI toxicity. For the duodenum, they recommended a V40 < 16% and a V45 < 2.6% to limit both acute and late toxicity [84].

Liu et al. reported on 68 patients treated with IMRT with an SIB approach with doses of 50, 60, and 70–80 Gy in 15–20 fractions. On multivariate analysis, a V45 of the duodenum was an independent predictor for grade 2+ GI toxicity. A V45 of 0.5 cm^3 was the optimal threshold to predict GI toxicity [85].

Role of Surgery in Initially Locally Advanced Unresectable Disease

Even some patients with locally advanced cancers can essentially receive neoadjuvant dose-escalated radiation and go on to margin-negative resections in this setting [62, 86]. In the University of Michigan Ben-Josef series, 12 of 50 patients (24%) receiving high-dose radiotherapy were able to undergo resection with good outcomes; 10 patients (83%) had R0 resection, and 5 patients (42%) had a major pathological response. The median survival in these patients was 32 months. They noted that residual imaging abnormalities next to blood vessels before surgery often represented just fibrotic tissue. Additionally, the surgery could be done safely after high-dose radiation [12]. With similar doses of radiation, Badiyan at Washington University also reported that 10/32 (32%) patients underwent resection and surgical resection was the only treatment factor which significantly impacted overall survival ($p = 0.005$). Two of the ten had a complete pathologic response and 9/10 had negative margins [22]. In the MCW series of Chatzizacharias et al., total neoadjuvant treatment was given to 96 patients with LAPC (45 Type A, 51 Type B). Forty-seven of the 96 patients (49%) were taken to surgery, and 40 (42%) underwent resection. Resected patients had a median overall survival of 38.9 months [25].

Conclusions

Locally advanced pancreas cancer is a diverse disease. Though the LAP07 trial did not confer a survival benefit with the addition of modest dose radiation, it creates an opportunity to seek further truths in the treatment of this difficult disease. Many questions remain. What features predict for resistance to both chemotherapy and radiation, and what features distinguish tumors with the propensity to spread early and widely vs. those that persist locally? What chemotherapy agents could be better coupled with radiation, and what radiation techniques could further improve outcomes by increasing local control and decreasing complications? Dose escalation studies using contemporary image-guided radiation may be an important therapeutic intervention for select patients with LAPC. Precision medicine with an investigation of biospecimens as well as imaging studies (radiomics) might help to predict which patients may benefit the most from intensive local therapy following effective systemic treatment.

Bibliography

1. Siegel RL, Miller KD, Jemal A. Cancer statistics, 2017. CA Cancer J Clin. 2017;67(1):7–30.
2. Schrag D. Optimizing treatment for locally advanced pancreas cancer: progress but no precision. JAMA. 2016;315(17):1837–8.
3. Evans DB, George B, Tsai S. Non-metastatic pancreatic cancer: resectable, borderline resectable, and locally advanced-definitions of increasing importance for the optimal delivery of multimodality therapy. Ann Surg Oncol. 2015;22(11):3409–13.
4. Huguet F, Andre T, Hammel P, Artru P, Balosso J, Selle F, et al. Impact of chemoradiotherapy after disease control with chemotherapy in locally advanced pancreatic adenocarcinoma in GERCOR phase II and III studies. J Clin Oncol. 2007;25(3):326–31.
5. Krishnan S, Rana V, Janjan NA, Varadhachary GR, Abbruzzese JL, Das P, et al. Induction chemotherapy selects patients with locally advanced, unresectable pancreatic cancer for optimal benefit from consolidative chemoradiation therapy. Cancer. 2007;110(1):47–55.
6. Hammel P, Huguet F, van Laethem JL, Goldstein D, Glimelius B, Artru P, et al. Effect of chemoradiotherapy vs chemotherapy on survival in patients with locally advanced pancreatic cancer controlled after 4 months of gemcitabine with or without erlotinib: the LAP07 randomized clinical trial. JAMA. 2016;315(17):1844–53.
7. Iacobuzio-Donahue CA, Fu B, Yachida S, Luo M, Abe H, Henderson CM, et al. DPC4 gene status of the primary carcinoma correlates with patterns of failure in patients with pancreatic cancer. J Clin Oncol. 2009;27(11):1806–13.
8. Ben-Josef E, Lawrence TS. Chemoradiotherapy for unresectable pancreatic cancer. Int J Clin Oncol. 2008;13(2):121–6.
9. Murphy JD, Adusumilli S, Griffith KA, Ray ME, Zalupski MM, Lawrence TS, et al. Full-dose gemcitabine and concurrent radiotherapy for unresectable pancreatic cancer. Int J Radiat Oncol Biol Phys. 2007;68(3):801–8.
10. Shinchi H, Takao S, Noma H, Matsuo Y, Mataki Y, Mori S, et al. Length and quality of survival after external-beam radiotherapy with concurrent continuous 5-fluorouracil infusion for locally unresectable pancreatic cancer. Int J Radiat Oncol Biol Phys. 2002;53(1):146–50.
11. Huguet F, Girard N, Guerche CS, Hennequin C, Mornex F, Azria D. Chemoradiotherapy in the management of locally advanced pancreatic carcinoma: a qualitative systematic review. J Clin Oncol. 2009;27(13):2269–77.
12. Ben-Josef E, Schipper M, Francis IR, Hadley S, Ten-Haken R, Lawrence T, et al. A phase I/II trial of intensity modulated radiation (IMRT) dose escalation with concurrent fixed-dose rate gemcitabine (FDR-G) in patients with unresectable pancreatic cancer. Int J Radiat Oncol Biol Phys. 2012;84(5):1166–71.
13. Crane CH. Improving long-term survival in patients with locally advanced pancreatic cancer via the delivery of definitive radiotherapy doses. Oncology (Williston Park). 2015;29(8):561–2, 6.
14. Crane CH. Hypofractionated ablative radiotherapy for locally advanced pancreatic cancer. J Radiat Res. 2016;57(Suppl 1):i53–i7.
15. Hammel PHF, Van Laethem JL, et al. Comparison of chemoradiotherapy (CRT) and chemotherapy (CT) in patients with a locally advanced pancreatic cancer (LAPC) controlled after 4 months of gemcitabine with or without erlotinib: final results of the international phase III LAP07 study. J Clin Oncol. 2013;31:LBA4003.
16. Jani A, Horowitz DP. Radiation therapy deviations in trial of locally advanced pancreatic cancer [corrected]. JAMA. 2016;316(13):1409.
17. Loehrer PJ Sr, Feng Y, Cardenes H, Wagner L, Brell JM, Cella D, et al. Gemcitabine alone versus gemcitabine plus radiotherapy in patients with locally advanced pancreatic cancer: an Eastern Cooperative Oncology Group trial. J Clin Oncol. 2011;29(31):4105–12.
18. Mukherjee S, Hurt CN, Bridgewater J, Falk S, Cummins S, Wasan H, et al. Gemcitabine-based or capecitabine-based chemoradiotherapy for locally advanced pancreatic cancer (SCALOP): a multicentre, randomised, phase 2 trial. Lancet Oncol. 2013;14(4):317–26.
19. Hurt CN, Falk S, Crosby T, McDonald A, Ray R, Joseph G, et al. Long-term results and recurrence patterns from SCALOP: a phase II randomised trial of gemcitabine- or capecitabine-based chemoradiation for locally advanced pancreatic cancer. Br J Cancer. 2017;116(10):1264–70.
20. Conroy T, Desseigne F, Ychou M, Bouche O, Guimbaud R, Becouarn Y, et al. FOLFIRINOX versus gemcitabine for metastatic pancreatic cancer. N Engl J Med. 2011;364(19):1817–25.
21. Christians KK, Tsai S, Mahmoud A, Ritch P, Thomas JP, Wiebe L, et al. Neoadjuvant FOLFIRINOX for borderline resectable pancreas cancer: a new treatment paradigm? Oncologist. 2014;19(3):266–74.
22. Badiyan SN, Olsen JR, Lee AY, Yano M, Menias CO, Khwaja S, et al. Induction chemotherapy followed by concurrent full-dose gemcitabine and intensity-modulated radiation therapy for borderline resectable and locally advanced pancreatic adenocarcinoma. Am J Clin Oncol. 2016;39(1):1–7.
23. Katz MH, Shi Q, Ahmad SA, Herman JM, Marsh Rde W, Collisson E, et al. Preoperative modified FOLFIRINOX treatment followed by capecitabine-based chemoradiation for borderline resectable pancreatic cancer: alliance for clinical trials in oncology trial A021101. JAMA Surg. 2016;151(8):e161137.
24. Faris JE, Blaszkowsky LS, McDermott S, Guimaraes AR, Szymonifka J, Huynh MA, et al. FOLFIRINOX in locally advanced pancreatic cancer: the Massachusetts General Hospital Cancer Center experience. Oncologist. 2013;18(5):543–8.

25. Chatzizacharias NA, Tsai S, Griffin M, Tolat P, Ritch P, George B, et al. Locally advanced pancreas cancer: staging and goals of therapy. Surgery. 2018;163:1053.
26. Paulson ES, Erickson B, Schultz C, Allen LX. Comprehensive MRI simulation methodology using a dedicated MRI scanner in radiation oncology for external beam radiation treatment planning. Med Phys. 2015;42(1):28–39.
27. Heerkens HD, Hall WA, Li XA, Knechtges P, Dalah E, Paulson ES, et al. Recommendations for MRI-based contouring of gross tumor volume and organs at risk for radiation therapy of pancreatic cancer. Pract Radiat Oncol. 2017;7(2):126–36.
28. Heerkens HD, van Vulpen M, van den Berg CA, Tijssen RH, Crijns SP, Molenaar IQ, et al. MRI-based tumor motion characterization and gating schemes for radiation therapy of pancreatic cancer. Radiother Oncol. 2014;111(2):252–7.
29. Reese AS, Lu W, Regine WF. Utilization of intensity-modulated radiation therapy and image-guided radiation therapy in pancreatic cancer: is it beneficial? Semin Radiat Oncol. 2014;24(2):132–9.
30. Huguet F, Goodman KA, Azria D, Racadot S, Abrams RA. Radiotherapy technical considerations in the management of locally advanced pancreatic cancer: American-French consensus recommendations. Int J Radiat Oncol Biol Phys. 2012;83(5):1355–64.
31. Bussels B, Goethals L, Feron M, Bielen D, Dymarkowski S, Suetens P, et al. Respiration-induced movement of the upper abdominal organs: a pitfall for the three-dimensional conformal radiation treatment of pancreatic cancer. Radiother Oncol. 2003;68(1):69–74.
32. Li XA, Liu F, Tai A, Ahunbay E, Chen G, Kelly T, et al. Development of an online adaptive solution to account for inter- and intra-fractional variations. Radiother Oncol. 2011;100(3):370–4.
33. Tai A, Liang Z, Erickson B, Li XA. Management of respiration-induced motion with 4-dimensional computed tomography (4DCT) for pancreas irradiation. Int J Radiat Oncol Biol Phys. 2013;86(5):908–13.
34. Taniguchi CM, Murphy JD, Eclov N, Atwood TF, Kielar KN, Christman-Skieller C, et al. Dosimetric analysis of organs at risk during expiratory gating in stereotactic body radiation therapy for pancreatic cancer. Int J Radiat Oncol Biol Phys. 2013;85(4):1090–5.
35. Cattaneo GM, Passoni P, Sangalli G, Slim N, Longobardi B, Mancosu P, et al. Internal target volume defined by contrast-enhanced 4D-CT scan in unresectable pancreatic tumour: evaluation and reproducibility. Radiother Oncol. 2010;97(3):525–9.
36. Prokesch RW, Chow LC, Beaulieu CF, Bammer R, Jeffrey RB Jr. Isoattenuating pancreatic adenocarcinoma at multi-detector row CT: secondary signs. Radiology. 2002;224(3):764–8.
37. Arvold ND, Niemierko A, Mamon HJ, Fernandez-del Castillo C, Hong TS. Pancreatic cancer tumor size on CT scan versus pathologic specimen: implications for radiation treatment planning. Int J Radiat Oncol Biol Phys. 2011;80(5):1383–90.
38. Godfrey DJ, Patel BN, Adamson JD, Subashi E, Salama JK, Palta M. Triphasic contrast enhanced CT simulation with bolus tracking for pancreas SBRT target delineation. Pract Radiat Oncol. 2017;7(6):e489–e97.
39. Qiu H, Wild AT, Wang H, Fishman EK, Hruban RH, Laheru DA, et al. Comparison of conventional and 3-dimensional computed tomography against histopathologic examination in determining pancreatic adenocarcinoma tumor size: implications for radiation therapy planning. Radiother Oncol. 2012;104(2):167–72.
40. Hall WA, Mikell JL, Mittal P, Colbert L, Prabhu RS, Kooby DA, et al. Tumor size on abdominal MRI versus pathologic specimen in resected pancreatic adenocarcinoma: implications for radiation treatment planning. Int J Radiat Oncol Biol Phys. 2013;86(1):102–7.
41. Koong AC, Mehta VK, Le QT, Fisher GA, Terris DJ, Brown JM, et al. Pancreatic tumors show high levels of hypoxia. Int J Radiat Oncol Biol Phys. 2000;48(4):919–22.
42. Von Hoff DD, Korn R, Mousses S. Pancreatic cancer – could it be that simple? A different context of vulnerability. Cancer Cell. 2009;16(1):7–8.
43. Park MS, Klotz E, Kim MJ, Song SY, Park SW, Cha SW, et al. Perfusion CT: noninvasive surrogate marker for stratification of pancreatic cancer response to concurrent chemo- and radiation therapy. Radiology. 2009;250(1):110–7.
44. Goldstein SD, Ford EC, Duhon M, McNutt T, Wong J, Herman JM. Use of respiratory-correlated four-dimensional computed tomography to determine acceptable treatment margins for locally advanced pancreatic adenocarcinoma. Int J Radiat Oncol Biol Phys. 2010;76(2):597–602.
45. Gabata T, Matsui O, Kadoya M, et al. Small pancreatic adenocarcinomas: efficacy of MR imaging with fat supression and gadolinium enhancement. Radiology. 1994;193:683–8.
46. Semelka RC, Kelekis NL, Molina PL, Sharp TJ, Calvo B. Pancreatic masses with inconclusive findings on spiral CT: is there a role for MRI? J Magn Reson Imaging. 1996;6(4):585–8.
47. Semelka R, editor. Abdominal-pelvic MRI. 2nd ed. Hoboken: John Wiley & Sons, INc.; 2006.
48. Ichikawa T, Erturk SM, Motosugi U, Sou H, Iino H, Araki T, et al. High-b value diffusion-weighted MRI for detecting pancreatic adenocarcinoma: preliminary results. AJR Am J Roentgenol. 2007;188(2):409–14.
49. Barral M, Taouli B, Guiu B, Koh DM, Luciani A, Manfredi R, et al. Diffusion-weighted MR imaging of the pancreas: current status and recommendations. Radiology. 2015;274(1):45–63.
50. Cuneo KC, Chenevert TL, Ben-Josef E, Feng MU, Greenson JK, Hussain HK, et al. A pilot study of diffusion-weighted MRI in patients undergoing neoadjuvant chemoradiation for pancreatic cancer. Transl Oncol. 2014;7(5):644–9.
51. Dalah E, Erickson B, Oshima K, Schott D, Hall WA, Paulson E, et al. Correlation of ADC with pathologi-

cal treatment response for radiation therapy of pancreatic cancer. Transl Oncol. 2018;11(2):391–8.

52. Ueno M, Niwa T, Ohkawa S, Amano A, Masaki T, Miyakawa K, et al. The usefulness of perfusion-weighted magnetic resonance imaging in advanced pancreatic cancer. Pancreas. 2009;38(6):644–8.
53. Akisik MF, Sandrasegaran K, Bu G, Lin C, Hutchins GD, Chiorean EG. Pancreatic cancer: utility of dynamic contrast-enhanced MR imaging in assessment of antiangiogenic therapy. Radiology. 2010;256(2):441–9.
54. Cui Y, Song J, Pollom E, Alagappan M, Shirato H, Chang DT, et al. Quantitative analysis of (18) F-Fluorodeoxyglucose positron emission tomography identifies novel prognostic imaging biomarkers in locally advanced pancreatic cancer patients treated with stereotactic body radiation therapy. Int J Radiat Oncol Biol Phys. 2016;96(1):102–9.
55. Chang JS, Choi SH, Lee Y, Kim KH, Park JY, Song SY, et al. Clinical usefulness of (1)(8) F-fluorodeoxyglucose-positron emission tomography in patients with locally advanced pancreatic cancer planned to undergo concurrent chemoradiation therapy. Int J Radiat Oncol Biol Phys. 2014;90(1):126–33.
56. Schellenberg D, Quon A, Minn AY, Graves EE, Kunz P, Ford JM, et al. 18Fluorodeoxyglucose PET is prognostic of progression-free and overall survival in locally advanced pancreas cancer treated with stereotactic radiotherapy. Int J Radiat Oncol Biol Phys. 2010;77(5):1420–5.
57. Hall WA, Heerkens HD, Paulson ES, Meijer GJ, Kotte AN, Knechtges P, et al. Pancreatic gross tumor volume contouring on computed tomography (CT) compared with magnetic resonance imaging (MRI): results of an international contouring conference. Pract Radiat Oncol. 2018;8(2):107–15.
58. Yamazaki H, Nishiyama K, Tanaka E, Koiwai K, Shikama N, Ito Y, et al. Dummy run for a phase II multi-institute trial of chemoradiotherapy for unresectable pancreatic cancer: inter-observer variance in contour delineation. Anticancer Res. 2007;27(4C):2965–71.
59. Dalah E, Moraru I, Paulson E, Erickson B, Li XA. Variability of target and normal structure delineation using multimodality imaging for radiation therapy of pancreatic cancer. Int J Radiat Oncol Biol Phys. 2014;89(3):633–40.
60. Ito Y, Okusaka T, Kagami Y, Ueno H, Ikeda M, Sumi M, et al. Evaluation of acute intestinal toxicity in relation to the volume of irradiated small bowel in patients treated with concurrent weekly gemcitabine and radiotherapy for locally advanced pancreatic cancer. Anticancer Res. 2006;26(5B):3755–9.
61. Kelly P, Das P, Pinnix CC, Beddar S, Briere T, Pham M, et al. Duodenal toxicity after fractionated chemoradiation for unresectable pancreatic cancer. Int J Radiat Oncol Biol Phys. 2013;85(3):e143–9.
62. Krishnan S, Chadha AS, Suh Y, Chen HC, Rao A, Das P, et al. Focal radiation therapy dose escalation improves overall survival in locally advanced pancreatic cancer patients receiving induction chemotherapy and consolidative chemoradiation. Int J Radiat Oncol Biol Phys. 2016;94(4):755–65.
63. Bittner MI, Grosu AL, Brunner TB. Comparison of toxicity after IMRT and 3D-conformal radiotherapy for patients with pancreatic cancer – a systematic review. Radiother Oncol. 2015;114(1):117–21.
64. Prasad S, Cambridge L, Huguet F, Chou JF, Zhang Z, Wu AJ, et al. Intensity modulated radiation therapy reduces gastrointestinal toxicity in locally advanced pancreas cancer. Pract Radiat Oncol. 2016;6(2):78–85.
65. Singh AK, Tierney RM, Low DA, Parikh PJ, Myerson RJ, Deasy JO, et al. A prospective study of differences in duodenum compared to remaining small bowel motion between radiation treatments: implications for radiation dose escalation in carcinoma of the pancreas. Radiat Oncol. 2006;1:33.
66. Herman JM, Chang DT, Goodman KA, Dholakia AS, Raman SP, Hacker-Prietz A, et al. Phase 2 multi-institutional trial evaluating gemcitabine and stereotactic body radiotherapy for patients with locally advanced unresectable pancreatic adenocarcinoma. Cancer. 2015;121(7):1128–37.
67. Moraru IC, Tai A, Erickson B, Li XA. Radiation dose responses for chemoradiation therapy of pancreatic cancer: an analysis of compiled clinical data using biophysical models. Pract Radiat Oncol. 2014;4(1):13–9.
68. Chauffert B, Mornex F, Bonnetain F, Rougier P, Mariette C, Bouche O, et al. Phase III trial comparing intensive induction chemoradiotherapy (60 Gy, infusional 5-FU and intermittent cisplatin) followed by maintenance gemcitabine with gemcitabine alone for locally advanced unresectable pancreatic cancer. Definitive results of the 2000-01 FFCD/SFRO study. Ann Oncol. 2008;19(9):1592–9.
69. Ceha HM, van Tienhoven G, Gouma DJ, Veenhof CH, Schneider CJ, Rauws EA, et al. Feasibility and efficacy of high dose conformal radiotherapy for patients with locally advanced pancreatic carcinoma. Cancer. 2000;89(11):2222–9.
70. Chung SY, Chang JS, Lee BM, Kim KH, Lee KJ, Seong J. Dose escalation in locally advanced pancreatic cancer patients receiving chemoradiotherapy. Radiother Oncol. 2017;123(3):438–45.
71. Rudra S, Jiang N, Rosenberg SA, Olsen JR, Parikh PJ, Bassetti MF, et al. High dose adaptive MRI guided radiation therapy improves overall survival of inoperable pancreatic cancer. Int J Radiat Oncol Biol Phys. 2017;99(2):E184.
72. de Geus SWL, Eskander MF, Kasumova GG, Ng SC, Kent TS, Mancias JD, et al. Stereotactic body radiotherapy for unresected pancreatic cancer: a nationwide review. Cancer. 2017;123(21):4158–67.
73. Petrelli F, Comito T, Ghidini A, Torri V, Scorsetti M, Barni S. Stereotactic body radiation therapy for locally advanced pancreatic cancer: a systematic review and pooled analysis of 19 trials. Int J Radiat Oncol Biol Phys. 2017;97(2):313–22.
74. Rosati LM, Kumar R, Herman JM. Integration of stereotactic body radiation therapy into the multidis-

ciplinary management of pancreatic cancer. Semin Radiat Oncol. 2017;27(3):256–67.
75. Kavanagh BD, Pan CC, Dawson LA, Das SK, Li XA, Ten Haken RK, et al. Radiation dose-volume effects in the stomach and small bowel. Int J Radiat Oncol Biol Phys. 2010;76(3 Suppl):S101–7.
76. Prior P, Tai A, Erickson B, Li XA. Consolidating duodenal and small bowel toxicity data via isoeffective dose calculations based on compiled clinical data. Pract Radiat Oncol. 2014;4(2):e125–31.
77. Verma J, Sulman EP, Jhingran A, Tucker SL, Rauch GM, Eifel PJ, et al. Dosimetric predictors of duodenal toxicity after intensity modulated radiation therapy for treatment of the para-aortic nodes in gynecologic cancer. Int J Radiat Oncol Biol Phys. 2014;88(2):357–62.
78. Xu KM, Rajagopalan MS, Kim H, Beriwal S. Extended field intensity modulated radiation therapy for gynecologic cancers: is the risk of duodenal toxicity high? Pract Radiat Oncol. 2015;5(4):e291–7.
79. Poorvu PD, Sadow CA, Townamchai K, Damato AL, Viswanathan AN. Duodenal and other gastrointestinal toxicity in cervical and endometrial cancer treated with extended-field intensity modulated radiation therapy to paraaortic lymph nodes. Int J Radiat Oncol Biol Phys. 2013;85(5):1262–8.
80. Murphy JD, Christman-Skieller C, Kim J, Dieterich S, Chang DT, Koong AC. A dosimetric model of duodenal toxicity after stereotactic body radiotherapy for pancreatic cancer. Int J Radiat Oncol Biol Phys. 2010;78(5):1420–6.
81. Bae SH, Kim MS, Cho CK, Kang JK, Lee SY, Lee KN, et al. Predictor of severe gastroduodenal toxicity after stereotactic body radiotherapy for abdominopelvic malignancies. Int J Radiat Oncol Biol Phys. 2012;84(4):e469–74.
82. Nakamura A, Shibuya K, Matsuo Y, Nakamura M, Shiinoki T, Mizowaki T, et al. Analysis of dosimetric parameters associated with acute gastrointestinal toxicity and upper gastrointestinal bleeding in locally advanced pancreatic cancer patients treated with gemcitabine-based concurrent chemoradiotherapy. Int J Radiat Oncol Biol Phys. 2012;84(2):369–75.
83. Huang J, Robertson JM, Ye H, Margolis J, Nadeau L, Yan D. Dose-volume analysis of predictors for gastrointestinal toxicity after concurrent full-dose gemcitabine and radiotherapy for locally advanced pancreatic adenocarcinoma. Int J Radiat Oncol Biol Phys. 2012;83(4):1120–5.
84. Cattaneo GM, Passoni P, Longobardi B, Slim N, Reni M, Cereda S, et al. Dosimetric and clinical predictors of toxicity following combined chemotherapy and moderately hypofractionated rotational radiotherapy of locally advanced pancreatic adenocarcinoma. Radiother Oncol. 2013;108(1):66–71.
85. Liu X, Ren G, Li L, Xia T. Predictive dosimetric parameters for gastrointestinal toxicity with hypofractioned radiotherapy in pancreatic adenocarcinoma. Onco Targets Ther. 2016;9:2489–94.
86. Combs SE, Habermehl D, Kessel K, Bergmann F, Werner J, Brecht I, et al. Intensity modulated radiotherapy as neoadjuvant chemoradiation for the treatment of patients with locally advanced pancreatic cancer. Outcome analysis and comparison with a 3D-treated patient cohort. Strahlenther Onkol. 2013;189(9):738–44.

Molecular Profiling in Pancreatic Ductal Adenocarcinoma

12

Ben George

Introduction

Pancreatic cancer (PC) is a highly lethal malignancy, and therapeutic advances over the last decade have translated into a survival benefit that can at best be characterized as modest. Approximately 53,670 people develop exocrine PC each year in the United States, and almost all are expected to die from the disease [1]. PC is expected to become the second leading cause of cancer-related mortality in the United States, second only to lung cancer in the next decade [1]. In the absence of validated predictive biomarkers to guide selection of therapy, clinical trial design in PC, over the last several decades, has defaulted to an "all-comers" approach. In clinical practice, it is well known that the inherent biology and response to treatment can be quite varied among patients with PC, arguing for their phenotypic/genotypic characterization, and biomarker-enriched treatment strategies.

Molecular Pathogenesis

A variety of precursor lesions have been described in the pancreas. These include pancreatic intraepithelial neoplasia (PanIN), intraductal papillary mucinous neoplasms (IPMNs), and mucinous cystadenomas (MCNs) [2]. PanIN gives rise to conventional ductal adenocarcinomas, and they are 13–100-fold more common than those arising from an IPMN or MCN [3]. IPMNs are macroscopically visible cystic neoplasms that arise in the mucin-producing main pancreatic duct or one of its branches, while MCNs are macroscopically visible cystic neoplasms that do not communicate with the pancreatic duct system.

A number of key experimental and epidemiological observations suggest that PC is a genetic disease: (i) a number of somatic alterations have been recurrently identified in PC, and many of these have also been identified in precursor lesions [4–6]; (ii) PCs are known to aggregate in some families, and the genetic basis for a subset of these has been well described [7–10]; and (iii) genetically engineered mouse models can recapitulate the full spectrum of pancreatic carcinogenesis and metastasis as seen in humans [11–13].

Historically, four major driver genes have been described in the development and progression of PC- one oncogene [*KRAS*] and three tumor suppressor genes [*CDKN2A*, *TP53*, and *SMAD4*]. KRAS is thought to be constitutively activated in 92–100% of PC patients, whereas TP53, SMAD4,

B. George (✉)
Division of Medical Oncology, Department of Medicine, The Medical College of Wisconsin, Milwaukee, WI, USA
e-mail: bgeorge@mcw.edu

S. Tsai et al. (eds.), *Management of Localized Pancreatic Cancer*,
https://doi.org/10.1007/978-3-319-98944-0_12

Table 12.1 Seminal next generation sequncing studies of PC

Author	Publication year	*N*	Methodology	Discovery
Jones, S [16]	2008	24	Exome sequencing	Core set of 12 cellular signaling pathways and processes
Collison, EA [18]	2011	2 datasets	Transcriptomic profiling	(i) Three subtypes—classical, quasi-mesenchymal (QM-PDA), and exocrine-like (ii) Prognostic value of subtypes
Biankin, AV [15]	2012	99	Whole genome sequencing, CNV analysis	(i) 16 significant mutated genes (ii) Frequent and diverse somatic aberrations in genes involved in axon guidance (SLIT/ROBO signaling)
Moffitt, RA [19]	2015	206	Transcriptomic profiling	(i) Basal and classical tumor subtypes (ii) Normal and activated stromal subtypes (iii) Prognostic and predictive values of the subtypes
Waddell, N [17]	2015	100	Whole genome sequencing, CNV analysis	(i) Four subtypes—stable, locally rearranged, scattered, unstable (ii) Predictive value of unstable subtype to platinum-based chemotherapy
Bailey, P [14]	2016	456	Whole genome sequencing, deep exome sequencing, CNV analysis, transcriptomic profiling	(i) Four subtypes—squamous, pancreatic progenitor, immunogenic, and aberrantly differentiated endocrine exocrine (ADEX) (ii) Identified 32 recurrently mutated genes grouped into 10 pathways

and CDKN2A have been reported to be inactivated in 74–83%, 31–33%, and 35–75% of patients, respectively [14–17]. While these individual genes play a pivotal role in pancreatic carcinogenesis, the recognition that derangements in multiple signaling pathways or cellular process was required for pancreatic carcinogenesis was the basis for early systematic attempts to identifying core pathways and processes involved in PC development [16]. Such attempts improved our understanding of PC pathogenesis substantially; however, the translated gain in therapeutic improvement was modest at best.

The overall dismal outcome associated with PCs, the lack of reliable predictive biomarkers to guide therapy, and the significant inter-/intratumoral heterogeneity emphasized the need for a unique, "tumor-specific," summative, biologic footprint to offer consistent prognostic and/or predictive information. Major advances in technology and bioinformatics have refined attempts at generating "expression signatures" or "tumor profiles" that reflect both tumor-specific genotypic and phenotypic information, in a granular fashion. Large-scale attempts have been made to generate genomic, epigenomic, transcriptomic, and proteomic profiles of PC, with the goal of identifying distinct prognostic and predictive signatures; some of the key attempts have been listed in Table 12.1. This chapter will attempt to summarize some of the key efforts in this field, as well as the opportunities and challenges of translating "OMICS" into routine clinical practice in a way that improves the lives of our patients.

The Genomic Landscape of PC

In an attempt to characterize the mutational landscape of PC, the Australian Pancreatic Cancer Genome Initiative (APGI) as part of the International Cancer Genome Consortium (ICGC) recruited and consented patients from participating institutions [17]. Whole genome sequencing and copy number variation (CNV) analysis was performed on 100 PCs with an epithelial cellularity of ≥40% (*n* = 75), complemented by cell lines derived from APGI participants (*n* = 25) to an average depth of 65× and compared to the germline (average depth 38×). A total of 857,971 somatic point mutations and small insertions/deletions were detected in the cohort; 7888 were non-silent mutations in 5424 genes. The average tumor mutational burden across the cohort was 2.64 per Mb (range 0.65–28.2 mutations per Mb). Chromosomal rearrangements leading to gene disruption were identified in genes well known to be important in PC (*TP53*, *SMAD4*, *CDKN2A*, *ARID1A*, and *ROBO2*) and new candidate drivers of PC carcinogenesis (*KDM6A* and *PREX2*).

Based on patterns of chromosomal structural variation, PCs were classified into four subtypes as below.

1. *Stable subtype* (20% of all samples) where tumor genomes contained ≤50 structural variation events and often exhibited widespread aneuploidy suggesting defects in cell cycle/mitosis. Prevalence of *TP53* mutations was slightly less than the rest of the cohort (61% versus a mean of 70% across all samples), while point mutation rates for *KRAS* and *SMAD4* were similar to the rest of the cohort.
2. *Locally rearranged subtype* (30% of all samples) where a significant focal event was identified on one or two chromosomes. Approximately one-third of locally rearranged genomes contained common focal amplifications in *KRAS*, *SOX9*, *GATA6*, *ERBB2*, *MET*, *CDK6*, *PIK3CA*, and *PIK3R3* but at low individual prevalence (1–2% of patients). The remaining local rearrangements involved complex genomic events such as breakage-fusion-bridge (*n* = 9) or chromothripsis (*n* = 15).
3. *Scattered subtype* (36% of all samples) where a moderate range of nonrandom chromosomal damage and < 200 structural variation events were detected.
4. *Unstable subtype* (14% of all samples) where tumors exhibited a large number of structural variation events (>200; maximum of 558); the scale of genomic instability suggested defects in DNA maintenance and thus a potential for therapeutic response to DNA-damaging agents. The majority of unstable tumors (10 of 14) fell within the top quintile of the *BRCA* signature [20]; further, the top quintile of the *BRCA* signature was associated with deleterious mutations in *BRCA1* (*n* = 2), *BRCA2* (*n* = 7), and *PALB2* (*n* = 2). The predictive value of this subtype was further reinforced when five patients with unstable genomes and/or a high *BRCA* mutational signature burden had excellent responses to platinum-based chemotherapy, while three patients who did not have these characteristics (off-genotype) did not respond.

Evolution of PC

It has been proposed that PC develops in a stepwise fashion, through a sequence of genetic alterations, with a relatively gradual evolutionary trajectory since these alterations are acquired independently [4–6, 21, 22]. However, the identification of clonally expanded precursor lesions that do not belong to the tumor lineage and a clinical phenotype that demonstrates aggressive metastatic potential argue against that theory [21, 23–26]. Notta et al. performed an in-depth analysis of over 100 whole genomes from purified primary and metastatic PCs using novel informatics tools, with a focus on DNA copy number (CN) changes, their associated rearrangements from tumor-enriched genomes, and mutational phenomena linked to rapid tumor progression, to reconcile these disparate theories [27]. They concluded that (i) most mutations accumulate when these tumors are still diploid, suggesting that a prolonged preneoplastic phase (assuming preneoplastic cells are diploid) predates the onset of invasive disease and that CN events are crucial for transformation; (ii) CN changes from chromothripsis appeared to be clonal (suggesting that such events were sustained early in tumorigenesis) and transformative; (iii) some PCs may not progress through a linear series of PanIN lesions; and (iv) If chromothripsis were indeed the transforming event in some PCs, a single event could confer a cell with both invasive and metastatic properties, suggesting a short latency period between invasion and metastasis.

Transcriptomic Classification of PC

Collison Classification

The first systematic attempt at molecular classification of PC was performed using gene expression profiling [18]. Intrinsically variable (standard deviation >0.8) genes in two gene expression microarray datasets (University of California San Francisco data set and Badea et al. [28]) obtained from resected PDA were identified. These two datasets were merged to increase power using the distance-weighted discrimination (DWD) method [29, 30], and nonnegative matrix factorization (NMF) analysis with consensus clustering [31] was performed to identify subtypes of the disease. This led to the development of a 62-gene signature *(PDAssigner) and identification of three PC subtypes which were* designated as classical, quasi-mesenchymal (QM-PDA), and exocrine-like. The classical subtype was characterized by high expression of adhesion-associated and epithelial genes, such as transmembrane protein 45B (TMEM45B), trefoil factor 1 (TFF1), and mucin 13 (MUC13); the QM-PDA subtype had high expression of mesenchyme-associated genes, such as absent in melanoma 2 (AIM2), glycoprotein m6b (GPM6B), and 5′-nucleotidase, ecto (NT5E); and the exocrine-like subtype had relatively high expression of tumor cell-derived digestive enzyme genes, such as regenerating islet-derived 1 beta (REG1B), pancreatic lipase-related protein 2 (PNLIPRP2), and cystic fibrosis transmembrane conductance regulator (CFTR). Further validation of the *PDAssigner* gene expression in three additional published PC gene expression datasets [32–34] also supported these three subtypes.

When 19 human PC cell lines (publicly available) and 15 mouse lines (derived from genetically engineered $TP53^{-/-}$ and $INK4A^{-/-16}$ models of PC) were analyzed using the 62 gene *PDAssigner*, representatives of the classical and QM-PDA subtypes were identified, but not the exocrine-like subtype, raising the possibility that the latter is an artifact of contaminating normal pancreas tissue adjacent to tumor.

The Collison classification was found to have both prognostic and predictive values. In a multivariate Cox regression model including stage and subtype, the subtype was an independent predictor of overall survival ($p = 0.024$) in the UCSF data set (where clinical information was available). Further, the QM-PDA subtype lines were more sensitive to gemcitabine than the classical subtype, while erlotinib was more effective in classical subtype cell lines demonstrating, perhaps, the predictive value of the Collison classification.

Thus, for the first time, the Collison classification demonstrated the feasibility of molecular classification of PC with limited, but promising prognostic and predictive utility.

Moffitt Classification

The complex interplay between tumor and stroma has been described as a hallmark of PC, further complicating attempts at elucidating its biology and non-druggable phenotype. Stromal ablation and reprogramming strategies have garnered tremendous attention in the evolution of PC treatment, validating the significance of stromal characterization as a key component of molecular classification [35–38]. Further, tumor material from metastatic sites is often mixed with cell types from the host organ, thus contributing to the "background noise" that needs to be factored in while evaluating gene expression profiling data. Moffitt and colleagues attempted to overcome these limitations by utilizing blind source separation with nonnegative matrix factorization (NMF) [20, 39, 40] to virtually micro-dissect primary and metastatic PC samples, thus generating and validating two tumor-specific as well as stromal-specific signatures [19].

NMF was employed to analyze gene expression in a cohort of microarray data from 145 primary and 61 metastatic PC tumors, 17 cell lines, 46 pancreas, and 88 distant site adjacent normal samples using Agilent (Agilent Technologies) human whole genome 4x44K DNA microarrays. These findings were validated utilizing RNA sequencing data performed on 15 primary tumors, 37 PC patient-derived xenografts (PDX), 3 cell lines, and 6 cancer-associated fibroblast (CAF) lines derived from deidentified patients with PC.

Independent of normal and stromal factors, two subtypes of PC, namely, "classical" and "basal-like," were identified. Patients with basal-like subtype tumors had a worse median overall survival of 11 months (44% 1-year survival) compared to 19 months (70% 1-year survival) for those with classical subtype tumors ($p = 0.007$), indicative of the prognostic effect of this classification. These subtypes and their prognostic value were independently validated within the ICGC PC microarray data set. Although basal-like subtype tumors had a worse prognosis, patients with basal-like subtype tumors demonstrated a trend toward better response to adjuvant therapy ($p = 0.072$); among these patients, adjuvant therapy provided a hazard ratio of 0.38 (95% CI 0.14–1.09), while in patients with classical subtype tumors, adjuvant therapy was associated with a hazard ratio of only 0.76 (95% CI 0.40–1.43). All cell lines ($p < 0.001$), as well as majority of metastatic samples ($p = 0.002$), analyzed in this study were classified as "basal-like," suggesting that cell line models represent only one subset of PC.

Consensus clustering divided tumor samples into two stromal subtypes, namely, "normal" and "activated"; both signatures were absent in PC cell lines, while many metastatic samples expressed them at low levels suggesting that these genes were not expressed by the tumor epithelial cells. Patients with an activated stroma subtype had a worse median survival of 15 months and 60% 1-year survival when compared to patients with a normal stroma subtype (median 24 months, 1-year 82%) indicative of the prognostic value of this classification.

Both "basal-like" and "classical" tumors were found within both "normal" and "activated" stroma subtypes; "classical" subtype tumors with "normal" stroma subtypes ($n = 24$) had the lowest hazard ratio of 0.39 (95% CI 0.21–0.73], while the "basal-like" subtype tumors with "activated" stroma subtypes ($n = 26$) had the highest hazard ratio of 2.28 (95% CI 1.34–3.87). Both classifications were independently associated with survival in a multivariate Cox regression model that included tumor subtypes, stromal subtypes, and clinical variables including gender, race, T stage, N stage, margin status, adjuvant therapy, histological grade, and age (stroma subtypes: $p = 0.037$, tumor subtypes: $p = 0.003$).

The investigators attempted to reconcile the Collison classification with their subtyping utilizing the published exemplar genes for "exocrine-like," "classical," and "quasi-mesenchymal" subtypes and found that (i) Collison's "classical" subtype had a significant overlap with Moffitt's "classical" subtype genes (20/22); (ii) the "quasi-mesenchymal" subtype appeared to be a mixed collection of genes from Moffitt's "basal-like" tumor (6/20) and stromal subtypes (6/20), perhaps, thus explaining the apparent mesenchymal-like gene expression that was observed; and (iii) Collison's "exocrine-like" genes overlapped with Moffitt's genes representing the exocrine pancreas (17/17); tumors in this cluster had an expression indistinguishable from adjacent normal samples from Moffit's data set, suggesting background contamination with adjacent normal pancreatic tissue in Collison's "exocrine-like" subtype.

In addition, by virtually excluding intrinsic, organ-specific contamination and focusing on tumor autonomous gene expression, the investigators established that intra-patient tumor heterogeneity between primary and metastatic sites was surprisingly low.

Bailey Classification

Bailey and colleagues performed a comprehensive, integrated genomic analysis of 456 PCs using a combination of whole genome and deep exome sequencing, along with gene copy number analysis to determine the mutational mechanisms and genomic events relevant in pancreatic carcinogenesis. Further, RNA expression profiling was used to define four subtypes (with distinct histopathological characteristics and prognosis) and the different transcriptional networks related to them. The four subtypes identified were (1) squamous, (2) pancreatic progenitor, (3) immunogenic, and (4) aberrantly differentiated endocrine exocrine (ADEX).

The squamous tumors were characterized by gene networks involved in inflammation, hypoxia response, metabolic reprogramming,

TGF-β signaling, MYC pathway activation, autophagy, upregulated expression of *TP63ΔN*, and its target genes as well as hypermethylation and concordant downregulation of genes that governed pancreatic endodermal cell-fate determination (*PDX1*, *MNX1*, *GATA6*, *HNF1B*, etc.).

The pancreatic progenitor class was defined by transcriptional networks containing transcription factors *PDX1*, *MNX1*, *HNF4G*, *HNF4A*, *HNF1B*, *HNF1A*, *FOXA2*, *FOXA3*, and *HES1* as well as gene programs regulating fatty acid oxidation, steroid hormone biosynthesis, drug metabolism, and *O*-linked glycosylation of mucins. Apomucins *MUC5AC* and *MUC1*, but not *MUC2* or *MUC6*, were preferentially co-expressed in pancreatic progenitor tumors and were consistent with PC-associated IPMN clustering within this class.

The ADEX class was a subclass of pancreatic progenitor tumors and defined by transcriptional networks that are important in later stages of pancreatic development and differentiation. The key networks identified included upregulation of (i) transcription factors *NR5A2*, *MIST1* (also known as *BHLHA15A*), and *RBPJL* and their downstream targets that are important in acinar cell differentiation and pancreatitis/regeneration and (ii) genes associated with endocrine differentiation and MODY (including *INS*, *NEUROD1*, *NKX2–2*, and *MAFA*).

The immunogenic class shared some of the characteristics of the pancreatic progenitor class but was associated with evidence of a significant immune infiltrate. B-cell signaling pathways, antigen presentation, $CD4^+$ T cell, $CD8^+$ T cell, and Toll-like receptor signaling pathways were associated with this subtype. Further, enrichment analysis identified upregulation of genes associated with nine different immune cell types and/or phenotypes. The upregulation of acquired tumor immune suppression pathways in this subtype inferred therapeutic opportunities with immune modulators.

There was significant overlap between this classification and Collison's subtyping, specifically (i) QM-PDA (Collison) and squamous (Bailey), (ii) classical (Collison) and pancreatic progenitor (Bailey), and (iii) exocrine-like (Collison) and ADEX (Bailey).

Epigenetic Classification

Aberrant DNA methylation is implicated in initiation and progression of several cancer types [41, 42]; hypermethylation of CpG islands and promoter regions is associated with transcriptional silencing of tumor suppressor genes [43], while hypomethylation is associated with overexpression of oncogenes [43] and genomic instability [44].

In an effort to define the genome-wide pattern of DNA methylation in PCs, Nones and colleagues captured the methylation profiles of 167 untreated resected PCs and compared them to a panel of 29 adjacent nontransformed pancreata using high-density arrays [45]. A total of 11,634 CpG sites associated with 3522 genes were significantly aberrantly methylated in PC and segregated PC from nonmalignant pancreas, regardless of tumor cellularity. Pathway analysis revealed that genes involved in key molecular mechanisms including cell adhesion, hedgehog signaling, stellate cell activation, TGF-β, integrin signaling, and WNT/NOTCH signaling were aberrantly methylated. Epigenetic alteration of genes involved in stellate cell activation and their putative role in modulating cross-talk between the tumor microenvironment and tumor cells indicated opportunities for new therapeutic interventions. Further, deep sequencing revealed that epigenetic inactivation of SLIT-ROBO signaling in PC constitutes an important, alternative mechanism to disrupting the axon guidance pathway.

Hypomethylation of *MET* and *ITGA2* was found to inversely correlate with their gene expression in patients with PC. The negative prognostic impact of MET and ITGA2 overexpression as well as the fact that both *MET* and *ITGA2* signals via *CDC42*, the key effector molecule that is normally suppressed by active SLIT-ROBO signaling, is suggestive of the important role of aberrant methylation in pancreatic carcinogenesis.

Integrated Analysis

The Cancer Genome Atlas Research Network performed an integrated, multi-platform, genomic, transcriptomic, and proteomic profiling of 150 PC specimens, including samples with characteristic low neoplastic cellularity [46].

Surgically resected PCs and matched germline DNA from whole blood were identified from 150 patients with mostly stage I–III PC; four patients with evidence of metastatic disease at diagnosis were excluded from survival analyses. The median follow-up of the remaining 146 patients was 676 days, and 71 of these were alive at last follow-up. The neoplastic cellularity ranged from 0% to 53% (median 18%) as judged by central pathology review and was evaluated independently using the ABSOLUTE algorithm [47].

This comprehensive analysis led to many crucial findings [46], as summarized below.

1. Depth of sequencing was critical to the detection of mutations and somatic copy number alterations (SCNAs) in low cellularity tumors, stressing the need for deep sequencing of low-purity samples to detect both clonal and subclonal alterations.
2. Many previously identified driver genomic alterations in PC were detected along with a new driver gene, *RREB1*.
3. Germline and somatic mutations in the DNA damage repair genes *BRCA2*, *PALB2*, and *ATM* were observed in 8% of samples, thus identifying a class of patients for whom platinum-based chemotherapy and/or PARP inhibition may provide therapeutic benefit. This data also emphasized the putative value of routine clinical testing for these germline variants in patients with PC, even in the absence of contributory family history.
4. 93% of PCs demonstrated a *KRAS* mutation, and 60% of *KRAS* wild-type tumors harbored alternative RAS-MAPK pathway-activating alterations, highlighting the significance of this pathway in this disease. Targetable genomic alterations were detected in 6/10 *KRAS* wild-type tumors.
5. Molecular classification of PCs based on gene expression into basal-like and classical subtypes was independent of tumor purity; samples classified as exocrine-like (Collison) QM-PDA (Collison), ADEX (Bailey), and immunogenic (Bailey) correlated with lower tumor purity. Among low-purity tumors, a higher estimated leukocyte fraction was associated with immunogenic subtype. Considering only the high-purity samples, the squamous subtype (Bailey) showed significant overlap with the basal-like samples (Moffitt), while the pancreatic progenitor (Bailey) and classical (Collison) subtypes largely overlapped with classical subtype defined by Moffitt. Thus, high-purity tumors could be consistently classified into a basal-like/squamous group and a classical/progenitor group, while the strong association of immunogenic and ADEX or exocrine-like subtypes with the low-purity samples likely reflected gene expression from nonneoplastic cells.
6. Analysis of protein expression with reverse-phase protein arrays (RPPA) in high-purity samples revealed prognostic subtypes, specifically, a group of tumors with improved prognosis and elevated RTK and MTOR signaling, suggesting a therapeutic opportunity.
7. Differential expression of the *EVADR*, *DEANR1*, and *GATA6-AS1* long noncoding RNA (lncRNAs) was associated with the classical subtype of PC.

Opportunities and Challenges

Robust and concerted attempts at molecular classification of PCs have yielded a wealth of data; however, there exists a chasm between such data and routine clinical practice that needs to be bridged rapidly. There are several hurdles that need to be overcome: (i) the prognostic and to some extent predictive utility of the various classification schemes have been established, but the "OMIC" platform of choice for translation into clinical practice remains unclear; (ii) limited availability of tumor material for

"OMICS"—in regular clinical practice, for example there is limited tumor material available from endoscopic ultrasound (EUS)-guided fine-needle aspiration (FNA) samples (in the neoadjuvant setting) or core biopsies in the metastatic setting; (iii) cost—the cost of NGS may not currently be justified by the limited treatment options available and the existing insurance reimbursement model; (iv) lack of robust Clinical Decision Support (CDS) and bioinformatic tools to reliably and effectively reconcile "OMIC" data into clinically actionable "capsules" for the practicing clinician; and (v) pragmatic barriers to expedited "OMIC" profiling/reporting, identification of actionable biomarkers, and enrollment in "personalized medicine" PC trials [48–54].

On the other hand, the significant technologic and bioinformatic advances that have been realized over the past decade provide a glimpse of the substantial promise of precision medicine in the treatment of PC. Specifically, identification of (i) substantial minority of patients with alterations in DNA damage repair genes and their likelihood of response to platinum/PARP therapy, (ii) RAS wild-type patients with actionable somatic alterations, and (iii) predictive "OMIC" profiles utilizing machine learning algorithms that may have immediate relevance in the therapeutic landscape of PC. Further refinement of the myriad "OMIC" strategies that are in various stages of development will likely transform the early detection, screening, diagnostic, and therapeutic options for this aggressive disease.

References

1. Jemal A, et al. Global cancer statistics. CA Cancer J Clin. 2011;61(2):69–90.
2. Matthaei H, et al. Cystic precursors to invasive pancreatic cancer. Nat Rev Gastroenterol Hepatol. 2011;8(3):141–50.
3. Winter JM, et al. 1423 pancreaticoduodenectomies for pancreatic cancer: a single-institution experience. J Gastrointest Surg. 2006;10(9):1199–210; discussion 1210–1
4. Hruban RH, et al. Progression model for pancreatic cancer. Clin Cancer Res. 2000;6(8):2969–72.
5. Moskaluk CA, Hruban RH, Kern SE. p16 and K-ras gene mutations in the intraductal precursors of human pancreatic adenocarcinoma. Cancer Res. 1997;57(11):2140–3.
6. Wilentz RE, et al. Loss of expression of Dpc4 in pancreatic intraepithelial neoplasia: evidence that DPC4 inactivation occurs late in neoplastic progression. Cancer Res. 2000;60(7):2002–6.
7. Hahn SA, et al. BRCA2 germline mutations in familial pancreatic carcinoma. J Natl Cancer Inst. 2003;95(3):214–21.
8. Jones S, et al. Exomic sequencing identifies PALB2 as a pancreatic cancer susceptibility gene. Science. 2009;324(5924):217.
9. Klein AP, et al. Prospective risk of pancreatic cancer in familial pancreatic cancer kindreds. Cancer Res. 2004;64(7):2634–8.
10. Rogers CD, et al. The genetics of FANCC and FANCG in familial pancreatic cancer. Cancer Biol Ther. 2004;3(2):167–9.
11. Bardeesy N, et al. Both p16(Ink4a) and the p19(Arf)-p53 pathway constrain progression of pancreatic adenocarcinoma in the mouse. Proc Natl Acad Sci U S A. 2006;103(15):5947–52.
12. Hingorani SR, et al. Trp53R172H and KrasG12D cooperate to promote chromosomal instability and widely metastatic pancreatic ductal adenocarcinoma in mice. Cancer Cell. 2005;7(5):469–83.
13. Skoulidis F, et al. Germline Brca2 heterozygosity promotes Kras(G12D) -driven carcinogenesis in a murine model of familial pancreatic cancer. Cancer Cell. 2010;18(5):499–509.
14. Bailey P, et al. Genomic analyses identify molecular subtypes of pancreatic cancer. Nature. 2016;531(7592):47–52.
15. Biankin AV, et al. Pancreatic cancer genomes reveal aberrations in axon guidance pathway genes. Nature. 2012;491(7424):399–405.
16. Jones S, et al. Core signaling pathways in human pancreatic cancers revealed by global genomic analyses. Science. 2008;321(5897):1801–6.
17. Waddell N, et al. Whole genomes redefine the mutational landscape of pancreatic cancer. Nature. 2015;518(7540):495–501.
18. Collisson EA, et al. Subtypes of pancreatic ductal adenocarcinoma and their differing responses to therapy. Nat Med. 2011;17(4):500–3.
19. Moffitt RA, et al. Virtual microdissection identifies distinct tumor- and stroma-specific subtypes of pancreatic ductal adenocarcinoma. Nat Genet. 2015;47(10):1168–78.
20. Alexandrov LB, et al. Signatures of mutational processes in human cancer. Nature. 2013; 500(7463):415–21.
21. Luttges J, et al. Allelic loss is often the first hit in the biallelic inactivation of the p53 and DPC4 genes during pancreatic carcinogenesis. Am J Pathol. 2001;158(5):1677–83.
22. Wilentz RE, et al. Inactivation of the p16 (INK4A) tumor-suppressor gene in pancreatic duct lesions: loss of intranuclear expression. Cancer Res. 1998;58(20):4740–4.

23. Chari ST, et al. Early detection of sporadic pancreatic cancer: summative review. Pancreas. 2015;44(5):693–712.
24. Cooper CS, et al. Analysis of the genetic phylogeny of multifocal prostate cancer identifies multiple independent clonal expansions in neoplastic and morphologically normal prostate tissue. Nat Genet. 2015;47(4):367–72.
25. Martincorena I, et al. Tumor evolution. High burden and pervasive positive selection of somatic mutations in normal human skin. Science. 2015;348(6237):880–6.
26. Ross-Innes CS, et al. Whole-genome sequencing provides new insights into the clonal architecture of Barrett's esophagus and esophageal adenocarcinoma. Nat Genet. 2015;47(9):1038–46.
27. Notta F, et al. A renewed model of pancreatic cancer evolution based on genomic rearrangement patterns. Nature. 2016;538(7625):378–82.
28. Badea L, et al. Combined gene expression analysis of whole-tissue and microdissected pancreatic ductal adenocarcinoma identifies genes specifically overexpressed in tumor epithelia. Hepato-Gastroenterology. 2008;55(88):2016–27.
29. Benito M, et al. Adjustment of systematic microarray data biases. Bioinformatics. 2004;20(1):105–14.
30. Herschkowitz JI, et al. Identification of conserved gene expression features between murine mammary carcinoma models and human breast tumors. Genome Biol. 2007;8(5):R76.
31. Brunet JP, et al. Metagenes and molecular pattern discovery using matrix factorization. Proc Natl Acad Sci U S A. 2004;101(12):4164–9.
32. Balagurunathan Y, et al. Gene expression profiling-based identification of cell-surface targets for developing multimeric ligands in pancreatic cancer. Mol Cancer Ther. 2008;7(9):3071–80.
33. Grutzmann R, et al. Gene expression profiling of microdissected pancreatic ductal carcinomas using high-density DNA microarrays. Neoplasia. 2004;6(5):611–22.
34. Pei H, et al. FKBP51 affects cancer cell response to chemotherapy by negatively regulating Akt. Cancer Cell. 2009;16(3):259–66.
35. Lee JJ, et al. Stromal response to hedgehog signaling restrains pancreatic cancer progression. Proc Natl Acad Sci U S A. 2014;111(30):E3091–100.
36. Olive KP, et al. Inhibition of hedgehog signaling enhances delivery of chemotherapy in a mouse model of pancreatic cancer. Science. 2009; 324(5933):1457–61.
37. Ozdemir BC, et al. Depletion of carcinoma-associated fibroblasts and fibrosis induces immunosuppression and accelerates pancreas Cancer with reduced survival. Cancer Cell. 2015;28(6):831–3.
38. Rhim AD, et al. Stromal elements act to restrain, rather than support, pancreatic ductal adenocarcinoma. Cancer Cell. 2014;25(6):735–47.
39. Alexandrov LB, et al. Deciphering signatures of mutational processes operative in human cancer. Cell Rep. 2013;3(1):246–59.
40. Biton A, et al. Independent component analysis uncovers the landscape of the bladder tumor transcriptome and reveals insights into luminal and basal subtypes. Cell Rep. 2014;9(4):1235–45.
41. Hansen KD, et al. Increased methylation variation in epigenetic domains across cancer types. Nat Genet. 2011;43(8):768–75.
42. Lao VV, Grady WM. Epigenetics and colorectal cancer. Nat Rev Gastroenterol Hepatol. 2011;8(12):686–700.
43. Irizarry RA, et al. The human colon cancer methylome shows similar hypo- and hypermethylation at conserved tissue-specific CpG island shores. Nat Genet. 2009;41(2):178–86.
44. Jones PA, Baylin SB. The fundamental role of epigenetic events in cancer. Nat Rev Genet. 2002;3(6):415–28.
45. Nones K, et al. Genome-wide DNA methylation patterns in pancreatic ductal adenocarcinoma reveal epigenetic deregulation of SLIT-ROBO, ITGA2 and MET signaling. Int J Cancer. 2014;135(5):1110–8.
46. Integrated Genomic Characterization of Pancreatic Ductal Adenocarcinoma. Cancer Cell. 2017;32(2):185–203.e13.
47. Carter SL, et al. Absolute quantification of somatic DNA alterations in human cancer. Nat Biotechnol. 2012;30(5):413–21.
48. Chantrill LA, et al. Precision medicine for advanced pancreas Cancer: the individualized molecular pancreatic Cancer therapy (IMPaCT) trial. Clin Cancer Res. 2015;21(9):2029–37.
49. Kim ES, et al. The BATTLE trial: personalizing therapy for lung cancer. Cancer Discov. 2011;1(1):44–53.
50. Le Tourneau C, et al. Designs and challenges for personalized medicine studies in oncology: focus on the SHIVA trial. Target Oncol. 2012;7(4):253–65.
51. Thompson AM, et al. Prospective comparison of switches in biomarker status between primary and recurrent breast cancer: the breast recurrence in tissues study (BRITS). Breast Cancer Res. 2010;12(6):R92.
52. Tran B, et al. Cancer genomics: technology, discovery, and translation. J Clin Oncol. 2012;30(6): 647–60.
53. Tsimberidou AM, Ringborg U, Schilsky RL. Strategies to overcome clinical, regulatory, and financial challenges in the implementation of personalized medicine. Am Soc Clin Oncol Educ Book. 2013:118–25.
54. Von Hoff DD, et al. Pilot study using molecular profiling of patients' tumors to find potential targets and select treatments for their refractory cancers. J Clin Oncol. 2010;28(33):4877–83.

Genetic Counseling for Pancreatic Cancer

13

Jennifer L. Geurts

Genetic Counseling and Risk Assessment

Genetic counseling and cancer risk assessment are the process of identifying, educating, and guiding individuals with a hereditary predisposition to cancer. Genetic counselors utilize pedigree analysis, lifestyle risk factor information, genetic testing, risk modeling algorithms, clinical findings, and/or molecular profiling to provide a comprehensive evaluation, including quantitative risk estimates when feasible. This information is then utilized by the treating providers to develop a management plan for early detection, prevention, risk reduction, and/or treatment of disease. Importantly, notification and communication tools for at-risk family members are included. Patient education regarding the hereditary impact of the condition is an essential element along with psychosocial assessment of coping with the information, which may result in referral to mental health professionals when appropriate.

Recommendations on the essential elements of genetic cancer risk assessment, counseling, and testing have been outlined by the National Society of Genetic Counselors [1]. Individuals with a personal or family history suggestive of an increased cancer risk should be referred for genetic assessment per National Comprehensive Cancer Network (NCCN) guidelines [2, 3]. Informed consent prior to genetic testing should include the purpose of the test, description of the genes being analyzed, potential results, implications for medical management, reproductive risks and review of the possible benefits, risks, alternatives, and limitations of testing [1, 4]. While the process of risk assessment often includes genetic testing, genetic counseling is often beneficial to patients even though genetic testing may not be completed. Reasons for not pursuing genetic testing include situations in which the patient is not the best candidate in the family to initiate testing, the testing is not clinically indicated, financial considerations, logistical barriers, fear of discrimination, and concern for adverse psychological effects [5–8].

The genetic testing approach typically involves an initial comprehensive evaluation in the individual with cancer when possible. Considering the numerous genes identified in association with pancreatic cancer (PC), it is reasonable to consider a large gene panel which includes all the genes of interest, rather than testing individual genes one by one. The gene panel testing approach has been shown to be more cost-effective, have faster turnaround times, and increase mutation detection rates [9, 10]. Current genetic testing strategies identify a germline mutation in less than a third of suspected hereditary cases [11–16]. The remaining two-thirds or

J. L. Geurts (✉)
Department of Surgery, The Medical College of Wisconsin, Milwaukee, WI, USA
e-mail: jgeurts@mcw.edu

S. Tsai et al. (eds.), *Management of Localized Pancreatic Cancer*,
https://doi.org/10.1007/978-3-319-98944-0_13

more without a causative mutation are considered to have a familial form of the disease. Familial pancreatic cancer (FPC) is defined as at least two first-degree relatives with PC; some authors are more inclusive and consider three or more relatives of any degree in this classification [17–19].

Although the NCCN provides breast/ovarian and colon cancer-directed genetic guidelines, no national guidelines exist which specifically address criteria for genetic testing in PC. A current study looking at individuals with PC and a previous history of malignancy found that 23% of germline mutation carriers did not meet NCCN Hereditary Breast and Ovarian Cancer or Lynch Syndrome test guidelines [20]. Recently, a large study analyzing tumor and germline DNA in advanced stage cancer found that 25% of PC patients carried a germline mutation [21]. These studies and others prompt consideration for genetic evaluation of all patents with PDAC (regardless of family history), due to newly recognized increased prevalence of germline mutations, emerging gene directed therapies for treatment, and options for early detection and prevention of cancer in at-risk family members.

Even with the advanced technology of the next-generation sequencing and its capacity for uncovering substantial genetic heterogeneity in PC, there is considerable missing heritability which highlights the need for new gene discovery in addition to novel genomic disease-causing mechanisms (i.e., epigenetics). For unexplained familial cases, there are significant challenges to clinical management of at-risk family members. In these cases, a Mendelian risk prediction model, PancPRO, has been developed to determine appropriate high-risk populations for targeted screening [22]. The model was validated using data from the National Familial Pancreatic Tumor Registry and considers age and family history of PC to predict development of the disease, in addition to the probability of carrying a mutation in a susceptibility gene. Subsequent validation in an Italian cohort showed that the tool is useful for identifying asymptomatic individuals who may benefit from screening for early detection of PC [23, 24].

Criteria for PC screening have been developed by the International Cancer of the Pancreas Screening (CAPS) Consortium and more recently the American College of Gastroenterology (ACG) [25, 26]. At this time, screening for PC is reserved for high-risk individuals as defined by a known hereditary cancer syndrome associated with PDAC or those with a family history suggestive of FPC. There is no clear consensus on the optimal screening modality, although MRI and/or EUS are considered preferable [27, 28]. Other considerations still debated include screening interval, age to start/stop screening, and management of abnormal findings [26]. Recommendations thus far have been based on evidence of increased risk and expert opinion rather than proven efficacy of screening. The numerous experienced centers represented in the CAPS Consortium, which is working to address this lack of data, have established a multidisciplinary approach performing screening in the setting of research protocols.

Hereditary Syndromes

PC is becoming more appreciated as a heritable disease as approximately 10% of all individuals with PC also have a first-degree relative with the disease [29, 30]. Several autosomal dominant inherited syndromes have been associated with PC to a variable degree represented in Table 13.1. The known syndromes display autosomal dominant inheritance with reduced penetrance. The most notable and earliest described associations include hereditary breast and ovarian cancer (HBOC) syndrome with a primary focus on the *BRCA2* gene, melanoma-pancreatic cancer syndrome due to mutations in the *CDKN2A* gene, and Peutz-Jeghers syndrome (PJS) which is caused by *SKT11* gene mutations. Subsequently, mutations in the mismatch repair genes (*MLH1*, *MSH2*, *MSH6*, and *PMS2*) causing Lynch syndrome and additional DNA double-strand break repair genes (*BRCA1*, *PALB2*, *ATM*) have demonstrated an increased risk for PC development. Each year, additional genes with varying degrees of preliminary evidence are identified lending to

Table 13.1 Syndromes associated with increased risk for pancreatic adenocarcinoma

Condition	Gene(s)	Relative ↑risk of PC
Peutz-Jeghers syndrome	*STK11*	72×
Melanoma-pancreatic cancer syndrome	*CDKN2A*	13×–34×
Hereditary breast and ovarian cancer syndrome	*BRCA1*, *BRCA2*	2×–10×
Other DNA repair genes	*ATM*, *PALB*	UNK
Lynch syndrome (HNPCC)	*MLH1*, *MSH2*, *MSH6*, *PMS2*	9×–11×
Familial adenomatous polyposis syndrome	*APC*	4×–5×
Li-Fraumeni syndrome	*TP53*	UNK
Hereditary pancreatitis	*PRSS1*, *SPINK1*	53×

UNK unknown

the growing list of PC predisposition genes. Due to the variable phenotypic expressivity, these syndromes are important to recognize as there are associations other than PC which may impact medical management implications for the patient and/or their family. For unaffected at-risk family members, modifications to general population screening guidelines may be made depending on the gene and cancer risk involved, including initiation of screening at an earlier age, use of alternative screening modalities, and increasing frequency of screening [2, 3]. Although single inherited gene mutations produce a major effect on cancer risk, disease penetrance is incomplete as there is considerable inter-family variability observed due to underlying genetic modifiers, environment, lifestyle, and other unknown factors [31, 32]. For this reason, individual risk estimates should consider the gene mutation in combination with the presentation and phenotype of the cancers present in the family.

Peutz-Jeghers Syndrome (PJS) Mutations in the *STK11* gene are the only known cause of PJS, a hamartomatous polyposis condition characterized by mucocutaneous pigmentation and cancer predisposition. In PJS the lifetime risk for any cancer type is up to 93% with a PC specific risk of 36% [33]. Due to the striking extra-pancreatic findings, this condition is easily recognizable, albeit rare occurring in anywhere from 1:8,300 to 1:280,000 live births [34]. In females, the risk for breast cancer is approximately 54%, and ovarian sex cord tumors with annular tubules are present in almost all affected individuals [33, 34]. Gastrointestinal cancers as a whole are the most common malignancy; additionally PJS polyps occur throughout the gastrointestinal tract and are a considerable source of morbidity [34].

Melanoma-Pancreatic Cancer Syndrome Nearly all PDAC shows somatic inactivation of the *CDKN2A* gene, supporting the role for this gene in PC risk. The *CDKN2A* gene is an important tumor suppressor which codes for two proteins, p16 (INK4) and p14 (ARF), both involved in cell cycle regulation. Germline mutations in the *CDKN2A* gene are associated with an increased risk for melanoma and PC. This condition is also referred to as familial atypical multiple mole melanoma-pancreatic cancer (FAMMM-PC). Some individuals with a *CDKN2A* mutation appear to only have an increased risk for melanoma. In the setting of a family history of PC and melanoma, the quoted PC risk for *CDKN2A* mutation carriers is 17% by the age of 75 [35]. However, this risk appears to be strongly influenced by genotype, ethnicity, personal risk factors, and family history of PC [36]. Smoking in *CDKN2A* mutation carriers appears to accelerate the risk for developing PC and other smoking-related cancers [37]. Importantly, *CDKN2A* gene mutations have been observed in families with only PC and no melanoma [38]. Mutations in *CDKN2A* appear to be the main susceptibility gene in Italian families with PC [39]. In most other populations, the presence of melanoma in the family history is a significant predictor of *CDKN2A* mutation. In families with melanoma and PC, the likelihood of a *CDKN2A* mutation is 11–40% [36, 40, 41].

Hereditary Breast and Ovarian Cancer (HBOC) Germline mutations in the *BRCA1* and *BRCA2* genes cause autosomal dominant HBOC. This syndrome is primarily associated with a high risk for breast cancer (50–80% lifetime risk) and ovarian cancer (20–40% lifetime risk) development [42–44]. However, there are also reports of a moderately increased risk for melanoma, prostate, pancreatic, gallbladder/bile duct, and colorectal cancer [43, 45]. Specific PC risk estimates for *BRCA2* carriers range from a 3.5- to 10-fold increased risk [45, 46]. The PC risk in *BRCA1* has been reported to be slightly less, around 2.5-fold increase over that of the general population [47].

Recent estimates predict the prevalence of *BRCA1/BRCA2* gene mutations in the general population to be 1:200 to 1:400 individuals. The combined carrier frequency is 1 in 40 for the Ashkenazi Jewish founder mutations: 185delAG in *BRCA1*, 5382insC in *BRCA1*, and 6174delT in *BRCA2*. These founder mutations may explain, in part, the increased incidence of PC in Jews. Approximately 6% of Ashkenazi Jewish individuals with pancreatic cancer, unselected for family history, are found to carry one of these founder mutations [48].

Some consider the recently described *PALB2* gene as part of the HBOC spectrum, as it is the partner and localizer of BRCA2 in the Fanconi anemia-DNA double-strand break repair pathway. Increased risk for breast cancer and PC is associated with mutations in the *PALB2* gene, but the exact risks for PC have not yet been established. The absolute risk for breast cancer in women with PALB2 mutations appears dependent on family history, with a 33% increased risk for those with no family history of breast cancer and a 58% elevated risk for those with a significant family history of breast cancer [49]. Studies of smaller, specific ethnic populations have suggested *PALB2* mutations are responsible for 0–4% of familial PC [50–54]. The relationship between HBOC and PC represents an example of how molecular genetics is beginning to provide insight on prognosis and precision therapeutics. Recently, several studies have reported an overall survival benefit when DNA cross-linking chemotherapy agents are used in BRCA-associated PC [55, 56]. In addition, there is hope for using these therapies in combination agents such as PARP inhibitors which play an important role in DNA break repair [57, 58]. When a tumor is deficient in homologous recombination due to *BRCA1*, *BRCA2*, or *PALB2* mutations, the addition of a PARP inhibitor leads to synthetic lethality [59].

Ataxia-Telangiectasia Mutated (ATM) The ATM protein is a member of the serine/threonine protein kinase family and is involved in DNA double-strand break repair. ATM is vital for genomic stability and cell response to DNA damage as it phosphorylates a variety of downstream proteins, including TP53, BRCA1, and CHEK2. Ataxia-telangiectasia is an autosomal recessive, childhood-onset lethal disease associated with progressive cerebellar ataxia, immunodeficiency, and increased cancer risk. In the heterozygous state, carriers of an *ATM* gene mutation have a four-fold increased risk of cancer. The reported carrier frequency of deleterious *ATM* variants in the general population is 0.5–1% [60, 61].

Families with FPC have been identified as having heterozygous *ATM* mutations; however, an estimate of PC risk has not been established. Various studies have identified heterozygous germline *ATM* mutations in PC cohorts, comprising 22–31% of the various hereditary gene mutations discovered thus far [15, 16, 62]. It has been estimated that carrying a single *ATM* mutation confers up to a 60% cumulative risk of breast cancer by age 80 in women and an increased risk for prostate cancer in men [63–65]. Additional cancer risks are unknown; this is an area of active study.

Lynch Syndrome Lynch syndrome, also known as hereditary nonpolyposis colorectal cancer (HNPCC), is the most common hereditary form of colon cancer. The population frequency of Lynch syndrome is approximately 1:370 individuals [66]. Lynch syndrome is caused by defects in the mismatch repair (MMR) genes which lead to tumor microsatellite instability (MSI). Lynch syndrome also confers an increased risk for extra-colonic cancer including, endometrial, ovarian, stomach, hepatobiliary tract, urinary tract, small bowel, and brain cancers. The pancreas-specific cancer risk in Lynch syndrome is up to 4% by age 70 [67]. Mutations in the MMR genes are thought to be an uncommon cause for inherited PC [68]. However, the recognition of this syndrome in PC has become increasingly important with the advent of immune checkpoint inhibition therapies. Pancreatic tumors with deficient mismatch repair have favorable response to this form of immunotherapy [69].

Familial Adenomatous Polyposis Familial adenomatous polyposis (FAP) syndrome is characterized by numerous (100 s–1000 s) colonic adenomas with a 100% risk for developing colorectal cancer without prophylactic surgical intervention. Extra-colonic risks include thyroid, hepatic, duodenal, and pancreas cancer. Few studies have addressed specific risk estimates for PC; a single study of 197 FAP families suggested a relative risk of approximately fourfold in this population [70]. FAP is caused by mutations in the *APC* gene and has an incidence of 1:6,000 to 1:13,000 live births [34].

Li-Fraumeni Syndrome Li-Fraumeni syndrome (LFS) is a highly penetrant, autosomal dominant cancer predisposition syndrome caused by mutations in the *TP53* gene. The *TP53* gene is a major tumor suppressor involved in many important pathways for cell cycle control, apoptosis, and DNA damage repair. The gene is commonly mutated in somatic cancer tissue including PC. The primary cancer risks in LFS include sarcoma, leukemia, brain, and breast cancers, while PC is only seen in approximately 1.3% of patients [71]. Although LFS is considered a rare condition, the true prevalence may be as high as 1:5,000 to 1:20,000 with a frequency of de novo mutation estimated between 7% and 20% [72–75].

Hereditary Pancreatitis Hereditary pancreatitis (HP) and cystic fibrosis (CF) are conditions which predispose to PC. These conditions lead to diffuse chronic inflammation and/or fibrotic changes in the gland, which convey the increased risk for cancer. Mutations in the *PRSS1* or *SPINK1* genes cause autosomal dominant HP, which displays a reduced penetrance. The lifetime risk for PC in this population has been estimated to be 40% and may be exacerbated by cigarette smoking and paternal inheritance of the disease [76, 77]. Mutations in the *CFTR* gene cause CF, an autosomal recessive condition associated with extensive pulmonary disease and pancreatic insufficiency with a 5.3-fold increased risk for PC [78].

Future Directions

The advent of the next-generation sequencing (NGS) technology has rapidly changed the understanding of hereditary risk for PC. Mutations in the *PALB2* and *ATM* genes were discovered by NGS as contributors to FPC; subsequent larger studies have confirmed their involvement as PC predisposition genes [14–16, 51, 79, 80]. However, prospective and retrospective studies on PC incidence in *ATM* and *PABL2* gene mutation carriers has yet to be completed. This research will be necessary to inform accurate cancer risks and early detection strategies for this population. The large amounts of data generated by NGS will allow FPC researchers to interrogate multiple genes involved in pathways such as the Fanconi anemia pathway and ATM/MRE11 pathway. These pathways have already produced candidates for hereditary risk in breast and ovarian cancer, such as the *NBN* gene and others [81, 82]. Researchers from the Czech Republic studied the *NBN* gene Slavic founder mutation c.657del5 (c.657_661delACAAA) in 241 unselected PC case and identified a mutation frequency of 2.07% which was significantly increased when compared to noncancer controls [83]. Single individuals with an *NBN* mutation and PC have been described in other NGS-based studies [15, 16]. The association between increased risk for breast cancer and *NBN* mutations has been demonstrated [84, 85]. Further research is necessary to clarify the risk of PC in *NBN* gene mutation carriers.

Several candidate genes have been individually reported in isolated families, including

BARD1, *BUB1B*, *CPA1*, *FANCC*, *FANCG*, *FANCM*, *PALLD*, and *RNASEL* [15, 16, 86, 87]. NGS and other advanced technologies will likely uncover several additional genetic factors of low to moderate penetrance that may have an additive effect on cancer risk. This polygenetic theory of inheritance challenges the traditional model of Mendelian genetics, where a single gene is thought to be causative. In addition, discovering and comprehending the effects epigenetics and intronic variants will lead to a new framework of understanding hereditary cancer in the future. Real challenges lie ahead to determine penetrance of these gene mutations and associated cancer risks. Large registries comprised of clinic laboratories and university researchers will be necessary to collect enough data to produce findings of clinical significance. Public efforts currently exist including PROMPT, ClinVar, and ENIGMA [88–90]. In addition, the vast amount of tumor sequencing currently underway will reveal information hidden in the germline that will be important to extract as it has implications to the patient and family beyond targeted cancer treatments.

References

1. Riley BD, Culver JO, Skrzynia C, Senter LA, Peters JA, Costalas JW, et al. Essential elements of genetic cancer risk assessment, counseling, and testing: updated recommendations of the National Society of Genetic Counselors. J Genet Couns. 2012;21(2):151–61.
2. Genetic/Familial high-risk assessment: colorectal: National Comprehensive Cancer Network (NCCN); 2017. Available from: https://www.nccn.org/professionals/physician_gls/pdf/genetics_colon.pdf.
3. Genetic/Familial high-risk assessment: breast and ovarian: National Comprehensive Cancer Network (NCCN); 2018. Available from: https://www.nccn.org/professionals/physician_gls/pdf/genetics_screening.pdf.
4. Robson ME, Bradbury AR, Arun B, Domchek SM, Ford JM, Hampel HL, et al. American Society of Clinical Oncology policy statement update: genetic and genomic testing for cancer susceptibility. J Clin Oncol. 2015;33:3660.
5. Hayden S, Mange S, Duquette D, Petrucelli N, Raymond VM. Large, prospective analysis of the reasons patients do not pursue BRCA genetic testing following genetic counseling. J Genet Couns. 2017;26(4):859–65.
6. Armstrong K, Calzone K, Stopfer J, Fitzgerald G, Coyne J, Weber B. Factors associated with decisions about clinical BRCA1/2 testing. Cancer Epidemiol Biomarkers Prev. 2000;9(11):1251–4.
7. Godard B, Pratte A, Dumont M, Simard-Lebrun A, Simard J. Factors associated with an individual's decision to withdraw from genetic testing for breast and ovarian cancer susceptibility: implications for counseling. Genet Test. 2007;11(1):45–54.
8. Kieran S, Loescher LJ, Lim KH. The role of financial factors in acceptance of clinical BRCA genetic testing. Genet Test. 2007;11(1):101–10.
9. Kurian AW, Hare EE, Mills MA, Kingham KE, McPherson L, Whittemore AS, et al. Clinical evaluation of a multiple-gene sequencing panel for hereditary cancer risk assessment. J Clin Oncol. 2014;32(19):2001–9.
10. Grant RC, Selander I, Connor AA, Selvarajah S, Borgida A, Briollais L, et al. Prevalence of germline mutations in cancer predisposition genes in patients with pancreatic cancer. Gastroenterology. 2015;148(3):556–64.
11. Haddad A, Kowdley GC, Pawlik TM, Cunningham SC. Hereditary pancreatic and hepatobiliary cancers. Int J Surg Oncol. 2011;2011:154673.
12. Hruban RH, Canto MI, Goggins M, Schulick R, Klein AP. Update on familial pancreatic cancer. Adv Surg. 2010;44:293–311.
13. Klein AP, Brune KA, Petersen GM, Goggins M, Tersmette AC, Offerhaus GJ, et al. Prospective risk of pancreatic cancer in familial pancreatic cancer kindreds. Cancer Res. 2004;64(7):2634–8.
14. Roberts NJ, Jiao Y, Yu J, Kopelovich L, Petersen GM, Bondy ML, et al. ATM mutations in patients with hereditary pancreatic cancer. Cancer Discov. 2012;2(1):41–6.
15. Chaffee KG, Oberg AL, McWilliams RR, Majithia N, Allen BA, Kidd J, et al. Prevalence of germ-line mutations in cancer genes among pancreatic cancer patients with a positive family history. Genet Med. 2018;20(1):119–27.
16. Hu C, Hart SN, Bamlet WR, Moore RM, Nandakumar K, Eckloff BW, et al. Prevalence of pathogenic mutations in cancer predisposition genes among pancreatic Cancer patients. Cancer Epidemiol Biomarkers Prev. 2016;25(1):207–11.
17. Brand RE, Lerch MM, Rubinstein WS, Neoptolemos JP, Whitcomb DC, Hruban RH, et al. Advances in counselling and surveillance of patients at risk for pancreatic cancer. Gut. 2007;56(10):1460–9.
18. Lynch HT, Brand RE, Deters CA, Shaw TG, Lynch JF. Hereditary pancreatic cancer. Pancreatology. 2001;1(5):466–71.
19. Hruban RH, Petersen GM, Goggins M, Tersmette AC, Offerhaus GJ, Falatko F, et al. Familial pancreatic cancer. Ann Oncol. 1999;10(Suppl 4):69–73.
20. Dudley B, Karloski E, Monzon FA, Singhi AD, Lincoln SE, Bahary N, et al. Germline mutation prevalence in individuals with pancreatic cancer and a history of previous malignancy. Cancer. 2018;124(8):1691–700.
21. Mandelker D, Zhang L, Kemel Y, Stadler ZK, Joseph V, Zehir A, et al. Mutation detection in

patients with advanced cancer by universal sequencing of cancer-related genes in tumor and normal DNA vs guideline-based germline testing. JAMA. 2017;318(9):825–35.
22. Wang W, Chen S, Brune KA, Hruban RH, Parmigiani G, Klein AP. PancPRO: risk assessment for individuals with a family history of pancreatic cancer. J Clin Oncol. 2007;25(11):1417–22.
23. Leonardi G, Marchi S, Falconi M, Zerbi A, Ussia V, de Bortoli N, et al. "PancPro" as a tool for selecting families eligible for pancreatic cancer screening: an Italian study of incident cases. Dig Liver Dis. 2012;44(7):585–8.
24. Del Chiaro M, Zerbi A, Capurso G, Zamboni G, Maisonneuve P, Presciuttini S, et al. Familial pancreatic cancer in Italy. Risk assessment, screening programs and clinical approach: a position paper from the Italian registry. Dig Liver Dis. 2010;42(9):597–605.
25. Syngal S, Brand RE, Church JM, Giardiello FM, Hampel HL, Burt RW. ACG clinical guideline: genetic testing and management of hereditary gastrointestinal cancer syndromes. Am J Gastroenterol. 2015;110(2):223–62. quiz 63.
26. Canto MI, Harinck F, Hruban RH, Offerhaus GJ, Poley JW, Kamel I, et al. International Cancer of the Pancreas Screening (CAPS) Consortium summit on the management of patients with increased risk for familial pancreatic cancer. Gut. 2013;62(3):339–47.
27. Langer P, Kann PH, Fendrich V, Habbe N, Schneider M, Sina M, et al. Five years of prospective screening of high-risk individuals from families with familial pancreatic cancer. Gut. 2009;58(10):1410–8.
28. Vasen HF, Wasser M, van Mil A, Tollenaar RA, Konstantinovski M, Gruis NA, et al. Magnetic resonance imaging surveillance detects early-stage pancreatic cancer in carriers of a p16-Leiden mutation. Gastroenterology. 2011;140(3):850–6.
29. Humphris JL, Johns AL, Simpson SH, Cowley MJ, Pajic M, Chang DK, et al. Clinical and pathologic features of familial pancreatic cancer. Cancer. 2014;120(23):3669–75.
30. Del Chiaro M, Zerbi A, Falconi M, Bertacca L, Polese M, Sartori N, et al. Cancer risk among the relatives of patients with pancreatic ductal adenocarcinoma. Pancreatology. 2007;7(5–6):459–69.
31. Mulligan AM, Couch FJ, Barrowdale D, Domchek SM, Eccles D, Nevanlinna H, et al. Common breast cancer susceptibility alleles are associated with tumour subtypes in BRCA1 and BRCA2 mutation carriers: results from the Consortium of Investigators of Modifiers of BRCA1/2. Breast Cancer Res. 2011;13(6):R110.
32. Barnes DR, Antoniou AC. Unravelling modifiers of breast and ovarian cancer risk for BRCA1 and BRCA2 mutation carriers: update on genetic modifiers. J Intern Med. 2012;271(4):331–43.
33. Giardiello FM, Brensinger JD, Tersmette AC, Goodman SN, Petersen GM, Booker SV, et al. Very high risk of cancer in familial Peutz-Jeghers syndrome. Gastroenterology. 2000;119(6):1447–53.
34. Lindor NM, McMaster ML, Lindor CJ, Greene MH. Concise handbook of familial cancer susceptibility syndromes – second edition. J Natl Cancer Inst Monogr. 2008;38:1–93.
35. Vasen HF, Gruis NA, Frants RR, van Der Velden PA, Hille ET, Bergman W. Risk of developing pancreatic cancer in families with familial atypical multiple mole melanoma associated with a specific 19 deletion of p16 (p16-Leiden). Int J Cancer. 2000;87(6):809–11.
36. Goldstein AM, Chan M, Harland M, Hayward NK, Demenais F, Bishop DT, et al. Features associated with germline CDKN2A mutations: a GenoMEL study of melanoma-prone families from three continents. J Med Genet. 2007;44(2):99–106.
37. Helgadottir H, Hoiom V, Jonsson G, Tuominen R, Ingvar C, Borg A, et al. High risk of tobacco-related cancers in CDKN2A mutation-positive melanoma families. J Med Genet. 2014;51(8):545–52.
38. Harinck F, Kluijt I, van der Stoep N, Oldenburg RA, Wagner A, Aalfs CM, et al. Indication for CDKN2A-mutation analysis in familial pancreatic cancer families without melanomas. J Med Genet. 2012;49(6):362–5.
39. Ghiorzo P, Fornarini G, Sciallero S, Battistuzzi L, Belli F, Bernard L, et al. CDKN2A is the main susceptibility gene in Italian pancreatic cancer families. J Med Genet. 2012;49(3):164–70.
40. Lynch HT, Brand RE, Hogg D, Deters CA, Fusaro RM, Lynch JF, et al. Phenotypic variation in eight extended CDKN2A germline mutation familial atypical multiple mole melanoma-pancreatic carcinoma-prone families: the familial atypical mole melanoma-pancreatic carcinoma syndrome. Cancer. 2002;94(1):84–96.
41. Bartsch DK, Langer P, Habbe N, Matthai E, Chaloupka B, Sina M, et al. Clinical and genetic analysis of 18 pancreatic carcinoma/melanoma-prone families. Clin Genet. 2010;77(4):333–41.
42. Chen S, Parmigiani G. Meta-analysis of BRCA1 and BRCA2 penetrance. J Clin Oncol. 2007;25(11):1329–33.
43. Phelan CM, Iqbal J, Lynch HT, Lubinski J, Gronwald J, Moller P, et al. Incidence of colorectal cancer in BRCA1 and BRCA2 mutation carriers: results from a follow-up study. Br J Cancer. 2014;110(2):530–4.
44. King MC, Marks JH, Mandell JB. Breast and ovarian cancer risks due to inherited mutations in BRCA1 and BRCA2. Science. 2003;302(5645):643–6.
45. Consortium TBCL. Cancer risks in BRCA2 mutation carriers. J Natl Cancer Inst. 1999;91(15):1310–6.
46. van Asperen CJ, Brohet RM, Meijers-Heijboer EJ, Hoogerbrugge N, Verhoef S, Vasen HF, et al. Cancer risks in BRCA2 families: estimates for sites other than breast and ovary. J Med Genet. 2005;42(9):711–9.
47. Thompson D, Easton DF. Cancer incidence in BRCA1 mutation carriers. J Natl Cancer Inst. 2002;94(18):1358–65.
48. Ferrone CR, Levine DA, Tang LH, Allen PJ, Jarnagin W, Brennan MF, et al. BRCA germline mutations in Jewish patients with pancreatic adenocarcinoma. J Clin Oncol. 2009;27(3):433–8.

49. Antoniou AC, Casadei S, Heikkinen T, Barrowdale D, Pylkas K, Roberts J, et al. Breast-cancer risk in families with mutations in PALB2. N Engl J Med. 2014;371(6):497–506.
50. Adank MA, van Mil SE, Gille JJ, Waisfisz Q, Meijers-Heijboer H. PALB2 analysis in BRCA2-like families. Breast Cancer Res Treat. 2011;127(2):357–62.
51. Jones S, Hruban RH, Kamiyama M, Borges M, Zhang X, Parsons DW, et al. Exomic sequencing identifies PALB2 as a pancreatic cancer susceptibility gene. Science. 2009;324(5924):217.
52. Harinck F, Kluijt I, van Mil SE, Waisfisz Q, van Os TA, Aalfs CM, et al. Routine testing for PALB2 mutations in familial pancreatic cancer families and breast cancer families with pancreatic cancer is not indicated. Eur J Hum Genet. 2012;20(5):577–9.
53. Stadler ZK, Salo-Mullen E, Sabbaghian N, Simon JA, Zhang L, Olson SH, et al. Germline PALB2 mutation analysis in breast-pancreas cancer families. J Med Genet. 2011;48(8):523–5.
54. Peterlongo P, Catucci I, Pasquini G, Verderio P, Peissel B, Barile M, et al. PALB2 germline mutations in familial breast cancer cases with personal and family history of pancreatic cancer. Breast Cancer Res Treat. 2011;126(3):825–8.
55. Golan T, Kanji ZS, Epelbaum R, Devaud N, Dagan E, Holter S, et al. Overall survival and clinical characteristics of pancreatic cancer in BRCA mutation carriers. Br J Cancer. 2014;111(6):1132–8.
56. James E, Waldron-Lynch MG, Saif MW. Prolonged survival in a patient with BRCA2 associated metastatic pancreatic cancer after exposure to camptothecin: a case report and review of literature. Anti-Cancer Drugs. 2009;20(7):634–8.
57. Bryant HE, Schultz N, Thomas HD, Parker KM, Flower D, Lopez E, et al. Specific killing of BRCA2-deficient tumours with inhibitors of poly(ADP-ribose) polymerase. Nature. 2005;434(7035):913–7.
58. Bhalla A, Saif MW. PARP-inhibitors in BRCA-associated pancreatic cancer. JOP. 2014;15(4): 340–3.
59. Helleday T. The underlying mechanism for the PARP and BRCA synthetic lethality: clearing up the misunderstandings. Mol Oncol. 2011;5(4):387–93.
60. Taylor AM, Byrd PJ. Molecular pathology of ataxia telangiectasia. J Clin Pathol. 2005;58(10):1009–15.
61. Swift M, Sholman L, Perry M, Chase C. Malignant neoplasms in the families of patients with ataxia-telangiectasia. Cancer Res. 1976;36(1):209–15.
62. Shindo K, Yu J, Suenaga M, Fesharakizadeh S, Cho C, Macgregor-Das A, et al. Deleterious germline mutations in patients with apparently sporadic pancreatic adenocarcinoma. J Clin Oncol: Official Journal of the American Society of Clinical Oncology. 2017;35(30):3382–90. https://doi.org/10.1200/JCO.2017.72.3502.
63. Meyer A, Wilhelm B, Dork T, Bremer M, Baumann R, Karstens JH, et al. ATM missense variant P1054R predisposes to prostate cancer. Radiother Oncol. 2007;83(3):283–8.
64. Pritchard CC, Mateo J, Walsh MF, De Sarkar N, Abida W, Beltran H, et al. Inherited DNA-repair gene mutations in men with metastatic prostate cancer. N Engl J Med. 2016;375(5):443–53.
65. Goldgar DE, Healey S, Dowty JG, Da Silva L, Chen X, Spurdle AB, et al. Rare variants in the ATM gene and risk of breast cancer. Breast Cancer Res. 2011;13(4):R73.
66. Hampel H, de la Chapelle A. The search for unaffected individuals with Lynch syndrome: do the ends justify the means? Cancer Prev Res (Phila). 2011;4(1):1–5.
67. Kastrinos F, Mukherjee B, Tayob N, Wang F, Sparr J, Raymond VM, et al. Risk of pancreatic cancer in families with Lynch syndrome. JAMA. 2009;302(16):1790–5.
68. Gargiulo S, Torrini M, Ollila S, Nasti S, Pastorino L, Cusano R, et al. Germline MLH1 and MSH2 mutations in Italian pancreatic cancer patients with suspected Lynch syndrome. Familial Cancer. 2009;8(4):547–53.
69. Hu ZI, Shia J, Stadler ZK, Varghese AM, Capanu M, Salo-Mullen E, et al. Evaluating mismatch repair deficiency in pancreatic adenocarcinoma: challenges and recommendations. Clin Cancer Res. 2018;24:1326.
70. Giardiello FM, Offerhaus GJ, Lee DH, Krush AJ, Tersmette AC, Booker SV, et al. Increased risk of thyroid and pancreatic carcinoma in familial adenomatous polyposis. Gut. 1993;34(10):1394–6.
71. Kleihues P, Schauble B, zur Hausen A, Esteve J, Ohgaki H. Tumors associated with p53 germline mutations: a synopsis of 91 families. Am J Pathol. 1997;150(1):1–13.
72. Chompret A, Brugieres L, Ronsin M, Gardes M, Dessarps-Freichey F, Abel A, et al. P53 germline mutations in childhood cancers and cancer risk for carrier individuals. Br J Cancer. 2000;82(12):1932–7.
73. Gonzalez KD, Buzin CH, Noltner KA, Gu D, Li W, Malkin D, et al. High frequency of de novo mutations in Li-Fraumeni syndrome. J Med Genet. 2009;46(10):689–93.
74. Gonzalez KD, Noltner KA, Buzin CH, Gu D, Wen-Fong CY, Nguyen VQ, et al. Beyond Li Fraumeni syndrome: clinical characteristics of families with p53 germline mutations. J Clin Oncol. 2009;27(8):1250–6.
75. Lalloo F, Varley J, Ellis D, Moran A, O'Dair L, Pharoah P, et al. Prediction of pathogenic mutations in patients with early-onset breast cancer by family history. Lancet (London, England). 2003;361(9363):1101–2.
76. Lowenfels AB, Maisonneuve P, Whitcomb DC. Risk factors for cancer in hereditary pancreatitis. International Hereditary Pancreatitis Study Group. Med Clin North Am. 2000;84(3):565–73.
77. Lowenfels AB, Maisonneuve P, Whitcomb DC, Lerch MM, DiMagno EP. Cigarette smoking as a risk factor for pancreatic cancer in patients with hereditary pancreatitis. JAMA. 2001;286(2):169–70.
78. Maisonneuve P, Marshall BC, Lowenfels AB. Risk of pancreatic cancer in patients with cystic fibrosis. Gut. 2007;56(9):1327–8.
79. Grant RC, Al-Sukhni W, Borgida AE, Holter S, Kanji ZS, McPherson T, et al. Exome sequencing identi-

fies nonsegregating nonsense ATM and PALB2 variants in familial pancreatic cancer. Hum Genomics. 2013;7:11.
80. Roberts NJ, Norris AL, Petersen GM, Bondy ML, Brand R, Gallinger S, et al. Whole genome sequencing defines the genetic heterogeneity of familial pancreatic cancer. Cancer Discov. 2016;6(2):166–75.
81. Pennington KP, Swisher EM. Hereditary ovarian cancer: beyond the usual suspects. Gynecol Oncol. 2012;124(2):347–53.
82. Castera L, Krieger S, Rousselin A, Legros A, Baumann JJ, Bruet O, et al. Next-generation sequencing for the diagnosis of hereditary breast and ovarian cancer using genomic capture targeting multiple candidate genes. Eur J Hum Genet. 2014;22(11):1305–13.
83. Borecka M, Zemankova P, Lhota F, Soukupova J, Kleiblova P, Vocka M, et al. The c.657del5 variant in the NBN gene predisposes to pancreatic cancer. Gene. 2016;587(2):169–72.
84. Seemanova E, Jarolim P, Seeman P, Varon R, Digweed M, Swift M, et al. Cancer risk of heterozygotes with the NBN founder mutation. J Natl Cancer Inst. 2007;99(24):1875–80.
85. Zhang B, Beeghly-Fadiel A, Long J, Zheng W. Genetic variants associated with breast-cancer risk: comprehensive research synopsis, meta-analysis, and epidemiological evidence. Lancet Oncol. 2011;12(5):477–88.
86. Bartsch DK, Fendrich V, Slater EP, Sina-Frey M, Rieder H, Greenhalf W, et al. RNASEL germline variants are associated with pancreatic cancer. Int J Cancer. 2005;117(5):718–22.
87. Bartsch DK, Krysewski K, Sina-Frey M, Fendrich V, Rieder H, Langer P, et al. Low frequency of CHEK2 mutations in familial pancreatic cancer. Familial Cancer. 2006;5(4):305–8.
88. Landrum MJ, Lee JM, Riley GR, Jang W, Rubinstein WS, Church DM, et al. ClinVar: public archive of relationships among sequence variation and human phenotype. Nucleic Acids Res. 2014;42(Database issue):D980–5.
89. Spurdle AB, Healey S, Devereau A, Hogervorst FB, Monteiro AN, Nathanson KL, et al. ENIGMA – evidence-based network for the interpretation of germline mutant alleles: an international initiative to evaluate risk and clinical significance associated with sequence variation in BRCA1 and BRCA2 genes. Hum Mutat. 2012;33(1):2–7.
90. Bajetta E, Rimassa L, Carnaghi C, Seregni E, Ferrari L, Di Bartolomeo M, et al. 5-Fluorouracil, dacarbazine, and epirubicin in the treatment of patients with neuroendocrine tumors. Cancer. 1998;83(2):372–8.

Medical Nutrition Therapy Throughout the Continuum of Care for Localized Pancreatic Cancers

14

Kara Sonntag

From the time of initial diagnosis of pancreatic cancer, proper nutrition is important for maintaining an acceptable level of quality of life. Nutrition therapy in pancreatic cancer focuses on adequate intake of calories, protein, and fluids in order to support strength and energy requirements. Nutrition interventions should be targeted at minimizing side effects of adjuvant treatments and helping patients prepare and recover from surgery. Primary goals of dietary interventions are to prevent or reverse malnutrition, maintain scheduled course of treatments without delays, navigate symptom management improving quality of life, enhance recovery after surgery, and prevent or treat macro- and micronutrient deficiencies.

Nutrition is an integral component of cancer care from the day of diagnosis, throughout treatments, extending into survivorship and end-of-life. Nutritional and dietetic professionals merge the science of oncology with the study of nutrition. It is the responsibility of the Registered Dietitian to manage nutrition-related symptoms of cancer and its treatment-related side effects. This is achieved by maximizing oral intake through nutritional guidance and education.

K. Sonntag (✉)
Froedtert Health, Food and Nutrition Services, Milwaukee, WI, USA
e-mail: kara.Sonntag@froedtert.com

The Role of the Pancreas in Digestion

In order for medical professionals to assess and treat patients with localized pancreatic cancers, it is imperative to understand the anatomy and physiology of the pancreas and its role in digestion. The pancreas comprised of two glands merged together into one organ. The tail of the pancreas is responsible for the endocrine function with the production of insulin, while the head of the pancreas is largely responsible for the exocrine actions.

The endocrine pancreas is composed of small groupings of cells, called the islets of Langerhans. Endocrine cells release hormones, primarily insulin and glucagon, into the bloodstream which help control blood glucose levels.

The normal flow of digestion starts when food is carried from the mouth to the stomach by the esophagus. In the stomach, digestive acids made by the stomach begin to break down the food. From the stomach, chyme (a thick fluid mass of partially digested food and gastric secretions) passes from the stomach directly into the first part of the small intestine (duodenum). In the duodenum, bile (which has been made in the liver and transported by the common bile duct) is combined with enzymes from the pancreas and enters the digestive system. Partially digested foods travel from the duodenum to the other parts of the small bowel, the

S. Tsai et al. (eds.), *Management of Localized Pancreatic Cancer*,
https://doi.org/10.1007/978-3-319-98944-0_14

jejunum, and ileum, where further digestion of food occurs. The ileum empties into the large intestine where water is reabsorbed and stool is eliminated through the anus.

The exocrine pancreas plays an integral role in the digestive process. The exocrine cells of the pancreas are responsible for secretion of digestive enzymes, electrolytes, and water into the duodenum in response to the presence of chyme. These exocrine cells release lipase, protease, and amylase into a series of small pancreatic ducts which drain into a large central duct. This main pancreatic duct extends the length of the pancreas and drains fluid produced by the exocrine cells into the duodenum via the common bile duct at the ampulla of Vater. Pancreatic secretions, intestinal secretions, and bile neutralize stomach acid to raise the pH of the contents in the duodenum which allows for improved digestion. The digestive enzymes are essential for processing food particles and fluids into smaller molecules that can be absorbed in the gastrointestinal tract.

As a tumor of the pancreas forms, these important functions can become hindered. Tumors in the head of the pancreas can result in pancreatitis, pain, and impaired release of digestive enzymes, resulting in digestive problems from the incomplete assimilation of food. When tumors upset the endocrine function of the pancreas, insulin and glucagon production are impaired potentially leading to the development of diabetes. Sixty percent to seventy percent of pancreatic cancer arise in the head of the pancreas [1]. Pancreatic cancers arise from the exocrine pancreas and account for 95% of pancreatic cancers [2]. Often, patients are already displaying nutrition-related concerns upon initial diagnosis of pancreatic cancer. These symptoms can range from jaundice, abdominal pain, weight loss, poor appetite, malabsorption and bowel changes, diabetes, and delayed gastric emptying. Medical nutritional therapy combined with medication management at initial diagnosis should focus on maximizing calorie and protein intake while minimizing symptoms.

Obtaining Initial Nutrition Assessment

Nutritional screening and assessment are critical components of care for cancer patients. Malnutrition is common and has been shown to be the cause of death in about 20% of patients with cancer [3]. Unintentional weight loss is common upon initial diagnosis of pancreatic cancer. A percentage of weight loss greater than 5% is associated with a greater surgical site infection rate, longer hospital stays, and increased morbidity and mortality [4]. Over 80% of pancreatic cancer patients report weight loss at the time of diagnosis, and over a third of these patients have lost greater than 10% of the initial body weight [5]. Cancer-associated cachexia is a severe disorder characterized by loss of body weight with specific depletion of skeletal muscle and adipose tissue. Cachexia is driven by a pathologic process of increased nutrient need combined with reduced food intake, metabolic changes, elevated energy expenditure, and excess catabolism and inflammation. It is also associated with increased morbidity and mortality, decreased response to therapy, escalated use of healthcare resources, and impaired quality of life [6]. However, proactive nutritional risk assessment is one way healthcare professionals can minimize negative outcomes.

The Academy of Nutrition and Dietetics (AND) utilizes the Nutrition Care Process (NCP) which is a four-step process for professionals to provide nutritional care to their patients [7]. Nutritional assessment is the first of the four steps which guides professionals in a systematic way to obtain and verify information needed to identify nutrition-related concerns. After a thorough assessment is completed, a nutritional diagnosis is assigned using standardized language to categorize patient-specific nutrition-related problems. This nutritional diagnosis guides the provider through the last two steps of nutritional intervention and monitoring and evaluation.

Nutritional screening and assessment parameters include patient medical history, food intake history, biochemical data, medication review, past allergies/intolerances, anthropometric data, and focused physical examinations. The patient's history and clinical diagnosis can be helpful to identify those at risk for malnutrition and inflammation. The history obtained should include pertinent medical and social information along with medications and supplement usage. The clinician will interview the patient and/or family member to obtain information on meal and snack patterns, adequacy of intake, food and nutrient tolerances, and barriers to nutritional adequacy such as nausea, vomiting, bowel changes, taste aversions, postprandial discomfort, anorexia, and early satiety. Biochemical data can be obtained through lab work and other pertinent medical tests and procedures. Anthropometric data includes current height and weight in addition to weight changes within a specific time frame. Nutrition-focused physical examinations embody a physical exam of muscle and adipose stores as well as the patient's oral cavity, eyes, hair, skin, and nails. The data compiled can direct dietetic professionals to determine the most appropriate nutritional diagnosis with subsequent interventions.

The Nutrition-Focused Physical Exam

The nutrition-focused physical exam is a way for nutrition practitioners to evaluate malnutrition in a tangible manor. Tangible manifestation of fat and muscle wasting helps classify the extent in which patients will be able to recover from adjuvant treatments, handle the demands of surgery, and resume an acceptable quality of life. Indications for performing the exam include criteria on weight loss and changes in energy intake, current diagnosis and chronic conditions, and procedures that place patients at high risk for malnutrition or nutritional deficiencies. Weight loss is documented and evaluated as weight change over time as a percentage lost from baseline. Hydration status and other clinical findings, such as edema and ascites, are taken into consideration when evaluating weight changes. Energy consumption is also reported as a percentage of consumption compared to typical intake over time [8].

The nutrition-focused physical assessment is composed of four main sections. Each site that is examined is ranked from 0 to 3 indicating extent of depletion (none to severe). Assessments of muscle stores include an evaluation of the muscle volume, as well as tone and functionality. It is important to know the muscles of the upper body are more susceptible to depletion secondary to nutritional deprivation, while the depletion of the muscles of the lower body may be secondary to inactivity. Assessment of subcutaneous fat is completed in conjunction with the muscle assessment. Loss of subcutaneous fat suggests an energy deficit and may be assessed by observing the areas where adipose tissue is typically stored. Assessment of fluid status is integral for several reasons. Fluid status must be assessed as malnutrition often causes edema related to oncotic pressure changes. In addition, weight changes can be distorted from ascites and/or edema.

In addition to the physical exam of the body, the practitioner should also carefully inspect parts of the body where high cell turnover occurs such as the mouth, tongue, skin, and hair. For example, the cellular turnover of the oral cavity is 3–5 days; therefore, vitamin and mineral deficiency may manifest early in the lips, tongue, gingival, or mucosa [9]. Other areas for the practitioner to evaluate are the patient's eyes, skin, hair, and nails. Table 14.1 reviews tips for evaluating specific areas of the body, while Fig. 14.1 reviews the exact sites for inspection.

Talking to the patient while performing the physical assessment can provide you with information pertinent to your findings. Take into consideration the information already obtained from the history and assessment noting that no two body types are alike and changes to physical composition can occur at different rates and affect different body sites. Therefore, asking the patient about the changes, they may have been noticing in their own body, regardless of changes on the scale can help formulate a more accurate physical assessment. This data helps to guide nutritional therapy at the initial visit while keeping in mind the upcoming planned course of treatment.

Table 14.1 Nutrition-focused physical exam tips for head-to-toe evaluation

Area of examination	Tips
Temporalis muscle	Usually one of the early signs of protein/calorie malnutrition Pay close attention to the pit of the temple for depression
Orbital region	Feel for cavernous look and less spongy response to light palpations
Buccal fat pad	Note if patient is not wearing dentures or does not have teeth Feel for sunken area between cheekbone and jawbone
Pectoralis major	Be certain patient is not slouching in chair or hunching forward Clavicles are typically more visible in males than females Note if you are able to scoop your fingers beneath the clavicle Assess the amount of stringy muscle fibers directly above and below the clavicle
Deltoid muscle	Pay attention to the degree of stringy striations around the base of the neck Glide hand over clavicle and acromion process to feel for protrusion
Trapezius muscle	Have patient sit up straight and push against your hand Evaluate for prominence of bones and depressions between them
Supraspinatus	Have patient sit up straight and push against your hand Evaluate for prominence of bones and depressions between them
Infraspinatus	Have patient sit up straight and push against your hand Evaluate for prominence of bones and depressions between them
Latissimus dorsi	Have patient sit up straight and push against your hand Evaluate for visible and concave depressions between the rib bones
Thoracic/lumbar region	Have patient sit up straight and push against your hand Evaluate for visible and concave depressions between the rib bones Assess with a gentle pinch the fat store just above the iliac crest
Triceps	Arm bent into a 90° angle Separate the muscle and fat by rolling fingers down the triceps area Assess depth to the pinch for amount of fat mass Men typically have less fat mass in this area than women
Interosseous muscle	Ask patient to make the "okay" sign with their forefinger and thumb Palpate the bulge as they pinch and release Notice indentations between the knuckles of the hand
Quadriceps muscle	Feel for wasting in each of the four muscle groups comprising the quadriceps The patient's knee should be bent with their heel on the bed or floor
Gastrocnemius muscle	Grasp the calf to determine if bulbous muscle is present To fully assess, you can ask the patient to flex and extend their toes
Edema/ascites	Press gently onto the ankle and chin bones and record how long it takes for impression to resolve Note how far the enema extends up the leg

Information adapted from Malone and Hamilton [10]

Nutrition Throughout Chemotherapy and Radiation Treatments

Chemotherapy and radiation are often used at various times to treat localized pancreatic cancer within the continuum of care. Each treatment modality is accompanied by possible nutrition-related side effects and fatigue which can compromise nutritional status. The nutritional goals while undergoing these treatments are to minimize nutrition-related side effects, reduce weight loss and catabolism, and preserve strength and energy to allow the patient to complete treatment without delays.

Chemotherapy is a systemic therapy which can affect cells throughout the entire body. Chemotherapy targets fast reproducing cells. Within the body, bone marrow, hair follicles, mucosal lining of the oral cavity, esophagus,

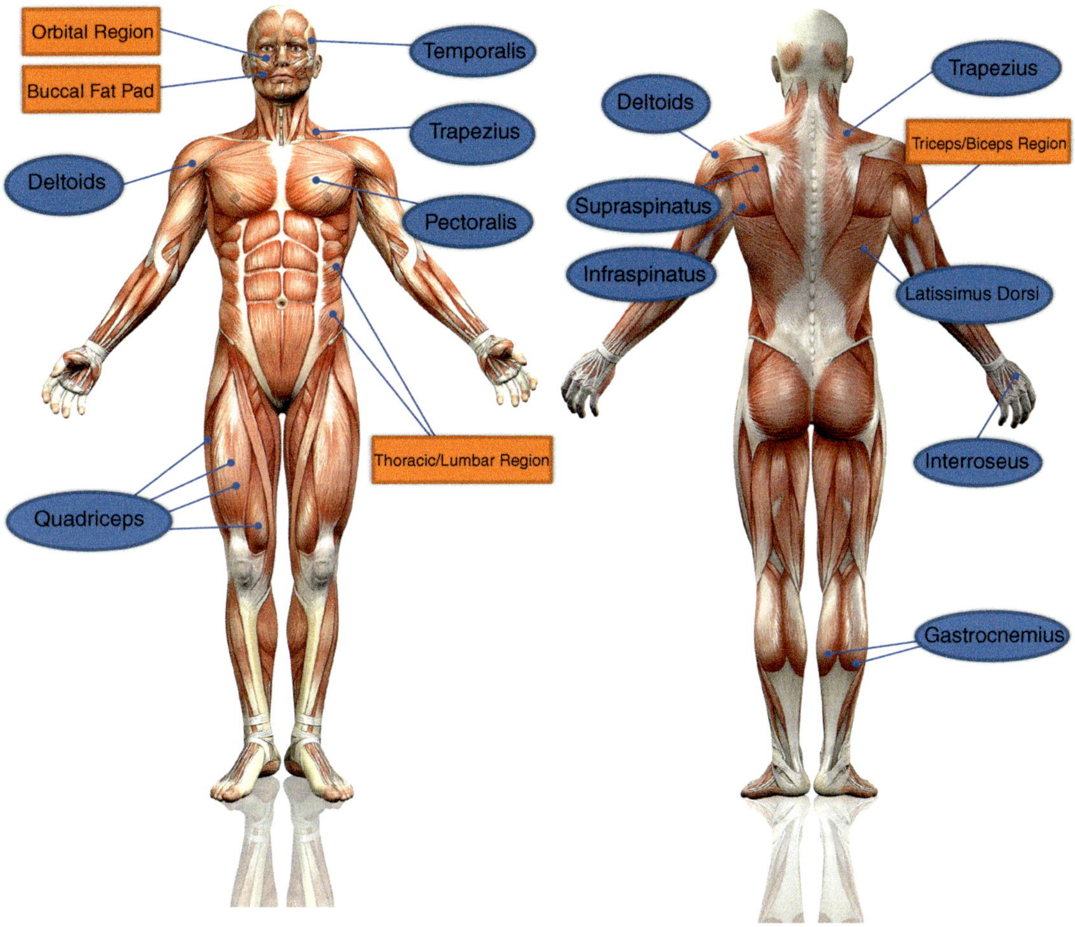

Fig. 14.1 Areas for inspection during a nutrition-focused physical exam

and GI tract are typically most at risk. Side effects of chemotherapy vary depending on the agent(s) used.

Radiation side effects may occur several weeks into treatments and continue to manifest for 2–4 weeks after treatment has completed. Side effects from radiation are generally limed to the specific site or treatment field but also include generalized fatigue. Symptoms may include decreased appetite, diarrhea, fatigue, nausea/vomiting, and weight loss.

Symptoms from cancer treatments can negatively impact a patient's quality of life. Inadequate management of these symptoms can result in a decline in a patient's nutritional status and potentially lead to malnutrition, which has been linked to poorer treatment outcomes [11]. Proper management of symptoms can positively impact tolerance of treatments, increase quality of life, and improved strength and energy. Most common side effects of treatments, both chemotherapy and radiation for pancreatic cancers, are nausea, vomiting, bowel pattern changes, anorexia, early satiety, and fatigue. Symptom management is a primary role of the nutritional professional in patients undergoing chemotherapy and radiation. Table 14.2 lists chemotherapy agents used for pancreatic cancers and common nutrition-related side effects, while Table 14.3 describes nutrition-related tips for management of these symptoms.

Table 14.2 Nutrition-related side effects of chemotherapy agents used for pancreatic cancers [1, 2]

Chemo agent	Trade name	Nausea	Diarrhea	Anorexia	Taste changes	Fatigue	Other
Gemcitabine	Gemzar	Low	X	X		X	
Fluorouracil	5-FU	Low	X			X	Mucositis
Capecitabine	Xeloda	Moderate	X			X	
Cisplatin	Platinol	Severe	X	X	X	X	
Oxaliplatin	Eloxatin	Moderate	X			X	Cold sensitivity
Nab-pacilataxel	Abraxane	Low				X	
Irinotecan	Camptosar	High	X-severe	X		X	
Folinic acid	Leucovorin	Low				x	

Elliott et al. [1]; Leser [11]

Table 14.3 Tips for nutritional management of treatment-related side effects [1, 2]

Side effect	Tips for management
Anorexia	Small frequent meals and snacks Eat nutrient dense foods Add calories and protein to favorite foods Make mealtimes pleasant Avoid drinking fluids 20 minutes prior to meals Consider light exercise to stimulate the appetite Utilize times when appetite is best
Early satiety	Small, frequent meals and snacks High-calorie and high-protein foods High-calorie, high-protein fluids between meals Avoid drinking fluids 20 minutes prior to meals Avoid high fiber which can cause bloating Don't lay down after eating
Constipation	Eat regular meals, snacks Increase fluid intake If allowed, increase fiber Drink hot beverages first thing in the morning Consider warm prune juice Increase physical activity, if approved by MD
Diarrhea	Limit/avoid insoluble fiber Add soluble fiber slowly Small, frequent meals and snacks Avoid greasy, fried, spicy foods Avoid caffeine and warm/hot beverages Avoid dairy products Avoid sweetened beverages BRAT (banana, white rice, applesauce, and white toast) foods with each meal If diarrhea is severe, consider rehydrating solution
Lactose intolerance	Avoid dairy products. Substitute almond milk or lactose-free products Try lactase enzyme supplement—amount needed depends on content of lactose consumed Try dairy products pretreated with lactase
Nausea	Try small, frequent meals and snacks—eat every 2–3 hours Consume liquids between meals Consider ginger ale or sucking on crystallized ginger Eat room temperature foods over extreme temperatures Suck on peppermint candies or try peppermint oils on wrists Avoid hard to digest foods—high-fiber, high-fat, greasy, and spicy foods Avoid favorite foods when nauseated Avoid strong odors Consider walking after mealtimes; do not lay down after eating
Sensitivity to cold	Choose warm or room temperature foods vs cold or frozen Be certain to use a towel or gloves to reach into the fridge or freezer to grab items to prepare Leave beverages at room temperature for at least 1 hour prior to drinking Lukewarm to hot beverages are better tolerated (hot cocoa vs chocolate milk) Purchase liquids that do not need to be refrigerated prior to consumption
Taste changes	Rinse mouth with baking soda solution (1 tbsp baking soda/1 tsp salt/1 quart water) before eating Use marinades and spices to mask other flavors Use plastic utensils if metallic taste Utilize flavors of foods tasting "normal or right" to season and mask offensive foods Utilize marinades and spices to disguise strange tastes Room temperature foods or chilled foods have less pungent flavors

Elliott et al. [1]; Leser [11]

Preoperative Medical Nutritional Therapy

Maximizing nutrition is vital to maintaining the strength one needs to cope with surgery after neoadjuvant treatment. Once surgery is determined as the next step in the plan of care, nutritional interventions can continue to support the patient to achieve positive outcomes. Weight loss prior to surgery is not typically advised or desired. Maintaining weight allows the protein and energy consumed to be stored for healing and recovery.

Reassessing the nutrition-focused physical exams is a helpful tool for practitioners to assess for and/or measure the extent of preoperative debilitation. This then can assist in predicting the level of post-op nutrition management the patient may require. It is important to compare the initial evaluations with the follow-up assessments in order to develop nutritional interventions to coincide with these changes. Debilitation prior to surgery negatively impacts the recovery process. One study showed that length of stay was significantly longer in patients who experienced significant preoperative weight loss compared to those who did not (17.0 days versus 10.0 days). Of patients who underwent nutritional assessment, 32% were classified as mild to moderately malnourished and 16% severely malnourished. Malnourished patients were hospitalized twice as long as well-nourished patients (15.8 days versus 7.6 days). Time taken to achieve adequate nutrition post-surgery was a factor in postoperative outcomes, with a positive correlation with length of stay, a negative correlation with postoperative weight change, and a greater risk of complications (52% versus 13%) [12]. Others have researched how inadequate preoperative nutrition status has been linked consistently to increases in postoperative complications and suboptimal surgical outcomes [13].

Enhanced Recovery After Surgery and Nutrition

Enhanced recovery after surgery (ERAS) and enhanced recovery protocols (ERPs) are interchangeable terminologies. The protocol components can be 17-plus interventions. Institutions often customize which interventions they implement depending on logistics, cost constraints, compliance, and resultant data. ERPs including immunonutrition and carbohydrate loading protocols have been shown to reduce length of stay, reduce 90-day readmissions, decrease post-op infection rates, decrease duration of bowel function return, and improve diet advancement [14].

Other non-nutritional components may include a selective or no bowel preparation, antibiotic prophylaxis, thromboprophylaxis, and reduction in premedication. A key component to the ERPs includes carbohydrate-rich, immunonutritional formulas which are consumed perioperatively. A majority of the studies have been conducted using IMPACT Advanced Recovery®. This provides a unique blend of arginine, omega-3 fatty acids, and nucleotides. These immunonutrients have been recommended by the Society of Critical Care Medicine and the American Society of Parenteral and Enteral Nutrition (ASPEN) to help support the nutritional requirements of major surgery patients. Arginine has been found to increase blood flow to surgical wounds and support the immune system. Omega-3 fatty acids show benefit in reducing inflammation, while nucleotides assist in rebuilding cells. Patients consume three cartons per day 5 days prior to surgery and for 5 days postoperatively. According to the American Society of Enhanced Recovery Implementation Guide, carbohydrate loading for patients with type 1 diabetes or delayed gastric emptying has been deemed not appropriate. Uncontrolled blood sugars may impair wound healing, increase risk of infection, increase inflammation, and potentiate cardiovascular and respiratory concerns. However, immunonutrition and the other components of the ERP can still be implemented for these individuals [16]. Figure 14.2 depicts the multiple components of the ERPs which can be implemented.

Nutritional professionals have a preoperative role of discussing what to expect nutritionally after surgery as one component to the ERPs [15]. This preadmission counseling discussion covers preoperative ingestion of immunonutrition and/or carbohydrate loading, typical postoperative diet progression, possible nutrition-related side effects of surgery (including exocrine pancreatic insuffi-

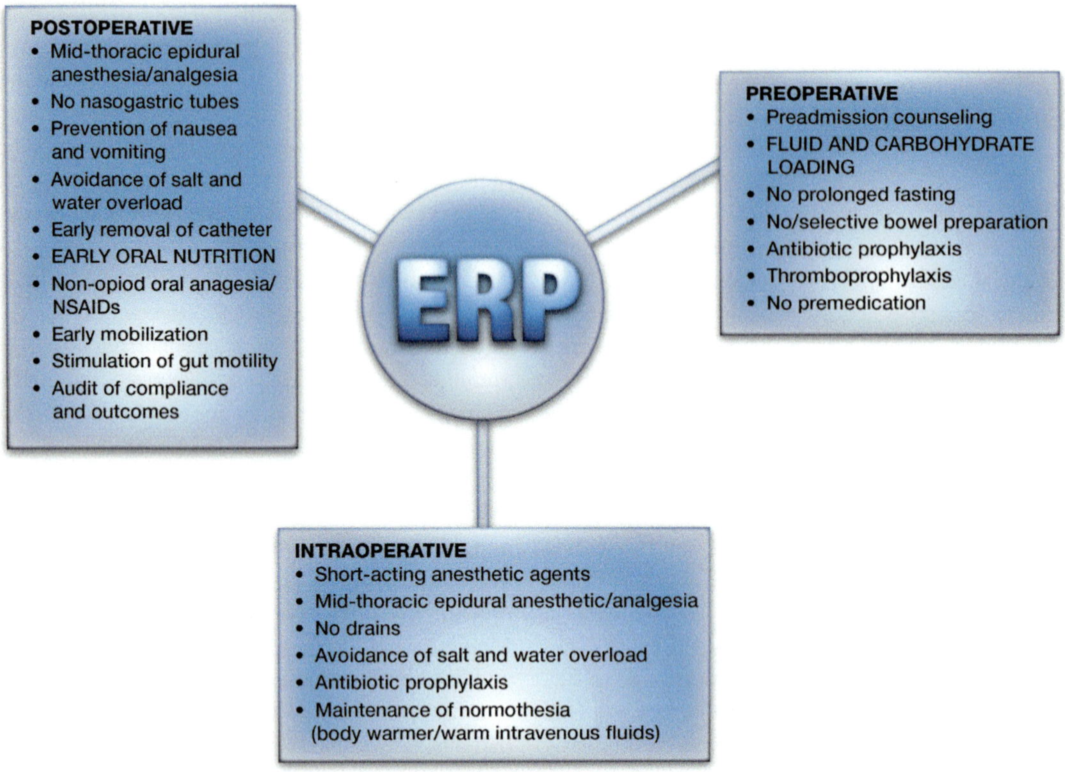

Fig. 14.2 Multiple components of the ERPs which can be implemented

ciency, delayed gastric emptying, and diabetes) early introduction of oral nutrition after surgery, possible nutritional support, and discharge diet information. Education is completed preoperatively to lessen the post-surgery burden on the patient which may increase retention. The institution's practice of immunonutrition and/or carbohydrate loading is also explained to the patient including rationale and goals of this practice including the patient's requirements. For review, Box 14.1 lists specific preoperative topics addressed by the Registered Dietitian.

Box 14.1 Preoperative nutrition-related education topics

- Preoperative immunonutrition
- Postoperative diet progression
- Possible nutrition-related side effects of surgery
  - Exocrine pancreatic insufficiency
  - Delayed gastric emptying
  - Diabetes/blood sugar management
- Possibility of nutritional support
- Early introduction of oral nutrition after surgery
- Post-op diet information
- High calorie/protein supplement use

Postoperative Nutritional Management

Pancreatic surgery affects both pancreatic function and the nutritional status of the patient. It is important to review the typical postoperative progression for diet advancement before discussing specific medical nutrition therapy interventions. Many facilities place a nasogastric tube during surgery which is set to low intermittent suction to prevent nausea and vomiting of gastric acids in the immediate postoperative period. This tube remains in place 1–2 days, while the patient is NPO or allowed only ice chips. Clamping trials typically begin around day 2–3. If the patient denies nausea or has signs of bowel function, the tube is then removed, and a clear liquid diet is initiated. If these items are tolerated, full liquids are started. Some institutions prefer to skip the full liquid step as this diet is typically high in fat and can cause gas and bloating. If this step is skipped, patients are started on selective foods from the hospital offerings which are most often well tolerated. Box 14.2 lists some of these foods which are low in fat and fiber and easily digested. If the patient still does not have complaints of nausea or vomiting, a solid diet of low-fat, low-fiber foods is initiated. Appendix 1 is a comprehensive review of the low-fat, low-fiber diet. Typical reintroduction of solid foods post-surgery can take 5–7 days.

Box 14.2 Well-tolerated foods for early introduction

- Banana
- Canned fruit
- Cream of Wheat®/Grits®/Farina®
- Rice Krispies®/Rice Chex®
- Plain Cheerios®
- Plain bagel
- English muffin
- White or sourdough bread/toast
- Scrambled egg
- Hard-cooked egg
- Pancakes
- Chicken noodle soup
- Noodles
- White rice
- White potatoes, mashed potatoes
- Grilled boneless chicken breast
- Baked white fish
- Turkey breast
- Pretzels
- Saltine crackers
- Graham crackers

Postoperative Nutritional Support

Because patients undergoing pancreaticoduodenectomy are often nutritionally depleted at the time of surgery, nutritional support is often considered. It is well documented that routine total parenteral nutrition is not beneficial and far inferior to enteral nutrition post-pancreatic surgery as it is associated with higher incidence of complications [17]. Total parenteral nutrition has been shown to have an increased rate of complications, longer duration to first bowel movement, and delay in resumption of general diet [18, 19]. Enteral nutrition support is preferred for reasons of better substrate utilization, prevention of mucosal atrophy, maintenance of gastrointestinal integrity, and immunocompetence while reducing complications and improving nutritional status [20]. The value of jejunostomy tube placement and utilization post-pancreaticoduodenectomy is still not without debate and should be addressed on a case-by-case basis. Research has shown both risks and benefits to the practice making the choice an unclear one. Some research shows that early postoperative enteral nutrition enhances immune function, reduces infections, and results in earlier return of bowel function decreasing overall length of stay [21]. Other studies have associated tube feedings with diarrhea, abdominal cramping, excess gas production, and delayed gastric emptying [22]. The differences in each individual's tolerance of preoperative chemotherapy, the wide spectrum of nutritional status at initial diagnosis, and ECOG/Karnofsky scores at time of surgery combined with the individualization of each surgery make this a complex topic to research. Individual approach should be taken in evaluating whether the patient may benefit from intraoperative jejunostomy placement. This is a multidisciplinary-based decision taking into account the exact surgery to be performed, patient's history of neoadjuvant treatment tolerance, and evaluating the functional and nutritional status of the patient leading up to surgery. Ongoing nutritional assessments and comparisons between preoperative nutrition-focused physical evaluations can help the nutritional professional recommend a preoperative malnutrition diagnosis highlighting which patients may benefit from surgically placed jejunostomies.

If a patient has a J-tube placed intraoperatively, feeds are typically started on post-op day 2 or 3 regardless of return of bowel function [23]. Most patients tolerate a semi-elemental formula well. Other institutions may start with a low-fiber, polymeric formula resulting in good tolerance overall. The feeds are started at a low rate of 10 ml/hr and advanced by 10–15 ml/hr daily to goal of 30–45 ml/hr. GI tolerance should be monitored as feedings are advanced. A complete elemental formula can be considered if patients develop severe, uncontrolled diarrhea. If oral intake is very poor (consistently <50% estimated needs), the rate of tube feeding can increase up to 50 ml/hr. The goal is for total calorie intake >80% of estimated needs prior to discharge including nutritional support and oral intake. While cycling the tube feedings is not recommended in the acute post-op phase (7–10 days), prior to discharge, patients may be cycled to <16-hour infusions. This provides the patient with freedom from the feedings in order to work on increasing oral intake and activity.

As previously mentioned, parenteral nutrition is not a standard of care for post-Whipple patients unless complications indicate its usage. Postoperative complications that may warrant the use of PN are prolonged ileus, pancreatic or anastomotic leak, diarrhea refractory to medication management (i.e., short bowel syndrome), GI fistulas, and large chylous leak [24].

Discharge Readiness

Nutritional status should be stable for at least 2 days prior to discharge. Calorie counts instituted in the hospital should result in patient meeting at least 80% of estimated protein and calorie needs through any combination of oral intake and nutrition support. Oral nutritional supplementation offered to the patient in the hospital should be emphasized to continue upon discharge. Patients and families are instructed to keep a weight, food, and bowel log including documentation of GI symptoms and medication intake. Prior to discharge, reeducation on the low-fat, low-fiber diet should also be completed.

Side Effect Management

The nutritional professional plays an intricate role in side effect management post-surgery. Common nutritional complications after pancreas surgery include gastroparesis or delayed gastric emptying, slow return of bowel function/post-op ileus, fat malabsorption, hyperglycemia, anastomotic leak, chylous leak, dumping syndrome, and fluid–electrolyte imbalances. The following section will discuss nutritional management of some of these complications.

Delayed Gastric Emptying

Delayed gastric emptying can be broadly defined as a disorder which slows or stops the movement of food from the stomach to the small intestines. Gastric emptying is regulated by volume of food, gastrin, gastric tone, and both nervous reflexes and hormonal feedback (stimulated by dietary fat) from the duodenum. The gastric tone of the proximal stomach influences liquid emptying, while the tone of the distal stomach is involved in the emptying of solids. All of these aforementioned functions are surgically compromised after a pancreaticoduodenectomy which makes delayed gastric emptying one of the most common complications after pancreatic resection. Further exacerbating gastric emptying is the decrease in gut motility associated with narcotic and opioid analgesic use. Other medications known to compromise gastric emptying include aluminum-containing antacids, anticholinergics, ondansetron, and several categories of antidepressants [24]. Pharmacists can help to review medications and consider alternatives; however, the benefits of the medications may outweigh the delay in gastric emptying.

Clinical symptoms of delayed gastric emptying include decreased appetite and anorexia, nausea and vomiting, bloating, fullness (especially in the morning after fasting overnight) early satiety, postprandial hypoglycemia, or fluctuating glucose levels in otherwise well-controlled patients. Meal pattern and structure directly impacts the degree of gastric emptying. Factors that slow gastric emptying include high-calorie and high-fat content, digestibility of foods consumed, osmolality of bolus, and meal volume [25]. Medical nutritional therapy can help manage delayed gastric emptying. Implementing small, frequent meals and snacks, increasing consumption of liquid calories, adhering to a low-fat, low-fiber diet, and chewing foods thoroughly are some of the dietary principles which can help with symptom management [24]. In addition to medical nutritional therapy, delayed gastric emptying can also be managed with scheduled prokinetic medications. Metoclopramide, 10 mg four times daily prior to meals, has been shown to improve symptoms of anorexia, nausea, and vomiting associated with this condition [1]. Diarrhea occurs infrequently at this dose; however, hyperactivity is common and responds to dose reductions. Erythromycin has also been used as a prokinetic agent however loses efficacy rather quickly and should not be used long term for risk of antibiotic resistance [24]. Liquid medications are also preferred and better tolerated. Tight glucose control is also important with patients struggling with delayed gastric emptying [24].

Exocrine Pancreatic Insufficiency

Depending on the type of surgical resection, risk of exocrine pancreatic insufficiency differs. Pancreaticoduodenectomy requires a circumferential dissection of the nerve plexus and interstitial cells of Cajal which potentially results in tonic inhibitory effects of the sympathetic nerves around the superior mesenteric artery causing diarrhea [20, 26]. Steatorrhea is 40% less common after distal pancreatectomy primarily because of the preservation of the celiac and SMA plexus and bilateral ganglions [26]. After pancreatic surgery, exocrine pancreatic insufficiency (EPI) and increased fecal fat excretion may increase by 38% [27], and over half of patients require enzyme supplementation [28, 29]. One of the more common symptoms of EPI is steatorrhea, which is subjective in nature and a poor measure of the degree of insufficiency. EPI has been found to begin to manifest when the pancreatic lipase is 5–10% of its normal output [26]. Supplementation can improve steatorrhea symptoms but does not necessarily indicate the proper absorption of nutrients or improvement in nutritional status [27, 30]. Malabsorption is multifactorial in origin. Dumping syndrome, decreased production of enzymes, accelerated transit time related to greater-sized food particles entering the jejunum, or a combination of the three makes this a somewhat challenging problem to address. No one solution can be the "catch all" for every patient. Sometimes, combinations of several treatments are required.

Pancreatic Enzymes

Pharmaceutical pancreatic enzymes contain lipase, protease, and amylase from porcine (pig) glands. Prescription enzyme preparations, mostly enteric coated beads, resist degradation by gastric acid and are absorbed after passage into the small bowel. If not coated, or capsules are opened prior to ingestion, gastric acid suppression is typically necessary to prevent the inactivation of lipase. Currently, there is no objective measurement for adequate enzyme supplementation nor are there specific dosing instructions for this population as each individual presents with their own particular clinical symptoms, altering degrees of steatorrhea, and varying fat levels in the diet. Therefore, individualized doses are recommended. Although there are no specific dosing instructions for this population, there are guidelines and recommendations to consider. Fat-based dosing provides sufficient lipase to digest a specific amount of fat consumed. Fat-based dosing is generally dosed at 1000–4000 units of lipase/1 g of dietary fat consumed. This is often best utilized when calculated per kilogram dose appears too high for a starting dose. Weight-based dosing is another method. This is either calculated at 500–2500 units of lipase/kg/meal or <10,000 units of lipase/kg/day [31]. Typically, per meal dosing is calculated first and then double-checked to make sure it does not exceed the per day allotment. The total daily dose should reflect approximately three meals plus one to two snacks per day; however take into consideration the individual eating pattern of the patient. Snack doses should be approximately half the dose of mealtime amounts or slightly less. If calculations result in an "in-between" dose, it is best to start lower and titrate up to avoid constipation.

Common reported side effects of enzymes include abdominal pain, nausea, bloating, flatulence, constipation (often from too high of a dose), and the more seldom occurrence of exacerbated diarrhea. It is important to determine if symptoms are caused by the medications or if adjustments in dose, timing, or brand may be beneficial. In order to improve tolerance and effectiveness, enzyme replacement is taken with food, not chewed or crushed, and not directly mixed with foods with a pH of greater than 4.5 [32]. These actions can disrupt the protective enteric coating resulting in early release of enzymes, irritation of oral mucosa, and/or loss of enzyme activity. Capsules can be opened and added to a small amount of acidic soft foods with a pH of 4.5 or less (applesauce or pureed canned pears) at room temperature. Open capsules should never be chewed. Restricting fat in the diet long term is recommended if symptoms (weight loss, steatorrhea) are poorly controlled on enzymes or if enzymes are not tolerated.

Several factors influence the effectiveness of enzymes. Compliance is the number one controllable variable related to the efficacy of medications. Timing of ingesting the enzymes is another. Preferred method of practice is to take with the first bite of foods and if prescribed more than one capsule to spread the dosing intermittently throughout the meal. Enzyme timing may take many adjustments since gastric emptying varies in individuals. The enzymes should be timed to be present when the food passes into the small intestines. Taking with fat-containing snacks will also increase effectiveness. Gastric acid environment is another component that can increase or decrease effectiveness of enzymes. Decreased bicarbonate secretion and increased gastric acidity may reduce enzyme activity by delaying the release of enzymes in the proximal duodenum. The enteric coatings of enzymes generally protect the enzyme until a pH of 6. If this does not occur early in the duodenum (which after surgery the duodenum is bypassed), adding proton pump inhibitors, H2 blockers, or bicarbonate tablets to raise the pH of gastric secretions can enhance enzyme effectiveness. In addition, slower gastric emptying can also decrease the usefulness of enzymes. A prokinetic agent is recommended for this issue.

Pancreatic enzymes are a porcine product. This may be a barrier to compliance for vegetarian, vegan, and Jewish patients. Their faith has exceptions for these situations; however, some patients choose to abide by their religious rules. There are a few kosher enzymes which are vegetarian-based over-the-counter supplements. Each pill is approximately 5000 lipase units, and therefore the number of pills required per meal is often quadrupled. The effectiveness of these supplements has not been reviewed.

Dumping Syndrome

Dumping syndrome can occur after a pancreaticoduodenectomy because of the destruction of the pylorus. The pylorus valve located at the base of the stomach periodically releases small amounts of chyme into the intestines. Without that value, there is no regulation of amounts of food particles passing into, in these cases, the jejunum. The result is a large amount of undigested food which is not prepared for proper absorption.

Dumping syndrome encompasses both gastrointestinal symptoms coupled with vasomotor responses. Classic gastrointestinal symptoms are feeling of fullness, bloating, crampy abdominal pain, and nausea which are all relieved by explosive diarrhea. The vasomotor responses include sweating, dizziness, lightheadedness, flushing, and palpitations. The timings of these symptoms classify dumping as early (within 15–60 minutes of eating) or late (2–3 hours after eating and is usually just vasomotor in etiology) [11]. The gastrointestinal symptoms are often related to the rapid pouring of concentrated sugars into the small intestines from the stomach which provokes an osmotic diuresis into the lumen of the intestines. Vasomotor symptoms are in response to sudden transfer of glucose to the small intestines resulting in a rapid production and release of serum insulin causing hypoglycemia accompanied by the aforementioned symptoms. Typically, the gastrointestinal symptoms are early onset, while the vasomotor symptoms occur as late onset. These symptoms decrease as the body adjusts to the new anatomy and learns what types of foods trigger episodes.

Dietary interventions for dumping syndrome include elimination of simple sugars, small, frequent meals and snacks, avoidance of liquids with meals, eating slowly, and chewing foods thoroughly. Lying down after eating can slow down gastric emptying. Avoiding high-fiber foods can also help control symptoms. Clear liquid and full liquid diets are generally not well tolerated if dumping syndrome occurs due to the amount of simple sugars included in these diets. Limiting portions to half cup at a time and diluting fruit juices and other drinks can reduce the symptoms on these restrictive diets. Table 14.4 discusses medical nutrition therapy tips for dumping syndrome. It is important for patients to keep a thorough log of food and fluids consumed in addition to symptom log to determine which diet principles will most be beneficial to initiate. As patients adjust to their new anatomy, diet liberalization should be explored.

Table 14.4 Medical nutritional therapy to treat dumping syndrome [1, 2]

Tips to try	Things to avoid
6–8 small meals and snacks Drink liquids between meals; stop drinking 30–45 minutes prior to meals and no liquids for 1 hour following meals Chew food well and slow down when eating Eat a high-protein source with every meal and snacks Control carbohydrate intake to three or less servings per meal Consume lower-fat, room temperature, or cold foods (avoid temperature extremes) Consume foods high in pectin content (bananas, apples, oatmeal, rice, potatoes) or try 1 tbsp pectin mixed in ¼ cup applesauce with meals	Avoid large amounts of simple sugars and high-calorie beverages Avoid insoluble fiber as they can increase movement through the GI system Limit milk and milk products if not well tolerated Lactose can be hard to break down

Mueller [24]; Leser [11]

Endocrine Insufficiency and Diabetes

Nutritional management of diabetes varies throughout the continuum of care. Altered endocrine function is often present at pancreatic cancer diagnosis with approximately 50% of patients presenting with diabetes or insulin resistance. Half of these patients have reported pancreatic cancer diagnosis within 3 years of diabetes onset [33–35]. Liberalizing diet restrictions is appropriate throughout adjuvant treatments as well as postoperatively with much more aggressive medication management since most patients experience limited oral intake. Early involvement of the diabetes management team can greatly improve blood sugar control during hospitalization. Blood sugar levels tend to elevate under the body's physical stress of surgery. Patients should be advised they may be on insulin to help control levels in the hospital, but this does not necessarily mean they will be on insulin long term. In 90.5% (19/21) of patients with preoperatively known diabetes managed with insulin, no change in endocrine function is observed post-surgery. In contrast, endocrine function improved in 68.1% (15/22) of patients with newly diagnosed diabetes. Forty percent (14/35) of patients with a preoperative normal oral glucose tolerance test (OGTT) or prediabetes experienced deterioration in endocrine function [36]. Several more recent papers report varying percentages of resolution from 30.7–65% [37]. Factors associated with either the deterioration or improvements of pancreatic endocrine functions are diverse. Experimental models have suggested fasting blood glucose impairment when >50% of beta cells are removed, while retrospective studies have shown of 25–44% of the pancreatic volume during a distal pancreatectomy can influence impairment [38–40]. Other factors include new onset-DM; size, location and differentiation of the tumor; the presence of pancreatitis; BMI, preoperative bilirubin, and C-peptide levels; and extent of surgery [36]. Patients leaving the hospital should be instructed on blood glucose monitoring and set up to meet with an endocrinologist if necessary. One study indicated that endocrine function at 1-week post-surgery was predictive of the level of function at 12 months [37]. However, others demonstrated a transient rise in endocrine dysfunction which resolved at 3 months and a 12% decrease in DM from 6 to 12 months [34, 41]. Resolution of diabetes occurred in 20–57% of patients after Whipple procedure [34, 40, 42].

Patients who have completed their course of treatments and obtained a relatively stable nutritional status will benefit from following the American Diabetic Association's guidelines for medical nutrition therapy. These diet principles include regularly scheduled meals and snacks, reduced simple sugars, and a diet balanced with lean proteins and complex carbohydrates.

Vitamin (A, D, E, K, B12) and Mineral (Iron, Calcium, Zinc, Selenium) Deficiencies

Vitamin deficiencies are common after pancreaticoduodenectomy due to resected small bowel, altered anatomy, and insufficient pancreatic enzymes. After resection, patients lose the absorptive capacity of the duodenum and function of the gastric antrum/pylorus valve, chyme entering the jejunal loop is altered in composition, pH changes occur, and reduced pancreatic enzyme excretion is prominent. In many patients, clinicians attempt to normalize physiology with acid-suppressing medications and enzyme supplementation; however, these practices do not appear to prevent micronutrient depletions [43]. Furthermore, studies on long-term survivors of pancreaticoduodenectomies confirm this population may be predisposed to trace elements and fat-soluble vitamin deficiencies. This appears to be independent of dietary intake and degree of pancreatic exocrine function [44]. Specific nutrients at risk are discussed in this section. Table 14.5 summarizes the specific nutrient, symptoms of deficiency, appropriate lab testing, and subsequent supplementation recommendations.

Fat-Soluble Vitamins

Diminished pancreatic enzyme function increases the risk of fat-soluble vitamin deficiencies especially with severe exocrine insufficiency [45]. Fat-soluble vitamins include vitamin A, E, D, and K. These deficiencies manifest as subclinical presentations requiring laboratory testing [45, 46]. Most studies have resulted in vitamin A within normal range for most patients. Vitamin E levels, while found to be significantly lower than control group in studies, are generally still within the reference ranges [43]. Very few studies have been conducted on vitamin K in this population.

Vitamin D and Calcium

Vitamin D levels are well-documented deficiencies in this population. One study documents patients were found to display normal serum corrected calcium levels; however, 11/37 (30%) had elevated parathyroid hormone levels suggesting a compensatory secondary hyperparathyroidism in order to maintain normal blood calcium levels [43]. These patients were also found to have significantly lower serum vitamin D levels which were associated with an increased parathyroid hormone level. This indicates stimulation of both absorption and mobilization of calcium from bones to maintain blood levels. Vitamin D supplementation can be timed with meals and enzymes to enhance absorption.

Iron and Anemias

A classic pancreaticoduodenectomy includes resection of the gastric antrum resulting in loss of intrinsic factor which is necessary for B12 absorption. This can lead to B12 deficiencies. The resection of the duodenum portion places further risk on iron and zinc deficiencies. Vitamin B6 is mainly absorbed in the proximal small bowel, of which the entire duodenum and approximately 20 cm of jejunum are typically lost after surgical resection. Vitamin B6 deficiency can

Table 14.5 Micronutrient recommendations for deficiencies post-pancreaticoduodenectomy

Nutrient	Test	Normal levels	Potential causes of deficiencies	Recommendations for treatment
Vitamin A	Plasma retinol[a]	0.3–1.2 mg/L	Loss of the exocrine pancreas Inadequate PERT	10,000–25,000 IU/day orally until clinical improvement (1–2 weeks)
Vitamin D	25-hydroxyvitamin D[a]	30–80 ng/mL	Loss of the exocrine pancreas Inadequate PERT	6000–10,000 IU/day orally for 8 weeks or until >30 ng/mL with maintenance dose of 3000–6000 IU/day
Vitamin E	Serum/plasma alpha-tocopherol	5.5–18.0 mg/L	Loss of the exocrine pancreas Inadequate PERT	100–400 IU/day orally and up to 800 IU/day for 3 months
Iron	Ferritin, transferrin, transferrin saturation, serum iron[a]	Ferritin: Male: 38–530 ng/mL Female: 12–340 ng/mL Transferrin: 200–400 mg/dL Transferrin saturation: 20–50% Serum iron: Males: 50–170 µg/dL Females: 30–160 µg/dL	Gastric acid suppression Resection of duodenum and jejunum	325 mg iron sulfate orally up to three times daily for up to 3 months and then reassess
Vitamin B12	MMA, homocysteine	MMA: 0.00–0.40 µmol/L Homocysteine: <11 mmol/L	SIBO Gastric acid suppression Decreased proteolytic enzyme production	100–1000 mcg/month IM Or 350–500 mcg/day oral
Folate	Red blood cell folate	>366 ng/mL	pH changes Alcoholism	1 mg/day orally and up to 5 mg/day for 1–3 months
Thiamine	Whole blood thiamine[a]	70–180 nmol/L	SIBO Alcoholism Previous Whipple surgery	
Calcium	Ionized calcium (consider parathyroid level)	1.11–1.30 mmol/L	Resection of the duodenum Vitamin D deficiency Malabsorption	1200–1500 mg elemental calcium daily orally via calcium citrate in divided doses; reassess in 3 months
Copper	Serum copper[a]	Male: 70–140 µg/dL Female: 80–155 µg/dL	Gastric acid suppression Resection of the duodenum Previous Whipple surgery	2–4 mg elemental copper orally daily or every other day or may require 2 mg IV daily × 5 days initially if severe malabsorption or symptomatic; follow by oral replacement, reassess levels in 4–6 weeks

(continued)

Table 14.5 (continued)

Nutrient	Test	Normal levels	Potential causes of deficiencies	Recommendations for treatment
Zinc	Serum/plasma zinc[a]	60–120 μg/dL	Resection of duodenum and jejunum Gastric acid suppression Pancreatic insufficiency Previous Whipple surgery	220 mg oral zinc sulfate daily × 4 weeks, then reassess; may require 60 mg elemental zinc orally twice daily; monitor copper status with prolonged therapeutic zinc supplementation
Selenium	Erythrocyte glutathione peroxidase, Serum/plasma selenium[a]	Glutathione peroxidase: >10.5 U/mL erythrocytes [9] Serum/plasma selenium: 23–190 μg/L	Resection of duodenum and jejunum Oxidative stress Previous Whipple surgery	100 μg/day IV selenium × 10–20 days or until normalized with a maintenance dose of 60 μg/day orally

Adapted with permissions from [1]
Van Arsdale and Goral [54]
[a]Levels can be altered with inflammation, check with C-reactive protein measurement

lead to normocytic, macrocytic, or sideroblastic anemias due to impairment of heme synthesis [47] and likely an under-recognized cause of anemias in this population. Micronutrient deficiencies including vitamin B6, vitamin B12, folic acid, zinc, copper, and iron are all known to cause cytopenias. Subclinical anemias are prevalent in long-term survivors of pancreaticoduodenectomy [47]. Patients who exhibit subclinical iron deficiencies are manifested by low serum ferritin, elevated transferrin, increased iron binding capacity, and decreased transferrin saturation [44]. Although true levels of iron deficiencies have not yet been clinically documented, biochemical signs of mild anemias are often reported and propose the question of supplementation use for subclinical anemias.

Zinc deficiency was reported in up to 68% of pancreas resection patients, predominantly post-Whipple, although almost all were asymptomatic [48]. In one study, despite normal intakes of zinc, 50% of post-pancreaticoduodenectomy patients showed deficiency [44]. Copper deficiencies have also been reported in patients with gastric and bowel resections [49].

Selenium

Selenium is an important dietary antioxidant shown to be important in anti-inflammatory processes as well as protecting against cardiac disease, infective, and neoplastic processes. Whipple patients are prone to selenium deficiency due to duodenal resection and oxidative stress. Studies have found significantly reduced serum selenium values in 57% (21/37) of long-term pancreaticoduodenectomy survivors compared to non-operated controls [44].

Summary

Nutrition is a fundamental component of overall health and wellness, and it also plays a large role during times of illness and stress caused by disease, treatments, and surgical procedures. Appropriate nourishment provides the body with the mechanisms it needs to maintain and improve health.

Pancreatic cancer is an aggressive malignancy with a poor overall prognosis. The disease itself and its treatments can cause significant nutritional impairments adversely impacting the quality of life. Many patients experience cachexia [50] ultimately experiencing a lower quality of life, increased morbidity and mortality, longer hospital stays, and a reduced response to treatment [5, 51–53]. Malnutrition (broadly defined as lack of proper nutrition, caused by not having enough to eat, not eating enough of the right things, or being unable to use the food that one does eat) impacts quality of life in many ways. Unfortunately, lack of discreet nutritional markers ceases to exist as a standard of practice leaving the extent of malnutrition in this population underreported throughout the continuum of care.

After completion of cancer treatments, some cancer survivors experience continued loss of weight and lean body mass. Lingering effects of treatments can compromise a patient's long-term quality of life. These lasting effects include continued anorexia and poor nutritional intake, continued taste/smell aversions, continued vitamin/mineral deficiencies, persistent fatigue, and chronic bowel issues. The primary nutrition goals for recovery and survivorship are to attain a healthy body weight, improve strength and physical abilities, and proactively manage long-term treatment-related side effects in order for patients to achieve an acceptable quality of life.

Appendix 1: Low-fat, low-fiber diet

Food category	Foods to choose	Foods to not eat
Meat and meat substitutes	Tender beef, pork, and lamb (choose cuts of round or loin) Skinless poultry Fish Shrimp, crab, lobster Eggs Low-fat tofu Tuna packed in water *Trim meat of visible fat prior to cooking* *Choose cooking methods without added fat such as baked, broiled, steamed, poached, or grilled*	Tough meats Gristle from meats Sausages or hot dogs Bacon Spare ribs Oysters Poultry skin Meat or fish packed in oil High-fat tofu Legumes (chickpeas, lentils, kidney beans, black beans, etc.)
Dairy/dairy substitutes	Skim or 1% milk Low-fat yogurts without fruit on the bottom/peach yogurt Low-fat ice creams/frozen yogurt/sherbet Pudding made with 1% milk Low-fat cheeses, low-fat cream cheese Rice milk Almond milk	Whole or 2% milk Full-fat yogurts Berry-containing yogurts Full-fat ice cream Ice cream with nuts Custard Milkshakes Hard cheeses

(continued)

Appendix 1 (continued)

Food category	Foods to choose	Foods to not eat
Breads, cereals, and grains	White bread or rolls Saltines, oyster crackers Graham crackers Waffles Pancakes Low-fat muffins without nuts Animal crackers Baked chips or pretzels Plain biscuits Refined cereals (Puffed Rice, Corn Flakes, Rice Krispies, Rice Chex, and Special K) Oatmeal, Farina, Cream of Wheat/Rice, Grits White rice White pastas Couscous	Any bread or muffin with nuts, seeds, coconut, or dried fruit Wheat or whole wheat breads Wheat crackers Cornbread Donuts Pastries Croissants or scones Popcorn Regular chips Wheat, bran, or whole grain cereals Cereals with nuts, seeds, coconut, dried fruits, or granola Granola Brown rice Whole wheat pasta Wild rice Buckwheat Quinoa
Fruits	Canned fruits except pineapple chunks Applesauce Bananas Fruit cocktail Fresh fruits that have been peeled (apples, pears, peaches, plums) Seedless melons (watermelon, cantaloupe, honeydew) Papaya Mango	Fresh fruits not listed on opposite column Dried fruits (prunes, raisins, figs, and dates) Berries of all kinds Pineapples Citrus fruits Skins of fruits Grapes Kiwi
Vegetables	Well-cooked or canned vegetables without seeds or skins Carrots (al dente) Beets Asparagus tips Green beans, wax beans Iceberg lettuce (1–2 slices) White potatoes without skin Tomato sauces	Raw vegetables Fried vegetables Vegetables with seeds or skins such as Bok Choy Broccoli Brussels sprouts Cabbage Cauliflower Collard greens Corn Cucumbers Eggplant Kale Mushrooms Onions Peas Peppers Pickles Sauerkraut Spinach Squash Yams
Soups	Broth-based soups Soups made with allowed vegetables above	Cream-based soups

Food category	Foods to choose	Foods to not eat
Beverages	Water Decaf coffee (limit to 1 cup per day) Herbal teas (limit to 1 cup per day) Fruit juices: apple, grape, or cranberry Flattened carbonated beverages	Prune juice Juice with pulp
Desserts/sweets	Angel food cake Sherbet Fruit ice Popsicles Gelatin Hard candies Marshmallows Jelly/jams without seeds	Any dessert with nuts, seeds, coconut, or dried fruit Pastries Pies Cakes Brownies Donuts
Fats	Low-fat or light: Mayonnaise Salad dressings Margarine	Lard Fried foods Avocados Olives Gravies Cream sauces Hollandaise sauce Tartar sauce Butter Hydrogenated oils such as palm oil, soybean oil, and corn oil

References

1. Elliott L, Molseed LL, McCallum PD, American Dietetic Association, editors. The clinical guide to oncology nutrition. 2nd ed. American Dietetic Association: Chicago, IL; 2006. p. 270.
2. Becker AE. Pancreatic ductal adenocarcinoma: risk factors, screening, and early detection. World J Gastroenterol. 2014;20(32):11182.
3. Ozola Zalite I, Zykus R, Francisco Gonzalez M, Saygili F, Pukitis A, Gaujoux S, et al. Influence of cachexia and sarcopenia on survival in pancreatic ductal adenocarcinoma: a systematic review. Pancreatology. 2015;15(1):19–24.
4. Loh KW, Vriens MR, Gerritsen A, Borel Rinkes IHM, van Hillegersberg R, Schippers C, et al. Unintentional weight loss is the most important indicator of malnutrition among surgical cancer patients. Neth J Med. 2012;70(8):365–9.
5. Gärtner S, Krüger J, Aghdassi AA, Steveling A, Simon P, Lerch MM, et al. Nutrition in pancreatic cancer: a review. Gastrointest Tumors. 2016;2(4):195–202.
6. Baracos VE, Martin L, Korc M, Guttridge DC, Fearon KCH. Cancer-associated cachexia. Nat Rev Dis Primers. 2018;4:17105.
7. Lacey K, Pritchett E. Nutrition care process and model: ADA adopts road map to quality care and outcomes management. J Am Diet Assoc. 2003;103(8):1061–72.
8. Mueller C, Compher C, Ellen DM. The American Society for Parenteral and Enteral Nutrition (A.S.P.E.N.) Board of Directors. A.S.P.E.N. clinical guidelines: nutrition screening, assessment, and intervention in adults. J Parenter Enter Nutr. 2011;35(1):16–24.
9. Radler DR, Lister T. Nutrient deficiencies associated with nutrition-focused physical findings of the oral cavity. Nutr Clin Pract. 2013;28(6):710–21.
10. Malone A, Hamilton C. The Academy of Nutrition and Dietetics/the American Society for Parenteral and Enteral Nutrition consensus malnutrition characteristics: application in practice. Nutr Clin Pract. 2013;28(6):639–50.
11. Leser M, Academy of Nutrition and Dietetics, American Dietetic Association, Oncology Nutrition Dietetic Practice Group. Oncology nutrition for clinical practice. 2013.
12. Garth AK, Newsome CM, Simmance N, Crowe TC. Nutritional status, nutrition practices and post-operative complications in patients with gastrointestinal cancer: nutrition status and post-operative outcomes. J Hum Nutr Diet. 2010;23(4):393–401.
13. Aida T, Furukawa K, Suzuki D, Shimizu H, Yoshidome H, Ohtsuka M, et al. Preoperative immunonutrition decreases postoperative complications by modulating prostaglandin E2 production and T-cell differentiation in patients undergoing pancreatoduodenectomy. Surgery. 2014;155(1):124–33.
14. Silvestri S, Franchello A, Deiro G, Galletti R, Cassine D, Campra D, et al. Preoperative oral immunonutrition

versus standard preoperative oral diet in well nourished patients undergoing pancreaticoduodenectomy. Int J Surg. 2016;31:93–9.
15. Braga M, Gianotti L, Vignali A, Carlo VD. Preoperative oral arginine and n-3 fatty acid supplementation improves the immunometabolic host response and outcome after colorectal resection for cancer. Surgery. 2002;132(5):805–14.
16. Majumder A, Fayezizadeh M, Neupane R, Elliott HL, Novitsky YW. Benefits of multimodal enhanced recovery pathway in patients undergoing open ventral hernia repair. J Am Coll Surg. 2016;222(6):1106–15.
17. Goonetilleke KS, Siriwardena AK. Systematic review of peri-operative nutritional supplementation in patients undergoing pancreaticoduodenectomy. JOP. 2006;7(1):5–13.
18. Liu C, Du Z, Lou C, Wu C, Yuan Q, Wang J, et al. Enteral nutrition is superior to total parenteral nutrition for pancreatic cancer patients who underwent pancreaticoduodenectomy. Asia Pac J Clin Nutr. 2011;20(2):154–60.
19. Park JS, Chung H-K, Hwang HK, Kim JK, Yoon DS. Postoperative nutritional effects of early enteral feeding compared with total parental nutrition in pancreaticoduodectomy patients: a prospective, randomized study. J Korean Med Sci. 2012;27(3):261.
20. Karagianni VT, Papalois AE, Triantafillidis JK. Nutritional status and nutritional support before and after pancreatectomy for pancreatic cancer and chronic pancreatitis. Indian J Surg Oncol. 2012;3(4):348–59.
21. Mahmoodzadeh H, Shoar S, Sirati F, Khorgami Z. Early initiation of oral feeding following upper gastrointestinal tumor surgery: a randomized controlled trial. Surg Today. 2015;45(2):203–8.
22. Nejat SN, Hosseini S. Comparing early oral feeding with traditional oral feeding in upper gastrointestinal surgery. Turk J Gastroenterol. 2010;21(2):119–24.
23. McClave SA, Taylor BE, Martindale RG, Warren MM, Johnson DR, Braunschweig C, et al. Guidelines for the provision and assessment of nutrition support therapy in the adult critically ill patient: Society of Critical Care Medicine (SCCM) and American Society for Parenteral and Enteral Nutrition (A.S.P.E.N.). J Parenter Enter Nutr. 2016;40(2):159–211.
24. Mueller CM, American Society of Parenteral and Enteral Nutrition, editors. The A.S.P.E.N. adult nutrition support core curriculum. 2nd ed. Silver Spring: A.S.P.E.N; 2012. p. 716.
25. Camilleri M, Parkman HP, Shafi MA, Abell TL, Gerson L. Clinical guideline: management of gastroparesis. Am J Gastroenterol. 2013;108(1):18–37.
26. Hackert T, Schütte K, Malfertheiner P. The pancreas: causes for malabsorption. Viszeralmedizin. 2014;30(3):6–6.
27. Sikkens ECM, Cahen DL, de Wit J, Looman CWN, van Eijck C, Bruno MJ. Prospective assessment of the influence of pancreatic cancer resection on exocrine pancreatic function: influence of pancreatic cancer resection on exocrine pancreatic function. Br J Surg. 2014;101(2):109–13.
28. Bock EA, Hurtuk MG, Shoup M, Aranha GV. Late complications after pancreaticoduodenectomy with pancreaticogastrostomy. J Gastrointest Surg. 2012;16(5):914–9.
29. Sikkens ECM, Cahen DL, van Eijck C, Kuipers EJ, Bruno MJ. The daily practice of pancreatic enzyme replacement therapy after pancreatic surgery: a northern European survey: enzyme replacement after surgery. J Gastrointest Surg. 2012;16(8):1487–92.
30. Lindkvist B, Phillips ME, Domínguez-Muñoz JE. Clinical, anthropometric and laboratory nutritional markers of pancreatic exocrine insufficiency: prevalence and diagnostic use. Pancreatology. 2015;15(6):589–97.
31. abbvie. Creon package insert. Abbvie; 2015.
32. Aptalis Pharma. ZENPEP package insert. Aptalis Pharma US, Inc; 2014.
33. Gupta S, Vittinghoff E, Bertenthal D, Corley D, Shen H, Walter LC, et al. New-onset diabetes and pancreatic cancer. Clin Gastroenterol Hepatol. 2006;4(11):1366–72.
34. Pannala R, Leirness JB, Bamlet WR, Basu A, Petersen GM, Chari ST. Prevalence and clinical profile of pancreatic cancer–associated diabetes mellitus. Gastroenterology. 2008;134(4):981–7.
35. Illés D, Terzin V, Holzinger G, Kosár K, Róka R, Zsóri G, et al. New-onset type 2 diabetes mellitus – a high-risk group suitable for the screening of pancreatic cancer? Pancreatology. 2016;16(2):266–71.
36. Roeyen G, Jansen M, Hartman V, Chapelle T, Bracke B, Ysebaert D, et al. The impact of pancreaticoduodenectomy on endocrine and exocrine pancreatic function: a prospective cohort study based on pre- and postoperative function tests. Pancreatology. 2017;17(6):974–82.
37. Kang MJ, Jung HS, Jang J-Y, Jung W, Chang J, Shin YC, et al. Metabolic effect of pancreatoduodenectomy: resolution of diabetes mellitus after surgery. Pancreatology. 2016;16(2):272–7.
38. Shirakawa S, Matsumoto I, Toyama H, Shinzeki M, Ajiki T, Fukumoto T, et al. Pancreatic volumetric assessment as a predictor of new-onset diabetes following distal pancreatectomy. J Gastrointest Surg. 2012;16(12):2212–9.
39. Ferrara MJ, Lohse C, Kudva YC, Farnell MB, Que FG, Reid-Lombardo KM, et al. Immediate post-resection diabetes mellitus after pancreaticoduodenectomy: incidence and risk factors. HPB. 2013;15(3):170–4.
40. Kang JS, Jang J-Y, Kang MJ, Kim E, Jung W, Chang J, et al. Endocrine function impairment after distal pancreatectomy: incidence and related factors. World J Surg. 2016;40(2):440–6.
41. Park JW, Jang J-Y, Kim E-J, Kang MJ, Kwon W, Chang YR, et al. Effects of pancreatectomy on nutritional state, pancreatic function and quality of life: quality of life after pancreatectomy. Br J Surg. 2013;100(8):1064–70.

42. Wu J-M, Ho T-W, Kuo T-C, Yang C-Y, Lai H-S, Chiang P-Y, et al. Glycemic change after pancreaticoduodenectomy: a population-based study. Medicine (Baltimore). 2015;94(27):e1109.
43. Armstrong T, Strommer L, Ruiz-Jasbon F, Shek FW, Harris SF, Permert J, et al. Pancreaticoduodenectomy for peri-ampullary neoplasia leads to specific micronutrient deficiencies. Pancreatology. 2007;7(1):37–44.
44. Armstrong T, Walters E, Varshney S, Johnson CD. Deficiencies of micronutrients, altered bowel function, and quality of life during late follow-up after pancreaticoduodenectomy for malignancy. Pancreatology. 2002;2(6):528–34.
45. Keim V, Klar E, Poll M, Schoenberg MH. Postoperative care following pancreatic surgery. Dtsch Arztebl Int. 2009;106(48):789–94.
46. Timofte D, Livadariu R, Bintintan V, Diaconu C, Ionescu L, Sandberg AA, et al. Metabolic disorders in patients operated for pancreatic cancer. Rev Med Chir Soc Med Nat Iasi. 2014;118(2):392–8.
47. Yasuda H, Fujiwara N, Ishizaki Y, Komatsu N. Anemia attributed to vitamin B6 deficiency in post-pancreaticoduodenectomy patients. Pancreatology. 2015;15(1):81–3.
48. Yu H-H, Yang T-M, Shan Y-S, Lin P-W. Zinc deficiency in patients undergoing pancreatoduodenectomy for periampullary tumors is associated with pancreatic exocrine insufficiency. World J Surg. 2011;35(9):2110–7.
49. Halfdanarson TR, Kumar N, Li C-Y, Phyliky RL, Hogan WJ. Hematological manifestations of copper deficiency: a retrospective review: hematological manifestations of copper deficiency. Eur J Haematol. 2008;80(6):523–31.
50. Mueller TC, Burmeister MA, Bachmann J, Martignoni ME. Cachexia and pancreatic cancer: are there treatment options? World J Gastroenterol. 2014;20(28):9361–73.
51. Kyle UG, Pirlich M, Lochs H, Schuetz T, Pichard C. Increased length of hospital stay in underweight and overweight patients at hospital admission: a controlled population study. Clin Nutr. 2005;24(1):133–42.
52. Bachmann J, Heiligensetzer M, Krakowski-Roosen H, Büchler MW, Friess H, Martignoni ME. Cachexia worsens prognosis in patients with resectable pancreatic cancer. J Gastrointest Surg. 2008;12(7):1193–201.
53. Fearon KCH, Baracos VE. Cachexia in pancreatic cancer: new treatment options and measures of success. HPB. 2010;12(5):323–4.
54. Van Arsdale S, Goral S. Nutrition therapy for total pancreatectomy and autologous islet cell transplant. Support Line. 2014;36(5):9–16.

15 Role of ^{18}F-Fluorodeoxyglucose Positron-Emission Tomography (FDG-PET) in the Management of Pancreatic Cancer

Chad A. Barnes, Michael Holt, and Susan Tsai

Introduction

A hallmark of cancer cells is the deregulated uptake of glucose in an effort to sustain the biosynthetic demands of rapid cellular proliferation [1, 2]. This metabolic process was first described by German physiologist Otto Warburg in the 1920s. In the seminal study, Warburg et al. observed a significant increase in glucose consumption and lactic acid production by cancer cells as compared to normal (non-cancerous) cells, despite aerobic conditions, suggesting an anomalous energy metabolism [3]. Subsequent investigators have corroborated this clinical observation and concluded that cancer cells have the ability to reprogram their energy metabolism such that they rely primarily on glucose catabolism for cellular energy production. In contrast, the energy pathway favored by normal tissue cells under aerobic conditions is the coupling of glycolysis with mitochondrial oxidative phosphorylation, as it yields an approximately 18-fold increase in energy production in comparison to glycolysis alone [2]. However, cancer cells are able to compensate by upregulating glucose transporters (GLUT) on the cell membrane, namely, GLUT1, resulting in an increased uptake of glucose into cells [2, 4].

Today, molecular imaging techniques such as integrated ^{18}F-fluorodeoxyglucose positron-emission tomography with computed tomography (FDG-PET/CT) have enabled the visualization and quantification of such cellular processes using molecular probes which mimic endogenous substrates metabolized by cells. FDG is a radioactive glucose analog which is imported into cells via GLUT. However, FDG is not completely metabolized upon entry into cells, in contrast to glucose, and accumulates proportionately to the amount of uptake and metabolic activity within cells [4]. This results in an increased accumulation of FDG within cells, particularly those which have high rates of glycolytic activity as cancers cells.

High levels of FDG uptake have been observed in several solid tumors and associated with poor survival outcomes [5–8]. This clinical observation has fueled the hypothesis that tumor FDG avidity on FDG-PET/CT may be a surrogate marker for tumor biology. Among patients with pancreatic cancer, tumor characteristics on FDG-PET/CT have been shown to closely correlate

C. A. Barnes
Department of Surgery, The Medical College of Wisconsin, Milwaukee, WI, USA

M. Holt
Department of Radiology, The Medical College of Wisconsin, Milwaukee, WI, USA

S. Tsai (✉)
Division of Surgical Oncology, Department of Surgery, The Medical College of Wisconsin, Milwaukee, WI, USA
e-mail: stsai@mcw.edu

S. Tsai et al. (eds.), *Management of Localized Pancreatic Cancer*,
https://doi.org/10.1007/978-3-319-98944-0_15

with clinical outcomes. For example, pancreatic cancers which have high levels of FDG uptake on pretreatment FDG-PET/CT imaging have been associated with more aggressive histologic tumor grade, early treatment failures, and poor survival outcomes, despite the receipt of multimodality therapy [8–14]. However, the role of FDG-PET/CT imaging in the management of pancreatic cancer has been somewhat limited and remains poorly defined. This chapter will review the use of FDG-PET/CT imaging as a prognostic tool among patients with pancreatic cancer.

FDG-PET/CT in the Staging of Pancreatic Cancer

At present, FDG-PET/CT is primarily utilized in the context of equivocal extra-pancreatic lesions on staging CT concerning for metastases or in select patients thought to be high risk for harboring occult metastases due to either a large primary tumor, significant elevation of serum carbohydrate antigen 19–9 (CA19–9), or the presence of suspicious lymph nodes on CT imaging. FDG-PET/CT has been shown to improve the detection of occult metastases in patients with pancreatic cancer. In a review including 65 patients with localized pancreatic cancer, clinical staging was performed using CT angiogram and FDG-PET/CT, and the sensitivities for detecting metastases were 57% and 61% using CT angiogram and FDG-PET/CT, respectively. However, when FDG-PET/CT was used in combination with CT angiogram, the sensitivity for detecting metastases increased to 87%. Importantly, the detection of occult metastatic disease with FDG-PET/CT altered the initial plan of care in 7 (11%) of the 65 patients [15]. Similarly, in a review of 71 patients with locally advanced pancreatic cancer who underwent FDG-PET/CT imaging as part of radiation therapy planning, FDG-PET/CT detected occult metastases in 19 (26%) patients which were not identified on CT imaging. In each of these 19 patients, the treatment modality and/or sequencing of therapies were influenced by the diagnosis of metastatic disease [16]. This underscores the importance of accurate staging of disease and the value of multimodality imaging, which may prevent the application of invasive therapies to patients who will derive little oncologic benefit yet endure the associated morbidity.

In the absence of suspected metastatic disease, the routine use of FDG-PET/CT is not recommended [17]. This is largely due to conflicting evidence that FDG-PET/CT imaging improves the accuracy of diagnosis of pancreatic cancer as compared to CT alone. A recent multi-institutional study including 550 patients with suspected pancreatic cancer found FDG-PET/CT to be superior to CT at diagnosing pancreatic cancer. In this study, all patients underwent both multidetector CT and FDG-PET/CT imaging as part of their diagnostic evaluation, and 261 (47%) of the 550 patients were found to have pancreatic cancer. Multidetector CT had a sensitivity and specificity of 88.5% and 70.6%, respectively, at diagnosing pancreatic cancer, whereas FDG-PET/CT had a sensitivity and specificity of 92.7% and 75.8%, respectively [18]. However, prior meta-analyses have demonstrated comparable diagnostic capabilities for CT and FDG-PET/CT [19, 20].

A meta-analysis including 65 studies demonstrated a pooled sensitivity and specificity of 91% and 85%, respectively, for diagnosing pancreatic cancer with conventional CT imaging. In addition, CT was determined to be superior to both magnetic resonance imaging (MRI) and ultrasound (US) at diagnosing pancreatic cancer; FDG-PET/CT was not evaluated in this study [19]. However, in later meta-analysis which included 35 studies, the pooled sensitivity and specificity were 90% and 76%, respectively, for diagnosing pancreatic cancer with FDG-PET/CT imaging. Therefore, the authors of this analysis concluded that FDG-PET/CT may not provide any additional benefit to CT at diagnosing pancreatic cancer. Interestingly, in the discussion of this analysis, the authors proposed the clinical utility of FDG-PET/CT may be disease prognostication, as several studies in the meta-analysis reported a correlation between tumor FDG avidity and survival outcomes [20].

Prognostic Value of Pretreatment FDG-PET/CT Imaging

Value of Pretreatment FDG-PET/CT

There is substantial evidence to suggest that tumor FDG avidity on FDG-PET/CT imaging may be prognostic of patient outcomes. Several parameters to quantify FDG uptake by tumor cells have been evaluated, including maximal standard uptake value (SUV), total lesion glycolysis (TLG), and metabolic tumor volume (MTV); however, SUV may be the most well studied. SUV is a semi-quantitative measure of FDG uptake which is determined by the equation: [region of interest activity (mCi/mL) x patient body weight (g)] / injected FDG dose [21]. The prognostic value of tumor SUV on FDG-PET/CT has been studied in a variety of cancers and shown to correlate with overall survival (OS) outcomes [5–8].

Data is evolving which suggests that pancreatic cancers with high SUVs on FDG-PET/CT may be associated with more aggressive tumor phenotypes and, subsequently, worse survival outcomes. For example, in a review of 102 patients with pancreatic cancer, SUV on pretreatment FDG-PET/CT directly correlated with pathologic tumor grade. The mean SUVs were 4.93, 6.47, and 7.29 for patients with well-, moderately, and poorly differentiated tumors, respectively. Further, the investigators observed an inverse relationship between maximal SUV and OS outcomes ($p = 0.002$) [9]. In another review including 42 patients with pancreatic cancer who underwent FDG-PET/CT imaging at diagnosis, there was a positive correlation between SUV and histologic grade, though this did not reach statistical significance. However, the investigators did observe a strong correlation between SUV and Ki-67 proliferative index (PI). The mean SUVs were 4.2, 6.0, and 8.6 for patients with low (≤ 5%), moderate (6% to 50%), and high (>50%) Ki-67 PI, respectively ($p < 0.001$) [11]. These findings suggest that SUV on FDG-PET/CT may be a surrogate marker for the biologic aggressiveness of pancreatic cancers. More compelling evidence to support this hypothesis may be the clinical observation that patients with higher SUVs experience worse survival outcomes as compared to patients with lower SUVs (Figs. 15.1 and 15.2). Table 15.1 summarizes studies which have demonstrated a correlation between tumor SUV on FDG-PET/CT and survival outcomes among patients with pancreatic cancer.

In a recent analysis of 105 patients with early-stage pancreatic cancer who underwent FDG-PET/CT imaging prior to resection, the investigators observed a significantly improved OS among patients with a low SUV (<5.1) as compared to those with a high SUV (>5.1). Of the 105 patients, the median OS of the 51 (49%) patients with low SUV was 28 months as compared to 16 months among the 54 (51%) patients with high SUV ($p = 0.036$) [8]. Similarly, in review of 128 patients with resected pancreatic cancer who underwent preoperative FDG-PET/CT imaging, the investigators used a cutoff of 6.0 to classify tumor SUV as either low (<6.0) or high (≥6.0). Of the 128 patients, the median OS of the 59 (46%) patients with low SUV was 37 months as compared to 18 months among the 69 (54%) patients with high SUV ($p < 0.001$) [14].

FDG-PET/CT has also been investigated among patients with advanced disease and similarly has demonstrated prognostic value. In a review of 69 patients with unresected, locally advanced pancreatic cancer treated with either chemotherapy, chemoradiation, or radiotherapy alone, the investigators observed a superior OS among patients with low SUV (≤5.5) as compared to those with high SUV (>5.5). In this study, FDG-PET/CT imaging was performed prior to the initiation of all therapies. Of the 69 patients, the median OS of the 34 (50%) patients with low SUV was 16.6 months as compared to 12.6 months among the 35 (50%) patients with high SUV ($p = 0.025$) [22]. These findings were consistent with a prior analysis which included 55 patients with unresected, locally advanced pancreatic cancer. In this study, patients were treated with chemotherapy and stereotactic body radiotherapy (SBRT). The investigators used the median SUV of 6.2 to classify patients

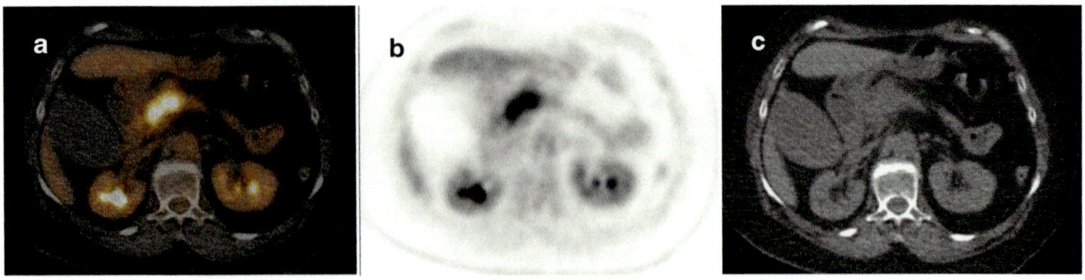

Fig. 15.1 FDG-PET/CT imaging of a 69-year-old female with a pancreatic head mass/neck and serum CA19–9 level of 933 U/mL. Axial fused FDG-PET/CT imaging (**a**) demonstrating increased FDG uptake throughout the pancreatic head/neck mass with a maximal SUV = 10.6. Axial FDG-PET (**b**) and noncontrast CT (**c**) are shown for comparison Endoscopic ultrasound-guided fine needle aspiration confirmed pancreatic cancer. The mass was staged as borderline resectable, and the patient was treated with neoadjuvant therapy prior to surgical resection. The patient developed recurrent disease 7 months from surgery and succumbed to her disease 19 months from initial pancreatic cancer diagnosis

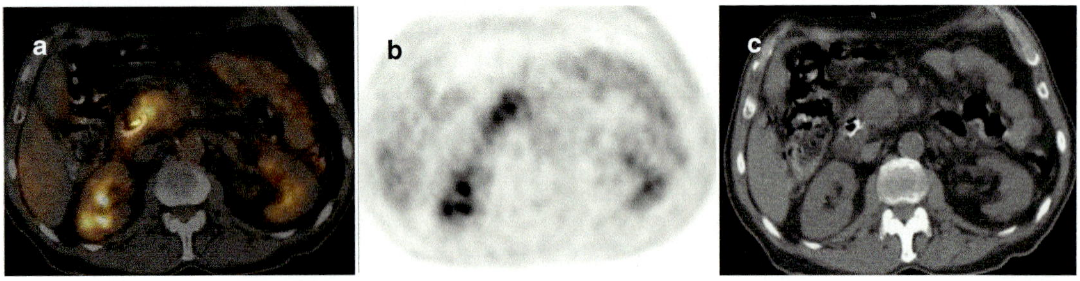

Fig. 15.2 FDG-PET/CT imaging of a 69-year-old male with a pancreatic head mass and significant elevation of serum CA19–9 level to 1775 U/mL. Axial fused FDG-PET/CT imaging (**a**) demonstrating heterogenous FDG uptake throughout the pancreatic head mass with a maximal SUV = 5.0. Axial FDG-PET (**b**) and noncontrast CT (**c**) are shown for comparison. Endoscopic ultrasound-guided fine needle aspiration confirmed pancreatic cancer. The mass was staged as borderline resectable and the patient treated with neoadjuvant therapy prior to surgical resection. The patient developed recurrent disease 28 months from surgery and succumbed to disease 54 months from initial pancreatic cancer diagnosis

as having either a low SUV (<6.2) or high SUV (≥6.2), and a superior OS was observed among patients with low SUV as compared to those with high SUV (15.3 vs 9.8 months, respectively; $p < 0.01$) [13].

Other Prognostic FDG-PET/CT Parameters

Volumetric parameters such as TLG and MTV have also been studied and shown to correlate with clinical outcomes among patients with pancreatic cancer [23]. MTV is the total volume of tumor with FDG uptake (usually over a set threshold), and TLG is derived by multiplying the MTV by the mean SUV. In contrast to maximal SUV which only measures FDG uptake in the region of the tumor with the highest level of metabolic activity, MTV and TLG provide a three-dimensional measure of total tumor burden and account for the metabolic heterogeneity among the different cell types comprising the tumor. High MTV and TLG values have been associated with worse survival outcomes among patients with pancreatic cancer. In an analysis of 55 patients with locally advanced pancreatic cancer treated with SBRT, the median MTV was 57.5 for all patients. Of the 55 patients, the median OS of patients with low MTV (<57.5) was 18.0 months as compared to 10.1 months among patients with high MTV (≥57.5; $p < 0.01$).

Table 15.1 Studies evaluating the impact of FDG-PET/CT on the survival of patients with pancreatic cancer

Author	Year	Number of patients	Cancer stage	Timing of image acquisition	SUV cutoffs	Median OS	*p*-value
Pimiento et al. [8]	2016	105	I and II	Pretreatment	<5.0 vs >5.0	28 vs 16 months	0.036
Yamamoto et al. [14]	2015	128	Resectable	Pretreatment	<6.0 vs ≥ 6.0	37 vs 18 months	<0.001
Wang et al. [22]	2015	69	Locally advanced	Pretreatment	≤ 5.5 vs >5.5	16.6 vs 12.6 months	0.025
Lee et al. [38]	2014	87	Resectable and borderline resectable	Pretreatment	≤ 4.7 vs >4.7	34.4 vs 20.6 months	0.03
Hwang et al. [39]	2012	165	I to IV	Pretreatment	≤ 4.1 vs >4.1	610 vs 229 days	<0.0001
Schellenberg et al. [13]	2010	55	Locally advanced	Following 1 cycle of chemotherapy, prior to SBRT	<6.2 vs ≥ 6.2	15.3 vs 9.8 months	<0.01
Sperti et al. [40]	2003	60	I, III, and IV	Pretreatment	≤ 4.0 vs >4.0	265 vs 178 days	0.005

Similarly, in a retrospective review of 122 patients with resected pancreatic cancer who underwent FDG-PET/CT imaging prior to surgery, patients were classified as low or high using the MTV and TLG median values of 15.7 and 57.7, respectively, as cutoffs. Of the 122 patients, the median OS of patients with high MTV and high TLG was 9.7 months as compared to 24.2 months among patients with low MTV and low TLG ($p < 0.001$). In the multivariable hazards analysis, the investigators observed that high MTV (HR: 2.72; $p < 0.001$), high TLG (HR: 2.79; $p < 0.001$), and elevated CA19–9 at diagnosis (HR: 2.65; $p = 0.006$) were independent factors associated with an increased risk of death. These data suggest the metabolic activity of pancreatic cancers on FDG-PET/CT at diagnosis is an important prognostic marker. When used in combination with CA19–9 level, which has been correlated with stage of disease, rates of resection, and survival outcomes, clinicians may be able to provide patients with highly accurate predictions of disease outcomes [24, 25].

FDG-PET/CT as a Predictor of Response to Therapy

Unfortunately, the vast majority of patients with resected pancreatic cancer will succumb to systemic disease recurrence. Among those who undergo up-front surgery followed by adjuvant therapy, the median time to first disease recurrence is approximately 13 months from the time of surgical resection [26, 27]. The timing and patterns of disease recurrence following neoadjuvant therapy and surgery are less clear; this is currently being investigated. Several predictors of disease recurrence have been identified, including positive resection margins, regional lymph node metastases, and perineural invasion – all determined upon pathologic review of surgically resected specimens [28]. At present, there are limited preoperative prognostic markers to stratify patients, with the exception of serum CA19–9 level. As such, identifying patients who are high risk for early treatment failures remains a major challenge in the management of patients with pancreatic cancer. Recent studies evaluating tumor FDG avidity on pretreatment FDG-PET/CT as a predictor of disease recurrence have demonstrated promising results. In a recent review of 46 patients with resected pancreatic cancer, patients with SUV < 6.0 ($n = 19$, 41%) experienced a median disease-free survival (DFS) of 25 months as compared to 13 months among patients with SUV ≥ 6.0 ($n = 27$, 59%; $p = 0.003$). In a multivariable hazards analysis, SUV ≥ 6.0 was associated with a 2.28-fold increased risk of disease recurrence (HR: 2.28; $p = 0.024$) [29].

FDG-PET/CT has been particularly successful at predicting early disease recurrences after surgery. For example, in a report including 128 patients with resected pancreatic cancer, the investigators observed an increased incidence of early (<6 months) postoperative recurrences among patients with SUV ≥ 6.0 as compared to those with SUV < 6.0 (49% vs 5%; $p < 0.001$). Of the 128 patients, the 3- and 5-year DFS rates and median DFS were 39.1%, 36.5%, and 23 months, respectively, for patients with SUV < 6.0, as compared to 13.0%, 13.0%, and 6 months among patients with SUV ≥ 6.0 ($p < 0.001$) [14]. Similarly, in a review of 56 patients treated with a surgery-first approach, 22 (39%) patients experienced disease recurrences within 6 months from surgery. The median SUV on pretreatment FDG-PET/CT among the 22 (39%) patients with early (<6 months) postoperative recurrences was 7.9 as compared to 4.2 among the 34 (61%) patients who did not experience an early recurrence ($p = 0.004$) [12]. This data suggests that patients with pancreatic cancers which demonstrate high FDG uptake on FDG-PET/CT may be at a higher risk for early disease recurrence due to aggressive tumor biology. This taken in the context of a significantly elevated CA19–9 should warrant careful consideration of the oncologic benefit of invasive therapies such as surgery (Figs. 15.1 and 15.3).

Among patients with unresected disease, pretreatment FDG-PET/CT SUV has been shown to be predictive of time to disease progression. In an analysis of 106 patients with unresected, stage II–IV pancreatic cancer who underwent initial

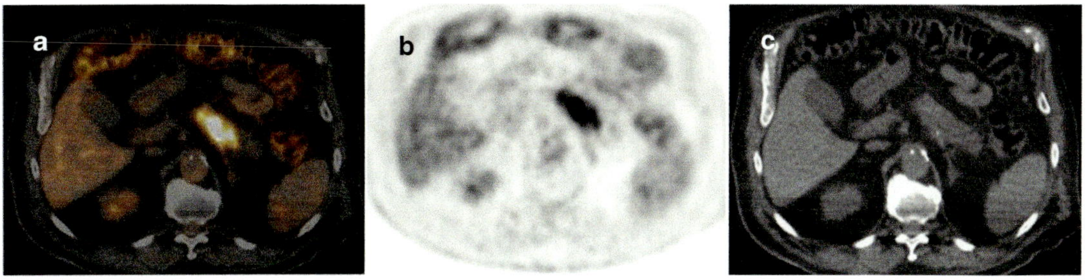

Fig. 15.3 FDG-PET/CT imaging of a 76-year-old male with a pancreatic body mass and serum CA19–9 level of 647 U/mL. Axial fused FDG-PET/CT imaging (**a**) demonstrating intense FDG uptake throughout the pancreatic body mass with a maximal SUV = 11.9. Axial FDG-PET (**b**) and noncontrast CT (**c**) are shown for comparison. Endoscopic ultrasound-guided fine needle aspiration confirmed pancreatic cancer. The mass was staged as resectable. The patient received neoadjuvant therapy prior to surgical resection and adjuvant therapy. The patient developed recurrent disease 8 months from surgery and succumbed to disease 17 months from initial pancreatic cancer diagnosis

staging with FDG-PET/CT, prior to the start of therapy, maximal SUV was shown to correlate with progression-free survival (PFS). Using a SUV cutoff of 4.93, the investigators observed that patients with SUV < 4.93 progressed at median of 385 days as compared to 204 days among patients with SUV > 4.93 [10]. Table 15.2 summarizes studies which have demonstrated a correlation between tumor SUV on FDG-PET/CT and disease progression in patients with pancreatic cancer.

Limitations of FDG-PET/CT

Though published data would suggest a pancreatic mass with a SUV greater than 2.0 to 4.0 on FDG-PET/CT is consistent with pancreatic cancer, differentiating benign inflammatory lesions from pancreatic cancers can be challenging [30, 31]. Similar to pancreatic cancer, inflammatory diseases of the pancreas such as acute/chronic pancreatitis may result in high levels of FDG uptake. A review of 47 patients with pancreatic lesions demonstrated that there is considerable overlap between the SUV ranges of patients with mass-forming pancreatitis (n = 14, 30%) and those with pancreatic cancer (n = 33, 70%). However, at both 1 hour and 2 hours post FDG injection, the SUVs of pancreatic cancers were generally higher than the SUVs of mass-forming pancreatitis (p = 0.001 and p = 0.012, respectively) [32]. In addition, the sensitivity of FDG-PET/CT at diagnosing pancreatic cancer has been shown to be significantly decreased among patients with elevated serum glucose levels, resulting in false negative studies [33]. As such, adequate glycemic control at the time of image acquisition is essential to accurately diagnose pancreatic cancers.

Future Directions

In recent years, integrated FDG-PET/MRI has emerged as an imaging modality for pancreatic cancer. FDG-PET/MRI may offer several potential advantages over FDG-PET/CT, as MRI produces superior imaging of soft tissue pathologies. In addition, the simultaneous acquisition of the FDG-PET and MRI results in optimal fusion of images and minimizes misregistration artifact associated with the sequential acquisition of FDG-PET and CT [34, 35]. Furthermore, FDG-PET/MRI is associated with an approximately 40% to 60% reduction in radiation exposure, which is particularly important among cancer patients who undergo frequent imaging for staging and/or surveillance purposes [34].

FDG-PET/MRI has been shown to be superior to FDG-PET/CT at differentiating pancreatic cancers from benign pancreatic lesions. In a review of 47 patients with pancreatic lesions, the diagnostic accuracy of FDG-PET/MRI at

Table 15.2 Studies evaluating the impact of FDG-PET/CT on disease progression in patients with pancreatic cancer

Author	Year	Number of patients	Cancer stage	Timing of image acquisition	SUV cutoffs	Time to progression	*p*-value
Pergolini et al. [29]	2017	46	Resectable	Pretreatment	<6.0 vs ≥ 6.0	25 vs 13 months	0.003
Pimeinto et al. [8]	2016	105	I and II	Pretreatment	<5.0 vs >5.0	14 vs 12 months	0.049
Chirindel et al. [10]	2015	106	II, III, and IV	Pretreatment	<4.93 vs >4.93	385 vs 204 days	0.01
Yamamoto et al. [14]	2015	128	Resectable	Pretreatment	<6.0 vs ≥ 6.0	23 vs 6 months	<0.001
Wang et al. [22]	2015	69	Locally advanced	Pretreatment	≤ 5.5 vs >5.5	9.6 vs 6.6 months	0.003
Lee et al. [38]	2014	87	Resectable and borderline resectable	Pretreatment	≤ 4.7 vs >4.7	12.9 vs 9.9 months	0.03
Schellenberg et al. [13]	2010	55	Locally advanced	Following one cycle of chemotherapy, prior to SBRT	<5.0 vs 5.0–10.0 vs >10.0	11.7 vs 8.0 vs 4.9 months	0.01

diagnosing pancreatic cancer was 93% and 90.7% for T1-weighted and T2-weighted fusion images, respectively, as compared to 88.4% for FDG-PET/CT [36]. Consistent with these findings, an analysis including 119 patients with pancreatic lesions reported a sensitivity, specificity, and accuracy of 99%, 82.6%, and 96.6%, respectively, at diagnosing pancreatic cancer with FDG-PET/MRI, as compared to 96.9%, 43.5%, and 86.6%, respectively, with FDG-PET/CT [37]. Despite preliminary data demonstrating improved diagnostic capabilities, FDG-PET/MRI has not been readily incorporated into clinical practice. This may be due to its limited availability, higher cost, and the specialized training required by technologists. Additionally, FDG-PET/MRI protocols for assessing pancreatic cancers have not been validated in the current literature.

Conclusion

The clinical utility of FDG-PET/CT in the management of patients with pancreatic cancer is evolving. Current data has demonstrated a strong correlation between tumor FDG avidity and clinical outcomes among patients with pancreatic cancer, suggesting the true value of FDG-PET/CT may be as prognostic tool, rather than diagnostic. Maximal SUV on FDG-PET/CT is an objective measure of tumor metabolic activity which may be a surrogate marker of tumor biology. Early insight into the biologic behavior of pancreatic cancers is extremely valuable information which may improve patient risk stratification and enable the delivery of more personalized and comprehensive treatment.

References

1. Pavlova NN, Thompson CB. The emerging hallmarks of cancer metabolism. Cell Metab. 2016;23(1):27–47.
2. Hanahan D, Weinberg RA. Hallmarks of cancer: the next generation. Cell. 2011;144(5):646–74.
3. Warburg O, Wind F, Negelein E. The metabolism of tumors in the body. J Gen Physiol. 1927;8(6):519–30.
4. Halbrook CJ, Lyssiotis CA. Employing metabolism to improve the diagnosis and treatment of pancreatic cancer. Cancer Cell. 2017;31(1):5–19.
5. Swisher SG, Erasmus J, Maish M, Correa AM, Macapinlac H, Ajani JA, Cox JD, Komaki RR, Hong D, Lee HK, Putnam JB Jr, Rice DC, Smythe WR, Thai L, Vaporciyan AA, Walsh GL, Wu TT, Roth JA. 2-Fluoro-2-deoxy-D-glucose positron emission tomography imaging is predictive of pathologic response and survival after preoperative chemoradiation in patients with esophageal carcinoma. Cancer. 2004;101(8):1776–85.
6. Kim JW, Oh JS, Roh JL, Kim JS, Choi SH, Nam SY, Kim SY. Prognostic significance of standardized uptake value and metabolic tumour volume on (1)(8)F-FDG PET/CT in oropharyngeal squamous cell carcinoma. Eur J Nucl Med Mol Imaging. 2015;42(9):1353–61.
7. Kim YH, Lee JA, Baek JM, Sung GY, Lee DS, Won JM. The clinical significance of standardized uptake value in breast cancer measured using 18F-fluorodeoxyglucose positron emission tomography/computed tomography. Nucl Med Commun. 2015;36(8):790–4.
8. Pimiento JM, Davis-Yadley AH, Kim RD, Chen DT, Eikman EA, Berman CG, Malafa MP. Metabolic activity by 18F-FDG-PET/CT is prognostic for stage I and II pancreatic cancer. Clin Nucl Med. 2016;41(3):177–81.
9. Ahn SJ, Park MS, Lee JD, Kang WJ. Correlation between 18F-fluorodeoxyglucose positron emission tomography and pathologic differentiation in pancreatic cancer. Ann Nucl Med. 2014;28(5):430–5.
10. Chirindel A, Alluri KC, Chaudhry MA, Wahl RL, Pawlik TM, Herman JM, Subramaniam RM. Prognostic value of FDG PET/CT-derived parameters in pancreatic adenocarcinoma at initial PET/CT staging. AJR Am J Roentgenol. 2015;204(5):1093–9.
11. Hu SL, Yang ZY, Zhou ZR, Yu XJ, Ping B, Zhang YJ. Role of SUV(max) obtained by 18F-FDG PET/CT in patients with a solitary pancreatic lesion: predicting malignant potential and proliferation. Nucl Med Commun. 2013;34(6):533–9.
12. Okamoto K, Koyama I, Miyazawa M, Toshimitsu Y, Aikawa M, Okada K, Imabayashi E, Matsuda H. Preoperative 18[F]-fluorodeoxyglucose positron emission tomography/computed tomography predicts early recurrence after pancreatic cancer resection. Int J Clin Oncol. 2011;16(1):39–44.
13. Schellenberg D, Quon A, Minn AY, Graves EE, Kunz P, Ford JM, Fisher GA, Goodman KA, Koong AC, Chang DT. 18Fluorodeoxyglucose PET is prognostic of progression-free and overall survival in locally advanced pancreas cancer treated with stereotactic radiotherapy. Int J Radiat Oncol Biol Phys. 2010;77(5):1420–5.
14. Yamamoto T, Sugiura T, Mizuno T, Okamura Y, Aramaki T, Endo M, Uesaka K. Preoperative FDG-PET predicts early recurrence and a poor prognosis after resection of pancreatic adenocarcinoma. Ann Surg Oncol. 2015;22(2):677–84.
15. Farma JM, Santillan AA, Melis M, Walters J, Belinc D, Chen DT, Eikman EA, Malafa M. PET/CT fusion

scan enhances CT staging in patients with pancreatic neoplasms. Ann Surg Oncol. 2008;15(9):2465–71.
16. Topkan E, Parlak C, Yapar AF. FDG-PET/CT-based restaging may alter initial management decisions and clinical outcomes in patients with locally advanced pancreatic carcinoma planned to undergo chemoradiotherapy. Cancer Imaging. 2013;13(3):423–8.
17. Network NCC. Pancreatic Adenocarcinoma 2017. Available from: http://www.nccn.org/professionals/physician_gls/pdf/pancreatic.pdf.
18. Ghaneh P, Hanson R, Titman A, Lancaster G, Plumpton C, Lloyd-Williams H, Yeo ST, Edwards RT, Johnson C, Abu Hilal M, Higginson AP, Armstrong T, Smith A, Scarsbrook A, McKay C, Carter R, Sutcliffe RP, Bramhall S, Kocher HM, Cunningham D, Pereira SP, Davidson B, Chang D, Khan S, Zealley I, Sarker D, Al Sarireh B, Charnley R, Lobo D, Nicolson M, Halloran C, Raraty M, Sutton R, Vinjamuri S, Evans J, Campbell F, Deeks J, Sanghera B, Wong WL, Neoptolemos JP. PET-PANC: multicentre prospective diagnostic accuracy and health economic analysis study of the impact of combined modality 18fluorine-2-fluoro-2-deoxy-d-glucose positron emission tomography with computed tomography scanning in the diagnosis and management of pancreatic cancer. Health Technol Assess. 2018;22(7):1–114.
19. Bipat S, Phoa SS, van Delden OM, Bossuyt PM, Gouma DJ, Lameris JS, Stoker J. Ultrasonography, computed tomography and magnetic resonance imaging for diagnosis and determining resectability of pancreatic adenocarcinoma: a meta-analysis. J Comput Assist Tomogr. 2005;29(4):438–45.
20. Rijkers AP, Valkema R, Duivenvoorden HJ, van Eijck CH. Usefulness of F-18-fluorodeoxyglucose positron emission tomography to confirm suspected pancreatic cancer: a meta-analysis. Eur J Surg Oncol. 2014;40(7):794–804.
21. Lin E, Alavi A. Pancreatic Cancer. PET and PET/CT: A Clinical Guide. 2nd ed. New York: Thieme; 2005. p. 190–5.
22. Wang SL, Cao S, Sun YN, Wu R, Chi F, Tang MY, Jin XY, Chen XD. Standardized uptake value on positron emission tomography/computed tomography predicts prognosis in patients with locally advanced pancreatic cancer. Abdom Imaging. 2015;40(8):3117–21.
23. Xu HX, Chen T, Wang WQ, Wu CT, Liu C, Long J, Xu J, Zhang YJ, Chen RH, Liu L, Yu XJ. Metabolic tumour burden assessed by (1)(8)F-FDG PET/CT associated with serum CA19-9 predicts pancreatic cancer outcome after resection. Eur J Nucl Med Mol Imaging. 2014;41(6):1093–102.
24. Aldakkak M, Christians KK, Krepline AN, George B, Ritch PS, Erickson BA, Johnston FM, Evans DB, Tsai S. Pre-treatment carbohydrate antigen 19-9 does not predict the response to neoadjuvant therapy in patients with localized pancreatic cancer. HPB (Oxford). 2015;17(10):942–52.
25. Katz MH, Varadhachary GR, Fleming JB, Wolff RA, Lee JE, Pisters PW, Vauthey JN, Abdalla EK, Sun CC, Wang H, Crane CH, Lee JH, Tamm EP, Abbruzzese JL, Evans DB. Serum CA 19-9 as a marker of resectability and survival in patients with potentially resectable pancreatic cancer treated with neoadjuvant chemoradiation. Ann Surg Oncol. 2010;17(7):1794–801.
26. Oettle H, Neuhaus P, Hochhaus A, Hartmann JT, Gellert K, Ridwelski K, Niedergethmann M, Zulke C, Fahlke J, Arning MB, Sinn M, Hinke A, Riess H. Adjuvant chemotherapy with gemcitabine and long-term outcomes among patients with resected pancreatic cancer: the CONKO-001 randomized trial. JAMA. 2013;310(14):1473–81.
27. Neoptolemos JP, Palmer DH, Ghaneh P, Psarelli EE, Valle JW, Halloran CM, Faluyi O, O'Reilly DA, Cunningham D, Wadsley J, Darby S, Meyer T, Gillmore R, Anthoney A, Lind P, Glimelius B, Falk S, Izbicki JR, Middleton GW, Cummins S, Ross PJ, Wasan H, McDonald A, Crosby T, Ma YT, Patel K, Sherriff D, Soomal R, Borg D, Sothi S, Hammel P, Hackert T, Jackson R, Buchler MW, European Study Group for Pancreatic C. Comparison of adjuvant gemcitabine and capecitabine with gemcitabine monotherapy in patients with resected pancreatic cancer (ESPAC-4): a multicentre, open-label, randomised, phase 3 trial. Lancet. 2017;389(10073):1011–24.
28. Groot VP, Rezaee N, Wu W, Cameron JL, Fishman EK, Hruban RH, Weiss MJ, Zheng L, Wolfgang CL, He J. Patterns, timing, and predictors of recurrence following pancreatectomy for Pancreatic ductal adenocarcinoma. Ann Surg. 2018;267(5):936.
29. Pergolini I, Crippa S, Salgarello M, Belfiori G, Partelli S, Ruffo G, Pucci A, Zamboni G, Falconi M. SUVmax after (18)fluoro-deoxyglucose positron emission tomography/computed tomography: a tool to define treatment strategies in pancreatic cancer. Dig Liver Dis. 2018;50(1):84–90.
30. Imdahl A, Nitzsche E, Krautmann F, Hogerle S, Boos S, Einert A, Sontheimer J, Farthmann EH. Evaluation of positron emission tomography with 2-[18F] fluoro-2-deoxy-D-glucose for the differentiation of chronic pancreatitis and pancreatic cancer. Br J Surg. 1999;86(2):194–9.
31. Delbeke D, Rose DM, Chapman WC, Pinson CW, Wright JK, Beauchamp RD, Shyr Y, Leach SD. Optimal interpretation of FDG PET in the diagnosis, staging and management of pancreatic carcinoma. J Nucl Med. 1999;40(11):1784–91.
32. Kato K, Nihashi T, Ikeda M, Abe S, Iwano S, Itoh S, Shimamoto K, Naganawa S. Limited efficacy of (18)F-FDG PET/CT for differentiation between metastasis-free pancreatic cancer and mass-forming pancreatitis. Clin Nucl Med. 2013;38(6):417–21.
33. Diederichs CG, Staib L, Glatting G, Beger HG, Reske SN. FDG PET: elevated plasma glucose reduces both uptake and detection rate of pancreatic malignancies. J Nucl Med. 1998;39(6):1030–3.
34. Matthews R, Choi M. Clinical utility of positron emission tomography magnetic resonance imaging

(PET-MRI) in gastrointestinal cancers. Diagnostics (Basel). 2016;6(3).
35. Yeh R, Dercle L, Garg I, Wang ZJ, Hough DM, Goenka AH. The role of 18F-FDG PET/CT and PET/MRI in pancreatic ductal adenocarcinoma. Abdom Radiol (NY). 2017.
36. Tatsumi M, Isohashi K, Onishi H, Hori M, Kim T, Higuchi I, Inoue A, Shimosegawa E, Takeda Y, Hatazawa J. 18F-FDG PET/MRI fusion in characterizing pancreatic tumors: comparison to PET/CT. Int J Clin Oncol. 2011;16(4):408–15.
37. Nagamachi S, Nishii R, Wakamatsu H, Mizutani Y, Kiyohara S, Fujita S, Futami S, Sakae T, Furukoji E, Tamura S, Arita H, Chijiiwa K, Kawai K. The usefulness of (18)F-FDG PET/MRI fusion image in diagnosing pancreatic tumor: comparison with (18)F-FDG PET/CT. Ann Nucl Med. 2013;27(6):554–63.
38. Lee JW, Kang CM, Choi HJ, Lee WJ, Song SY, Lee JH, Lee JD. Prognostic value of metabolic tumor volume and total lesion glycolysis on preoperative (1)(8)F-FDG PET/CT in patients with pancreatic cancer. J Nucl Med. 2014;55(6):898–904.
39. Hwang JP, Lim I, Chang KJ, Kim BI, Choi CW, Lim SM. Prognostic value of SUVmax measured by Fluorine-18 Fluorodeoxyglucose positron emission tomography with computed tomography in patients with pancreatic cancer. Nucl Med Mol Imaging. 2012;46(3):207–14.
40. Sperti C, Pasquali C, Chierichetti F, Ferronato A, Decet G, Pedrazzoli S. 18-Fluorodeoxyglucose positron emission tomography in predicting survival of patients with pancreatic carcinoma. J Gastrointest Surg. 2003;7(8):953–9; discussion 959-960.

The New Bench for the Academic Surgeon: Precision Medicine

16

Gwen Lomberk and Raul Urrutia

Introduction

During the last three decades, significant advances have been made in the field of pancreatic cancer. Notable among them is the realization of the contribution of genomics and epigenomics [1] to the progression of the disease; the discovery of new treatment regimens based on the combination of neoadjuvant therapy, surgery, and radiation [2]; the creation of a large number of animal models [3]; new radiographic modalities for diagnosis and treatment [4]; as well as the testing of a large number of targeted therapies [5]. Thus, although this falls short of the ultimate goal for every pancreatic cancer investigator to defeat this dismal disease, the field has progressed in the right direction with small yet steady improvements. Most of these changes have taken place because of the unprecedented partnership among patients, patient advocates, scientists, and philanthropists, who together have increased both the awareness and the funding for studies on this disease. This stimulus to the field has prepared many investigators, both conceptually and methodologically, to begin capturing and applying new developments from other areas of science to the study of pancreatic cancer, as well as create solutions that are specific for this disease. Many of these solutions are establishing part of the arsenal that has become the new revolution in medical practice and clinical research, namely, precision medicine. This specialty found its developmental roots in the race for sequencing the human genome. In fact, the engineering tools used to crack this code, specifically next-generation sequencing together with bioinformatics and data analytics, function as the current engine of precision medicine. According to the definition provided at the launch of the National Precision Medicine Initiative in 2015, this discipline represents "an emerging approach for disease treatment and prevention that takes into account individual variability in genes, environment, and lifestyle for each person [6]." Thus, precision medicine centers have been formed within most of the top US academic institutions. In addition, several national reference laboratories for precision medicine offer tools, services, and assays, primarily for the management of cancer. In fact, the critical value of "clinical utility" for precision medicine has been proven to exist due to the cancer field. Precision medicine offers, for the first time, the ability to interrogate patients,

G. Lomberk
Division of Research, Departments of Surgery and Pharmacology and Toxicology, The Medical College of Wisconsin, Milwaukee, WI, USA

R. Urrutia (✉)
Departments of Surgery and Biochemistry, The Medical College of Wisconsin, Milwaukee, WI, USA
e-mail: rurrutia@mcw.edu

S. Tsai et al. (eds.), *Management of Localized Pancreatic Cancer*,
https://doi.org/10.1007/978-3-319-98944-0_16

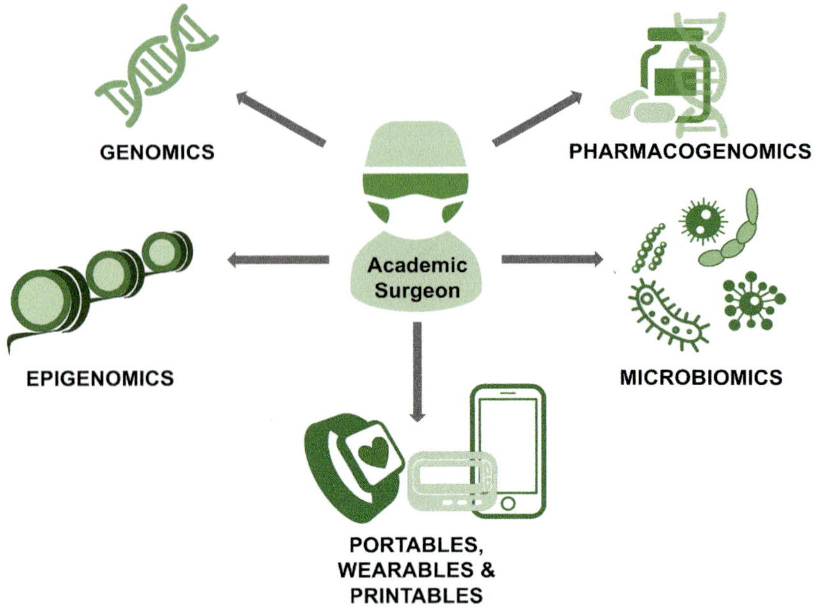

Fig. 16.1 Precision medicine as the new bench for the academic surgeon. The academic surgeon holds the possibility to play a key role in precision medicine through combining the methodologies of genomics, epigenomics, pharmacogenomics, and microbiome, as well as the acquisition of clinical data with printables, wearables, and portables

at the level of their germline as well as their cancer tissue, with the highest precision tools available to science. Although cell and animal models continue to be utilized for research, precision medicine is imparting us with the tools to study humans directly, with the immense advantages that this giant step forward signifies. Thus, this chapter will review the new branches of science that assemble the arsenal of tools for precision medicine, how they can address individual variations in genes, environment, and lifestyle for each of our patients, and the emergence of precision medicine as a "new bench" for academic surgeons (Fig. 16.1).

At the Beginning of the Journey Toward Precision Medicine, We Found the Genes

The significant efforts devoted to the Human Genome Project were based on the rationale of the time that if DNA held the code of life, determining the DNA sequence of an entire human would reveal a "Rosetta stone" to unlock the state of health and disease, as well as to change the "sick" phenotype into a more normal one. However, according to the expectations of many, the Human Genome Project did not find a single genome but rather the confirmation that humans vary quite frequently in DNA sequences. Humans have differences in common, as well as rare genomic variants in coding and noncoding regions, along with additional structural differences in genes, copy number variation, and repetitive sequences. In fact, it was soon realized that some of these differences prevent or protect from diseases, while others predispose to them. Moreover, human genomes are diverse not only in their germline DNA, but somatic DNA changes are present that confer differences in normal and diseased organs as well. In fact, the field of pancreatic cancer benefited from advances in the utilization of genomics in both germline and somatic DNA. At the level of somatic DNA, many of the initial discoveries are indebted to the Johns Hopkins group of Hruban et al., who together outlined the cancer progression model for pancreatic cancer [7]. This group and others were also key in detecting that specific germline alterations give rise to familial pancreatic cancer [8]. Interestingly, these pioneering discoveries were made before the latest advances in massive parallel sequencing or next-generation sequencing began, which determines the entire genome of an individual at a lower cost than many clinical diagnostic procedures. Moving forward several years from now, sophisticated methods of analyses have been implemented to allow one to reach conclusions of significant medical value. For instance, using exon panels or genome-wide methodologies, such as whole exome sequencing or whole genome sequencing from blood or peripheral blood mononuclear cells, the complete genomic makeup of an individual's germline DNA can be obtained, offering new possibilities. For instance, in the case of familial pancreatic cancer, the conclusion that someone was a carrier of a familial form of the disease used to be based solely on family history, showing the generations of affected individuals. However, though useful at the beginning, this approach did not clearly reflect the reality of the disease. Today, it is known that approximately 4% of patients diagnosed with apparent sporadic pancreatic cancer carry germline genomic variants in cancer driver genes in addition to the 5–10% occurrence with a family history of the disease [9]. Importantly, some of these variants may help to predict whether some of these patients will be more sensitive to a particular type of therapy (e.g., *BRCA* genes being more sensitive to radiation and platinum-based compounds [10]). As a result, the ability to obtain this refined knowledge is opening the question as whether genomic testing should be offered to individuals upon diagnosis, since the results can potentially inform disease management as well as aid the genetic counseling of these patients and their families.

It is noteworthy that the current implementation of precision medicine is not a significant undertaking. Whole exome sequencing (WES) is a methodology that uses probes to capture the protein-coding regions of the genome (exons) and sequence them [11]. Subsequently, the genes may contain alterations, now referred to with the terminology of genomic variants, as a known pathogenic one (e.g., KrasG12D), a variant of unknown significance (VUS), or a gene of unknown significance (GUS) [12]. VUS are those variants in which the amino acid substitution falls within a gene, for which significant information exists in relationship to the phenotype but has never been proven to be pathogenic. For instance, a mutation in Kras that involves a residue adjacent to a known pathogenic one, without existing proof to support the same conclusion for this new variant, would be classified as a VUS. In essence, GUS is similar, although it relates to variants in genes that have not been previously found to be associated with disease causation. Similar criteria are applied for both germline and somatic testing [13]. Whole genome sequencing (WGS) can provide the same data as WES along with an extensive amount of more information, as it reveals the remaining 99% of the genome that is not exposed with WES. In addition, the technique behind WGS is better than WES, since it does not implement a capture step, which sometimes creates artifacts or dissimilar representation of variants [11]. Another aspect for which WGS is superior to WES is its information on copy number and structural aberrations, while WES is suboptimal. With the release of the Illumina sequencers, the HiSeq X and NovaSeq 6000, the price of WGS has recently decreased significantly and promises to become even more affordable in the near future [14]. In addition to these approaches, narrower focused gene panels and arrays have acquired more rapid application to the clinic because these methods can select disease-specific pathways, are easy to process at a bioinformatics level, and, therefore, are valued at much lower cost [15]. Currently, there are institutional precision medicine centers and national reference laboratories that can provide all these services. Thus, the question is what type of information can be obtained with these methodologies. While there is a general agreement that gene panels represent a fast, reimbursable, and informative way to interrogate the potentially pathogenic genomic profile of patients and tumors, ultimately the best possible result for any of these genomic techniques is what is referred to as an "actionable variant." An "actionable variant" would offer insight that can be harnessed for immediate benefit with currently available medical options. For instance, tumors with mutations in DNA repair pathways are likely to be more sensitive to chemoradiation [16], thereby influencing the neoadjuvant and adjuvant therapies that potentially would be more effective for the patient carrying such a mutation. Similarly, a tumor with a mutation in a particular gene, for which drugs are being tested in clinical trials, can designate a patient to be eligible to participate, thereby providing additional benefits, including intangibles such as hope, which increase quality of life.

Novel molecular assays are rapidly entering the clinical domain of research-based monitoring in oncology, as well as other screening and diagnostics purposes, for which the aforementioned genomic techniques are at the core. A new form of effective and promising diagnosis is the liquid biopsy, in which investigators perform assays on cell-free circulating DNA in blood, or genetic material released by tumor cells, to detect mutations that would identify the presence of malignancy [17]. Another methodology, though more cumbersome, is to isolate circulating tumor cells from blood to subsequently obtain a genomic profile. In fact, the use of circulating DNA as a noninvasive biomarker in the clinical diagnosis and prognosis of pancreatic cancer is gaining significant momentum. Initial work focused on measuring the presence of Kras mutation in cell-free DNA. While this approach has provided a great proof of principle in support of the methodology and procedures, its limited sensitivity has not permitted advancement in patient management [18]. A more promising discovery was recently pioneered by Cohen and colleagues, in which a combined assessment of serum markers with circulating free DNA led to the development of the CancerSEEK assay that can diagnose eight cancer types, including pancreatic cancer with a median sensitivity of 70% and specificity >99% [19]. Another useful application of technology for cell-free DNA evaluation originated from studies out of the Mayo Clinic [20], which culminated in the development of Cologuard®, which is an FDA-approved, multi-target stool DNA test based on detecting an altered gene signature shed from cancer cells into the stool. Notably, although this assay is commercialized for colon cancer screening, the test reveals altered DNA released from any cancerous cell located within the aerodigestive and gastrointestinal tract from the mouth to the anus, and therefore follow-up studies are evaluating whether pancreatic, esophageal, stomach, lung, and hepatobiliary cancers are also revealed by the assay [21]. Further areas of prominent development are involved in the search for indicators that facilitate patient management based on prognosis, by monitoring disease-free survival through novel circulating markers, such as DNA, RNA, and protein, which are present in exosomes [22, 23]. Thus, genomics has completely changed the field of pancreatic cancer in terms of the future diagnosis, prognosis, and treatment of this disease. Furthermore, this discipline has paved the way for the establishment of other core elements of precision medicine, including pharmacogenomics, epigenomics, and microbiomics.

Pharmacogenomics: Own Your Drug Response

Just as humans have significant variation in the whole genome, it follows that pathways that are utilized in metabolism also differ. In fact, metabolisms for many molecules, including food products such as sugars, are significantly affected by genomic variants, which can range from the subtle to the complex metabolic disease state, resulting in genetically influenced metabotypes [24]. Not surprisingly, therefore, variations in genes that encode for enzymes participating in drug metabolism can have a significant impact on the way humans react to drugs. From anesthesia used to operate, opiates for controlling pain, anticlotting agents, chemotherapy, and radiation, patient sensitivity is influenced by enzymes, which by nature are encoded by genes that vary their potential response to treatments. This concept forms the basis of pharmacogenomics. Genomic variation can impact drug functionality at the level of either pharmacokinetics, including the absorption, distribution, metabolism, and/or elimination of a drug, or pharmacodynamics, such that the drug target or associated biological pathways are modified to alter drug effects [25]. Thus, by studying and taking into consideration these variations, pharmacogenomics has the ability to influence all aspects of patient management. Based on this knowledge, many centers around the world have incorporated pharmacogenomics testing into clinical care [25]. Thus, although in the early stages, pharmacogenomics promises to be an essential component of the future practice of pancreatic cancer surgery and treatment [26].

The fact that the arsenal of potentially beneficial therapeutic drugs is growing at a rapid speed presents evolving pharmacogenomics considerations. Besides new chemotherapeutic combinations, most efforts of pharmaceutical and academic institutions are directed to develop targeted therapies. In fact, success in this area has already been achieved with the development of epidermal growth factor receptor (EGFR) inhibitors which effectively target cancers, alone or in combination with other therapies [27]. In this regard, it is important to highlight that most of the drugs developed by pharma in the last decades were targeted to signaling enzymes and cell cycle inhibitors. However, this trend has recently changed to increase the development of epigenomic inhibitors, because they can reverse a pathogenetic inherited trait coming from the environment, and immunotherapeutics, which seek to harness the immune system to generate an antitumor response. However, little is known about the pharmacogenomics of these new drugs, which if approached properly, will provide more justification for pharmacogenomics testing. Furthermore, since genes are also regulated by epigenomic-based mechanisms, variations in the epigenomics of genes, such as drug-metabolizing enzymes, present an additional layer of complexity to develop a new field, pharmacoepigenomics [28]. Lastly, another metabolic pathway that can have gene variations is that involved in the response to radiation, which is considered as a variation of pharmacogenomics, better known as the field of radiogenomics. This field is populated by our historical radiotherapeutics partners focused on two complementary directions, namely, the study of genetic variation associated with response to radiation (radiation genomics) or reference to the correlation between cancer imaging features and gene expression (imaging genomics) [29]. Without a doubt, pharmacogenomics is anticipated to have a promising future with increasing benefits. For instance, all variations in drug-metabolizing enzymes can be filtered from WES and WGS, even from babies undergoing sequencing for other reasons, and those individuals will grow with the knowledge of their genome-based drug response profile for the rest of their lives. Thus, looking at the patient as a whole, and not solely as a "tumor carrier," pharmacogenomics can significantly impact numerous aspects of patient care from decisions for improving drug and radiation sensitivity as well as resistance to efforts for managing clotting or pain, as well as other symptoms.

Environment–Gene Interactions: The Role of Epigenomics

For many years, investigators, particularly in the area of genetic epidemiology, have been discussing the concept of gene–environment interactions. However, it required quite some time to truly define the term "environment" from a mechanistic point of view. In other words, the persistent question was how, molecularly, the environment changes gene programs, how it can be measured, and whether the deleterious environmental insults can be reverted. One of the major clues to this challenge came with the incorporation of concepts and methodologies from epigenomics. The term epigenetics was coined by Conrad Waddington in 1942 [30], which was more than 10 years before the publication of the structure of DNA responsible for the basis of genetic inheritance [31]. Today, epigenetics is understood as a form of inheritance that is independent of the coding capacity of DNA [1]. In other words, a gene can be either silenced or induced, and this pattern can be altered without being mutated. The broader term, epigenomics, refers to the collective epigenetic changes across many genes in a cell or entire organism. Therefore, it becomes essential to define what comprises the epigenome and how it can generate changes in the response of genes to the environment, without any alteration in the underlying base compositions of these genes. The epigenome is molecularly more complex than the genome, and its function is to regulate the former. The epigenome is formed by chromatin, which is composed of the DNA, small and large noncoding RNAs frequently associated to it, histones, as well as other regulatory proteins, which together transmit the messages from the environment to the nucleus where the result is a change in gene expression [1]. The key to understanding how the epigenome works in this context is to first get familiar with the concept of "marks." Marks are posttranslational modifications that are deposited onto DNA, RNA molecules, or associated proteins (e.g., histones) in response to an environmental stimulus. Certain marks instruct to either activate or silence the expression of genes located in this marked region of the nucleus by regulating the production of messenger RNA (mRNA). The marks are generated by a variety of molecular machinery specialized for this purpose. Protein complexes, referred to as writers, readers, and erasers, are responsible for depositing, reading and interpreting, and, when necessary, erasing the mark, respectively. For example, an inflammatory molecule present in the tumor microenvironment can bind to its corresponding receptor at the tumor cell surface, transmit the signal through the cytoplasm with a cascade of protein interactions and modifications, and eventually transmit to the nucleus where the activation or inactivation of writers, readers, and erasers occurs to modulate the expression of entire gene networks (e.g., a drug resistance pathway). To utilize one epigenomic pathway as an example for clarifying this concept, a stimulus can ultimately travel to the nucleus and activate DNA methyltransferases (writers), which will methylate DNA [32]. The methylated DNA will be interpreted as a command for gene silencing by methyl-binding proteins (readers), such as MeCP2. Once this signal either terminates or this change needs to be reversed, DNA is demethylated by Ten-eleven translocation (TET) enzyme (erasers). Thus, in this manner, instructions from the external environment are passed all the way to the nucleus of cells.

The second important consideration is the way that modifications of epigenome become inherited, similar to the inheritance of genomic variations, so that the resultant phenotype is indefinitely propagated from mother cells to their progeny. One of the most widely accepted mechanisms for inheritance of marks on the DNA and proteins comes from the discovery of the semiconservative replication of DNA [33]. Old models focus on the duplication of DNA as only representing the nucleic acid molecules. However, today it is known that proteins and RNAs are also at the replication fork. In addition, when the DNA is duplicated, the marks that were present in the region are also duplicated onto the nascent chromatin fiber. While the mechanisms are not fully elucidated, it is believed that the existing parental chromatin supplies half of the histones for the replicated DNA, and these clusters of parental chromatin may inform the propagation of histone marks to reestablish the epigenomic state [34]. In this manner, a cell with epigenomic changes will propagate these alterations, and if these epigenomic modifications lead to a more aggressive phenotype, then the progeny of this cell will also carry a more aggressive phenotype.

Fortunately, a large number of methodologies are now available to measure how the environment has changed the epigenome of a tumor or an individual. Similar to genomic methodologies, epigenomics can be studied in either a panel format or in genome-wide versions. For instance, various methodologies to measure DNA methylation exist, from methylated DNA immunoprecipitation (MeDIP), which is an immunoprecipitation-based methodology, to arrays which contain an extensive representation of the modifiable regions of DNA, as well as bisulfite modification of DNA to convert unmodified cytosines and protect methylated cytosines followed by next-generation sequencing, to define with high precision the genome-wide alterations in DNA methylation caused by an environmental stimulus [32]. Correspondingly, immunoprecipitation-based methodologies, known as chromatin immunoprecipitation or ChIP, combined with next-generation sequencing are employed specific to histone marks and chromatin machinery (writers, readers, and erasers) to map the genome-wide landscape of these epigenomic pathways [35]. The most advanced approaches involve the integration of many of these methodologies, which requires extensive resources in bioinformatics and data analytics [36].

Genomics and epigenomics research has led to the recent discovery that there is more than one subtype of pancreatic cancer with defined changes in histone and DNA marks that are congruent with gene silencing or activation [37–40]. These studies indicate that the basal subtype demonstrates more malignant behavior than the classical phenotype, opening an interesting avenue of investigation for clinical trials, which will seek to determine a priori the subtype of pancreatic cancer affecting the patient to potentially govern treatment management. Gene expression patterns in all of these studies were measured by RNA-seq, one of the most useful methodologies to survey the entire repertoire of RNAs, whether coding, noncoding, or foreign. This technique is also important when analyzing posttranscriptional RNA editing, a recently described phenomenon [41]. In this process, a particular RNA can be edited by specialized enzymes, thereby altering its sequence from the original one encoded by its mother gene. In this case, while a genomic mutation could be identified by WES or WGS, this mutation potentially may be fixed during posttranscriptional editing or vice versa. Without integrated information, the practitioner can have inaccurate information to manage the patient. Furthermore, RNA-seq plays a key role in the identification of novel markers in the form of small and large noncoding RNAs, as well as the profiling of tumor-produced exosomes for the same purpose. Therefore, the combination of methods for characterizing DNA methylation, histone marks, writers, readers, erasers, and a plethora of different RNA species is promoting significant advancement both mechanistically and translationally, at a speed that is by far faster than in previous decades.

The Environment as a Symbiosis: The Microbiome

Another important way that the environment can modify the state of a patient or the treatment of a tumor is through the microbiome. The microbiome is the collective group of microorganisms that normally colonize and live in equilibrium with humans. An extremely large number and even unknown types of microorganisms are present in all mucosa and in many organs [42]. In fact, today, less is known about the microbiome than is known about space or the sea. These organisms influence many physiological functions, a fact that was ignored until very recently, and in fact, the microbiome has been labeled as an extra human organ [43]. The microbiome plays a significant role in human health, and thus, not surprisingly, microbes can also promote disease, including cancer, when in a state of dysbiosis. While studies investigated the role of the pathogen *Helicobacter pylori* (*H. pylori*) in pancreatic cancer without conclusive evidence, some other investigations on dysbiosis of oral bacteria have found an association with higher risk for pancreatic cancer [44]. Thus, the microbiome may serve as a future source of biomarkers for pancreatic disease. Additionally, the microbiome can modify the quality of life and, potentially, even the treatment of pancreatic cancer, though studies in this area are currently underrepresented. Moreover, it seems inevitable that the microbiome will be different in a postoperative pancreatic cancer patient, yet how these changes contribute to the post-Whipple symptoms of patients and, thereby, their quality of life remains poorly understood. Recent reports have supported that the microbiome can also modulate the response to drugs, in particular some chemotherapeutic compounds [45]. Lastly, the effect of small lipid molecules produced by the microbiome to the whole organism is unknown. It would not be surprising that these substances influence paraneoplastic symptoms and, in this manner, alter quality of life. Thus, more studies of this type are necessary and represent a great opportunity for research in our field. In fact, we are optimistic that incorporating more microbiome studies to the field of pancreatic cancer research will soon generate exciting benefits for both science and medicine.

More Than Toys: Printables, Wearables, Portables, and the Importance of Data

More than genomics, the integrated data from numerous sources, including many from nongenomic origins, is potentially the most valuable and priceless output of any precision medicine efforts. Since its inception, the world of precision medicine was made possible by revolutionary developments in engineering, namely, advanced sequencing technologies and computational biology. In fact, from these efforts, an independent line of biomedical engineering research was launched that aims at designing novel precision medicine tools and services, as well as a whole collection of epidemiological research, which is based on obtaining better and more information (more precision) to help patient management. This new area of clinical research will generate the need for additional studies to measure the outcome of these precision medicine technologies, which are not necessarily genomic in nature. The invention of many non-genomic tools, such as portable and wearable biosensors, for precision medicine will require research collaborations with companies or academic departments of biomedical engineering. This extensive amount of information is now populating large warehouses in the most prestigious genomic centers, which is primed for data mining as an important nascent career in clinical research. Interestingly, society already depends on several types of implantable devices, such as insulin pumps, which are equipped with electronic monitoring. Gathering this data from consented patients, using apps that capture and transmit information from these pumps to a research center, may provide useful knowledge about how to improve this type of therapy and beyond [46]. In a similar manner, data can be gathered on any number of measurements via a wearable-/portable-based route for transmitting research information [47]. In addition, from the field of engineering and of direct interest to pancreatic surgeons are printables. For instance, several institutions around the world have implemented the use of 3D printing for reconstructing models of the individual cases of pancreatic cancer, based on imaging, before surgery, so that the intervention can be planned with better anatomical precision [48]. However, printables are not limited to surgical planning. Several institutions are investing in research on 3D bioprinting for a growing number of tissues and organs, such as blood vessels, liver, and cartilage, for grafting, as well as other manipulations that can help expand surgical options and improve outcomes. Through bioprinting, features can be engineered to recreate tissues and organs down to the minute shape, structure, and architecture in a precise, detailed, or even personalized manner, and therefore, this evolving technology is expected to offer one of the most efficient, convenient, and dependable ways to biofabricate tissue constructs [49]. Thus, technological devices will continue advancing capabilities for not only data collection and monitoring but also tissue engineering and beyond to provide real-time precision medicine.

Modeling Pancreatic Cancer in Cells and Animals: A Scientific Approach Reinforced by Precision Medicine

Precision medicine has brought a renaissance in clinical research by bringing advanced tools and concepts from basic science to interrogate humans rather than exclusively animal models. In many ways, the level and speed at which this change is occurring is unprecedented. Advancements in genomics, epigenomics, microbiome, pharmacogenomics, and the invention of new tools have directly expanded the capabilities of clinical research. In fact, for those institutions that have highly equipped precision medicine centers, there are no limitations for a practicing surgeon with academic aspirations to pursue research along this path, which functions in partnership with members of these centers, through collaborative arrangements or fee-for-services. Surgeons contribute to the development of new models, which represent a novel way to more directly interrogate human pancreatic tumors. Most conspicuous among these models are patient-derived xenografts, which can be done in several species, including the mouse [50] and chick embryo chorioallantoic membrane [51]. The concept of the xenograft was to create an avatar of a patient's tumor to determine tumor properties and test new methods. Today, xenografts are used prevalently in the field to discover new markers for diagnosis and prognosis, as well as novel therapeutic targets. In addition, these models have been utilized to evaluate therapy sensitivity. Another direct extension of the avatar concept has been the creation of patient-derived organoids, with the literal meaning "organ-like," which grow autonomously in vitro under conditions that allow cells to self-organize into structures recapitulating the complex three-dimensional organization of pancreatic cancer [52]. This self-renewing source of patient-derived cells allows investigators to implement genetic and chemical manipulations, serving a similar purpose as xenografts in a more rapid and potentially less expensive manner. Thus, models of pancreatic cancer have offered additional precision medicine tools at the hands of a surgeon, not only for helping his or her patients but also as a foundational approach to an academic research career. If the transformational manner and exquisite speed at which our ability to interrogate humans follows a similar trend as seen in recent years, these tools will prime the field to accelerate pancreatic cancer research and reach more robust conclusions.

The Concept of Team Science in Precision Medicine: A Place for the Pancreatic Surgeon and New Educational Opportunities

Among many paradigms that precision medicine has changed, the culture of the research team has shifted from the concept where a single Principal Investigator, in a pyramidal manner, directs a group of people, who generally had similar, or less, knowledge. More than ever, precision medicine has emphasized the advantages of team science implementation in biomedical research [53]. This approach leverages the diverse expertise of investigators from different fields to address complex health challenges through collaborative efforts. Together, a team composed of individuals with knowledge in many of the "omics" and data analytics along with engineers gives ample opportunities for a surgeon to better understand the patient condition, as well as to advance academic careers [54]. Surgeons have exquisite access to the patients, along with their tissue, which can be investigated by many of the methodologies for precision medicine (Fig. 16.1). Thus, it becomes critical to meditate on how they can better prepare to benefit from these possibilities. One solution is to integrate more concepts of precision medicine in residency research and fellowships, as well as create certificate and master programs in complementary areas to this field. Without a doubt, however, since the participation in precision medicine research does not need to be bench-intensive, the most useful background will be in bioinformatics and data analytics to speak the common language of the field.

Concluding Remarks

Whether from the bench to the bedside or from the bedside to the bench, translational research promises to advance the field of pancreatic cancer. However, the emergence of precision medicine has further evolved many research paradigms. Importantly, this research requires, in large part, team sciences. As a result of this approach, surgeons have a privileged position within the team with the firsthand opportunity to obtain tumors and develop human-to-mouse avatar models or organoids. By participating in and collaborating with scientists from precision medicine centers, their door opens the possibilities to do research in genomics, epigenomics, pharmacogenomics, radiomics, microbiome, and bioinformatics. An immersion into research based on precision medicine does not even require the principal investigator to have a bench. Thus, we believe that this translational research path represents a unique opportunity for pancreatic cancer researchers, in particular, the academic surgeon, to embrace an emerging concept of a new bench in scientific research, the bench embodied by precision medicine.

References

1. Lomberk GA, Urrutia R. The triple code model for pancreatic cancer: crosstalk among genetics, epigenetics, and nuclear structure. Surg Clin North

Am. 2015;95(5):935–52. https://doi.org/10.1016/j.suc.2015.05.011.
2. Tsai S, Erickson BA, Dua K, Ritch PS, Tolat P, Evans DB. Evolution of the management of resectable pancreatic cancer. J Oncol Pract. 2016;12(9):772–8. https://doi.org/10.1200/JOP.2016.015818.
3. Guerra C, Barbacid M. Genetically engineered mouse models of pancreatic adenocarcinoma. Mol Oncol. 2013;7(2):232–47. https://doi.org/10.1016/j.molonc.2013.02.002.
4. Coté GA, Smith J, Sherman S, Kelly K. Technologies for imaging the normal and diseased pancreas. Gastroenterology. 2013;144(6):1262–1271.e1261. https://doi.org/10.1053/j.gastro.2013.01.076.
5. Amanam I, Chung V. Targeted therapies for pancreatic cancer. Cancer. 2018;10(2):36.
6. Garrido P, Aldaz A, Vera R, Calleja MA, de Álava E, Martín M, Matías-Guiu X, Palacios J. Proposal for the creation of a national strategy for precision medicine in cancer: a position statement of SEOM, SEAP, and SEFH. Clin Transl Oncol. 2017;20:443. https://doi.org/10.1007/s12094-017-1740-0.
7. Hruban RH, Goggins M, Parsons J, Kern SE. Progression model for pancreatic cancer. Clin Cancer Res. 2000;6(8):2969.
8. Klein AP, Hruban RH, Brune KA, Petersen GM, Goggins M. Familial pancreatic cancer. Cancer J (Sudbury, Mass). 2001;7(4):266–73.
9. Pihlak R, Valle JW, McNamara MG. Germline mutations in pancreatic cancer and potential new therapeutic options. Oncotarget. 2017;8(42):73240–57. https://doi.org/10.18632/oncotarget.17291.
10. Hollis RL, Churchman M, Gourley C. Distinct implications of different BRCA mutations: efficacy of cytotoxic chemotherapy, PARP inhibition and clinical outcome in ovarian cancer. Onco Targets Ther. 2017;10:2539–51. https://doi.org/10.2147/OTT.S102569.
11. Warr A, Robert C, Hume D, Archibald A, Deeb N, Watson M. Exome sequencing: current and future perspectives. G3 (Bethesda). 2015;5(8):1543–50. https://doi.org/10.1534/g3.115.018564.
12. Richards S, Aziz N, Bale S, Bick D, Das S, Gastier-Foster J, Grody WW, Hegde M, Lyon E, Spector E, Voelkerding K, Rehm HL, On behalf of the ACMG Laboratory Quality Assurance Committee. Standards and guidelines for the interpretation of sequence variants: a joint consensus recommendation of the American College of Medical Genetics and Genomics and the Association for Molecular Pathology. Genet Med. 2015;17(5):405–24. https://doi.org/10.1038/gim.2015.30.
13. Li MM, Datto M, Duncavage EJ, Kulkarni S, Lindeman NI, Roy S, Tsimberidou AM, Vnencak-Jones CL, Wolff DJ, Younes A, Nikiforova MN. Standards and guidelines for the interpretation and reporting of sequence variants in cancer: a joint consensus recommendation of the Association for Molecular Pathology, American Society of Clinical Oncology, and College of American Pathologists. J Mol Diagn. 2017;19(1):4–23. https://doi.org/10.1016/j.jmoldx.2016.10.002.
14. Watson M. Illuminating the future of DNA sequencing. Genome Biol. 2014;15(2):108. https://doi.org/10.1186/gb4165.
15. Servant N, Roméjon J, Gestraud P, La Rosa P, Lucotte G, Lair S, Bernard V, Zeitouni B, Coffin F, Jules-Clément G, Yvon F, Lermine A, Poullet P, Liva S, Pook S, Popova T, Barette C, Prud'homme F, Dick J-G, Kamal M, Le Tourneau C, Barillot E, Hupé P. Bioinformatics for precision medicine in oncology: principles and application to the SHIVA clinical trial. Front Genet. 2014;5:152.
16. Gavande NS, VanderVere-Carozza PS, Hinshaw HD, Jalal SI, Sears CR, Pawelczak KS, Turchi JJ. DNA repair targeted therapy: the past or future of cancer treatment? Pharmacol Ther. 2016;160:65–83. https://doi.org/10.1016/j.pharmthera.2016.02.003.
17. Crowley E, Di Nicolantonio F, Loupakis F, Bardelli A. Liquid biopsy: monitoring cancer-genetics in the blood. Nat Rev Clin Oncol. 2013;10(8):472–84. https://doi.org/10.1038/nrclinonc.2013.110.
18. Le Calvez-Kelm F, Foll M, Wozniak MB, Delhomme TM, Durand G, Chopard P, Pertesi M, Fabianova E, Adamcakova Z, Holcatova I, Foretova L, Janout V, Vallee MP, Rinaldi S, Brennan P, McKay JD, Byrnes GB, Scelo G. KRAS mutations in blood circulating cell-free DNA: a pancreatic cancer case-control. Oncotarget. 2016;7(48):78827–40. https://doi.org/10.18632/oncotarget.12386.
19. Cohen JD, Li L, Wang Y, Thoburn C, Afsari B, Danilova L, Douville C, Javed AA, Wong F, Mattox A, Hruban RH, Wolfgang CL, Goggins MG, Dal Molin M, Wang T-L, Roden R, Klein AP, Ptak J, Dobbyn L, Schaefer J, Silliman N, Popoli M, Vogelstein JT, Browne JD, Schoen RE, Brand RE, Tie J, Gibbs P, Wong H-L, Mansfield AS, Jen J, Hanash SM, Falconi M, Allen PJ, Zhou S, Bettegowda C, Diaz L, Tomasetti C, Kinzler KW, Vogelstein B, Lennon AM, Papadopoulos N. Detection and localization of surgically resectable cancers with a multi-analyte blood test. Science. 2018;359:926.
20. Ahlquist DA, Zou H, Domanico M, Mahoney DW, Yab TC, Taylor WR, Butz ML, Thibodeau SN, Rabeneck L, Paszat LF, Kinzler KW, Vogelstein B, Bjerregaard NC, Laurberg S, Sørensen HT, Berger BM, Lidgard GP. Next-generation stool DNA test accurately detects colorectal cancer and large adenomas. Gastroenterology. 2012;142(2):248–e226. https://doi.org/10.1053/j.gastro.2011.10.031.
21. Cotter TG, Burger KN, Devens ME, Simonson JA, Lowrie KL, Heigh RI, Mahoney DW, Johnson DH, Ahlquist DA, Kisiel JB. Long-term follow-up of patients having false positive multi-target stool DNA tests after negative screening colonoscopy: the LONG-HAUL cohort study. Cancer Epidemiol Biomarkers Prev. 2017;26(4):614–21. https://doi.org/10.1158/1055-9965.EPI-16-0800.
22. Krantz BA, Reilly EM. Biomarker based therapy in pancreatic ductal adenocarcinoma: an emerging reality? Clin Cancer Res. 2018;24:2241–50.
23. Qiu J, Yang G, Feng M, Zheng S, Cao Z, You L, Zheng L, Zhang T, Zhao Y. Extracellular vesicles as media-

tors of the progression and chemoresistance of pancreatic cancer and their potential clinical applications. Mol Cancer. 2018;17(1):2. https://doi.org/10.1186/s12943-017-0755-z.

24. Kastenmüller G, Raffler J, Gieger C, Suhre K. Genetics of human metabolism: an update. Hum Mol Genet. 2015;24(R1):R93–R101. https://doi.org/10.1093/hmg/ddv263.
25. Relling MV, Evans WE. Pharmacogenomics in the clinic. Nature. 2015;526(7573):343–50. https://doi.org/10.1038/nature15817.
26. Krell J, Frampton AE, Jiao LR, Stebbing J. Can pharmacogenomics guide effective anticancer therapy in pancreatic ductal adenocarcinoma? Pharmacogenomics. 2012;13(9):977–9. https://doi.org/10.2217/pgs.12.73.
27. Mishra R, Hanker AB, Garrett JT. Genomic alterations of ERBB receptors in cancer: clinical implications. Oncotarget. 2017;8(69):114371–92. https://doi.org/10.18632/oncotarget.22825.
28. Ingelman-Sundberg M, Gomez A. The past, present and future of pharmacoepigenomics. Pharmacogenomics. 2010;11(5):625–7. https://doi.org/10.2217/pgs.10.59.
29. Bai HX, Lee AM, Yang L, Zhang P, Davatzikos C, Maris JM, Diskin SJ. Imaging genomics in cancer research: limitations and promises. Br J Radiol. 2016;89(1061):20151030. https://doi.org/10.1259/bjr.20151030.
30. Waddington CH. The epigenotype. 1942. Int J Epidemiol. 2012;41(1):10–3. https://doi.org/10.1093/ije/dyr184.
31. Watson JD, Crick FC. Molecular structure of nucleic acids: a structure for deoxyribose nucleic acid. JAMA. 1993;269(15):1966–7. https://doi.org/10.1001/jama.1993.03500150078030.
32. Li E, Zhang Y. DNA methylation in mammals. Cold Spring Harb Perspect Biol. 2014;6(5):a019133. https://doi.org/10.1101/cshperspect.a019133.
33. Chagin VO, Stear JH, Cardoso MC. Organization of DNA replication. Cold Spring Harb Perspect Biol. 2010;2(4):a000737. https://doi.org/10.1101/cshperspect.a000737.
34. Campos EI, Stafford JM, Reinberg D. Epigenetic inheritance: histone bookmarks across generations. Trends Cell Biol. 2014;24(11):664–74. https://doi.org/10.1016/j.tcb.2014.08.004.
35. Furey TS. ChIP-seq and beyond: new and improved methodologies to detect and characterize protein-DNA interactions. Nat Rev Genet. 2012;13(12):840–52. https://doi.org/10.1038/nrg3306.
36. Angelini C, Costa V. Understanding gene regulatory mechanisms by integrating ChIP-seq and RNA-seq data: statistical solutions to biological problems. Front Cell Dev Biol. 2014;2:51. https://doi.org/10.3389/fcell.2014.00051.
37. Bailey P, Chang DK, Nones K, Johns AL, Patch AM, Gingras MC, Miller DK, Christ AN, Bruxner TJ, Quinn MC, Nourse C, Murtaugh LC, Harliwong I, Idrisoglu S, Manning S, Nourbakhsh E, Wani S, Fink L, Holmes O, Chin V, Anderson MJ, Kazakoff S, Leonard C, Newell F, Waddell N, Wood S, Xu Q, Wilson PJ, Cloonan N, Kassahn KS, Taylor D, Quek K, Robertson A, Pantano L, Mincarelli L, Sanchez LN, Evers L, Wu J, Pinese M, Cowley MJ, Jones MD, Colvin EK, Nagrial AM, Humphrey ES, Chantrill LA, Mawson A, Humphris J, Chou A, Pajic M, Scarlett CJ, Pinho AV, Giry-Laterriere M, Rooman I, Samra JS, Kench JG, Lovell JA, Merrett ND, Toon CW, Epari K, Nguyen NQ, Barbour A, Zeps N, Moran-Jones K, Jamieson NB, Graham JS, Duthie F, Oien K, Hair J, Grutzmann R, Maitra A, Iacobuzio-Donahue CA, Wolfgang CL, Morgan RA, Lawlor RT, Corbo V, Bassi C, Rusev B, Capelli P, Salvia R, Tortora G, Mukhopadhyay D, Petersen GM, Munzy DM, Fisher WE, Karim SA, Eshleman JR, Hruban RH, Pilarsky C, Morton JP, Sansom OJ, Scarpa A, Musgrove EA, Bailey UM, Hofmann O, Sutherland RL, Wheeler DA, Gill AJ, Gibbs RA, Pearson JV, Waddell N, Biankin AV, Grimmond SM. Genomic analyses identify molecular subtypes of pancreatic cancer. Nature. 2016;531(7592):47–52. https://doi.org/10.1038/nature16965.
38. Raphael BJ, Hruban RH, Aguirre AJ, Moffitt RA, Yeh JJ, Stewart C, Robertson AG, Cherniack AD, Gupta M, Getz G, Gabriel SB, Meyerson M, Cibulskis C, Fei SS, Hinoue T, Shen H, Laird PW, Ling S, Lu Y, Mills GB, Akbani R, Loher P, Londin ER, Rigoutsos I, Telonis AG, Gibb EA, Goldenberg A, Mezlini AM, Hoadley KA, Collisson E, Lander E, Murray BA, Hess J, Rosenberg M, Bergelson L, Zhang H, Cho J, Tiao G, Kim J, Livitz D, Leshchiner I, Reardon B, Van Allen E, Kamburov A, Beroukhim R, Saksena G, Schumacher SE, Noble MS, Heiman DI, Gehlenborg N, Kim J, Lawrence MS, Adsay V, Petersen G, Klimstra D, Bardeesy N, Leiserson MDM, Bowlby R, Kasaian K, Birol I, Mungall KL, Sadeghi S, Weinstein JN, Spellman PT, Liu Y, Amundadottir LT, Tepper J, Singhi AD, Dhir R, Paul D, Smyrk T, Zhang L, Kim P, Bowen J, Frick J, Gastier-Foster JM, Gerken M, Lau K, Leraas KM, Lichtenberg TM, Ramirez NC, Renkel J, Sherman M, Wise L, Yena P, Zmuda E, Shih J, Ally A, Balasundaram M, Carlsen R, Chu A, Chuah E, Clarke A, Dhalla N, Holt RA, Jones SJM, Lee D, Ma Y, Marra MA, Mayo M, Moore RA, Mungall AJ, Schein JE, Sipahimalani P, Tam A, Thiessen N, Tse K, Wong T, Brooks D, Auman JT, Balu S, Bodenheimer T, Hayes DN, Hoyle AP, Jefferys SR, Jones CD, Meng S, Mieczkowski PA, Mose LE, Perou CM, Perou AH, Roach J, Shi Y, Simons JV, Skelly T, Soloway MG, Tan D, Veluvolu U, Parker JS, Wilkerson MD, Korkut A, Senbabaoglu Y, Burch P, McWilliams R, Chaffee K, Oberg A, Zhang W, Gingras M-C, Wheeler DA, Xi L, Albert M, Bartlett J, Sekhon H, Stephen Y, Howard Z, Judy M, Breggia A, Shroff RT, Chudamani S, Liu J, Lolla L, Naresh R, Pihl T, Sun Q, Wan Y, Wu Y, Jennifer S, Roggin K, Becker K-F, Behera M, Bennett J, Boice L, Burks E, Carlotti Junior CG, Chabot J, Pretti da Cunha Tirapelli D, Sebastião dos Santos J, Dubina M, Eschbacher J, Huang M, Huelsenbeck-Dill L, Jenkins R, Karpov A, Kemp R, Lyadov V, Maithel S, Manikhas G, Montgomery E, Noushmehr H,

Osunkoya A, Owonikoko T, Paklina O, Potapova O, Ramalingam S, Rathmell WK, Rieger-Christ K, Saller C, Setdikova G, Shabunin A, Sica G, Su T, Sullivan T, Swanson P, Tarvin K, Tavobilov M, Thorne LB, Urbanski S, Voronina O, Wang T, Crain D, Curley E, Gardner J, Mallery D, Morris S, Paulauskis J, Penny R, Shelton C, Shelton T, Janssen K-P, Bathe O, Bahary N, Slotta-Huspenina J, Johns A, Hibshoosh H, Hwang RF, Sepulveda A, Radenbaugh A, Baylin SB, Berrios M, Bootwalla MS, Holbrook A, Lai PH, Maglinte DT, Mahurkar S, Triche TJ Jr, Van Den Berg DJ, Weisenberger DJ, Chin L, Kucherlapati R, Kucherlapati M, Pantazi A, Park P, Saksena G, Voet D, Lin P, Frazer S, Defreitas T, Meier S, Chin L, Kwon SY, Kim YH, Park S-J, Han S-S, Kim SH, Kim H, Furth E, Tempero M, Sander C, Biankin A, Chang D, Bailey P, Gill A, Kench J, Grimmond S, Johns A, Cancer Genome I, Postier R, Zuna R, Sicotte H, Demchok JA, Ferguson ML, Hutter CM, Mills Shaw KR, Sheth M, Sofia HJ, Tarnuzzer R, Wang Z, Yang L, Zhang J, Felau I, Zenklusen JC. Integrated genomic characterization of pancreatic ductal adenocarcinoma. Cancer Cell. 2017;32(2):185–203.e113. https://doi.org/10.1016/j.ccell.2017.07.007.

39. Moffitt RA, Marayati R, Flate EL, Volmar KE, Loeza SGH, Hoadley KA, Rashid NU, Williams LA, Eaton SC, Chung AH, Smyla JK, Anderson JM, Kim HJ, Bentrem DJ, Talamonti MS, Iacobuzio-Donahue CA, Hollingsworth MA, Yeh JJ. Virtual microdissection identifies distinct tumor- and stroma-specific subtypes of pancreatic ductal adenocarcinoma. Nat Genet. 2015;47(10):1168–78. https://doi.org/10.1038/ng.3398.
40. Nicolle R, Blum Y, Marisa L, Loncle C, Gayet O, Moutardier V, Turrini O, Giovannini M, Bian B, Bigonnet M, Rubis M, Elarouci N, Armenoult L, Ayadi M, Duconseil P, Gasmi M, Ouaissi M, Maignan A, Lomberk G, Boher J-M, Ewald J, Bories E, Garnier J, Goncalves A, Poizat F, Raoul J-L, Secq V, Garcia S, Grandval P, Barraud-Blanc M, Norguet E, Gilabert M, Delpero J-R, Roques J, Calvo E, Guillaumond F, Vasseur S, Urrutia R, de Reyniès A, Dusetti N, Iovanna J. Pancreatic adenocarcinoma therapeutic targets revealed by tumor-stroma cross-talk analyses in patient-derived xenografts. Cell Rep. 2017;21(9):2458–70. https://doi.org/10.1016/j.celrep.2017.11.003.
41. Xu X, Wang Y, Liang H. The role of A-to-I RNA editing in cancer development. Curr Opin Genet Dev. 2018;48:51–6. https://doi.org/10.1016/j.gde.2017.10.009.
42. The Human Microbiome Project C. Structure, function and diversity of the healthy human microbiome. Nature. 2012;486(7402):207–14. https://doi.org/10.1038/nature11234.
43. Baquero F, Nombela C. The microbiome as a human organ. Clin Microbiol Infect. 2012;18:2–4. https://doi.org/10.1111/j.1469-0691.2012.03916.x.
44. Zambirinis CP, Pushalkar S, Saxena D, Miller G. Pancreatic cancer, inflammation and microbiome. Cancer J (Sudbury, Mass). 2014;20(3):195–202. https://doi.org/10.1097/PPO.0000000000000045.
45. Bashiardes S, Tuganbaev T, Federici S, Elinav E. The microbiome in anti-cancer therapy. Semin Immunol. 2017;32:74–81. https://doi.org/10.1016/j.smim.2017.04.001.
46. Klonoff DC, Ahn D, Drincic A. Continuous glucose monitoring: a review of the technology and clinical use. Diabetes Res Clin Pract. 2017;133:178–92. https://doi.org/10.1016/j.diabres.2017.08.005.
47. Triantafyllidis AK, Koutkias VG, Chouvarda I, Adami I, Kouroubali A, Maglaveras N. Framework of sensor-based monitoring for pervasive patient care. Healthc Technol Lett. 2016;3(3):153–8. https://doi.org/10.1049/htl.2016.0017.
48. Zheng Y-x, Yu D-f, Zhao J-g, Wu Y-l, Zheng B. 3D printout models vs. 3D-rendered images: which is better for preoperative planning? J Surg Educ. 2016;73(3):518–23. https://doi.org/10.1016/j.jsurg.2016.01.003.
49. Zhang YS, Yue K, Aleman J, Moghaddam KM, Bakht SM, Yang J, Jia W, Dell'Erba V, Assawes P, Shin SR, Dokmeci MR, Oklu R, Khademhosseini A. 3D bioprinting for tissue and organ fabrication. Ann Biomed Eng. 2017;45(1):148–63. https://doi.org/10.1007/s10439-016-1612-8.
50. Hidalgo M, Amant F, Biankin AV, Budinská E, Byrne AT, Caldas C, Clarke RB, de Jong S, Jonkers J, Mælandsmo GM, Roman-Roman S, Seoane J, Trusolino L, Villanueva A. Patient derived xenograft models: an emerging platform for translational cancer research. Cancer Discov. 2014;4(9):998–1013. https://doi.org/10.1158/2159-8290.CD-14-0001.
51. Rovithi M, Avan A, Funel N, Leon LG, Gomez VE, Wurdinger T, Griffioen AW, Verheul HMW, Giovannetti E. Development of bioluminescent chick chorioallantoic membrane (CAM) models for primary pancreatic cancer cells: a platform for drug testing. Sci Rep. 2017;7:44686. https://doi.org/10.1038/srep44686.
52. Baker LA, Tiriac H, Clevers H, Tuveson DA. Modeling pancreatic cancer with organoids. Trends Cancer. 2016;2(4):176–90. https://doi.org/10.1016/j.trecan.2016.03.004.
53. Steer CJ, Jackson PR, Hornbeak H, McKay CK, Sriramarao P, Murtaugh MP. Team science and the physician–scientist in the age of grand health challenges. Ann N Y Acad Sci. 2017;1404(1):3–16. https://doi.org/10.1111/nyas.13498.
54. Boland GM, Meric-Bernstam F. The role of surgeons in building a personalized medicine program. J Surg Oncol. 2015;111(1):3–8. https://doi.org/10.1002/jso.23684.

Index

S. Tsai et al. (eds.), *Management of Localized Pancreatic Cancer*,
https://doi.org/10.1007/978-3-319-98944-0